Edited by
GRAHAM THORNICROFT

Measuring Mental Health Needs
Second edition

GASKELL

Dedication

This book is dedicated to the memory of Marion Beeforth, who worked tirelessly for the interests, rights and needs of people with mental health problems.

Gaskell is an imprint of the Royal College of Psychiatrists
17 Belgrave Square, London SW1X 8PG

British Library Cataloguing-in-Publication Data
A catalogue record for this book is available from
the British Library.
ISBN 1-901242-60-9

Printed by Bell & Bain Limited, Glasgow, UK.

Contents

Contributors ix

Foreword *Sir Douglas Black* xiii

Preface *Graham Thornicroft* xv

Part I Definitions and targets for needs assessment

1 Defining mental health needs *John Wing,* 1
  Chris R. Brewin and Graham Thornicroft

2 Health targets *Rachel Jenkins and Bruce Singh* 22

Part II Measuring population needs

3 Population surveys of morbidity and need 43
  Rachel Jenkins and Howard Meltzer

4 Commissioners' information requirements 59
  on mental health needs and commissioning for
  mental health services *Andrew Stevens, James Raftery*
  and Richard A. Mendelsohn

5 Measuring (relative) need for mental health care 84
  services *Roy Carr-Hill*

6 Assessing demand for care at district level using 110
  a psychiatric case register *Mirella Ruggeri,*
  Francesco Amaddeo and Michele Tansella

7 Assessing the need for psychiatric services at 125
  district level: using the results of community surveys
  Paul Bebbington and Sian Rees

Part III Choosing among needs: priorities and costs

8 Setting priorities during the development of local 144
  psychiatric services *Elaine Murphy*

9 The Care Programme Approach: prioritising 159
  according to need in policy and practice
  Jonathan Bindman and Gyles Glover

10 Local catchment areas for needs-led mental health 171
  services *Geraldine Strathdee and Graham Thornicroft*

11   Needs from a user perspective   *Marion Beeforth*   190
      and Helen Wood
12   Costing psychiatric interventions   *Jennifer Beecham*   200
      and Martin Knapp

Part IV Evaluating the ability of psychiatric services to meet needs

13   Assessing systems of care for the long-term mentally ill   225
      in urban settings   *M. Susan Ridgely, Howard H. Goldman*
      and Jospeh P. Morrissey
14   Auditing the use of psychiatric beds   *Bernard Audini*   241
      and Richard Duffett

Part V Methods for assessing individual needs

15   The Cardinal Needs Schedule: a standardised   261
      research instrument for measuring individual needs
      Austin Lockwood and Max Marshall
16   Measuring individual needs for care and services   273
      Chris R. Brewin
17   The Camberwell Assessment of Need (CAN)   291
      Mike Slade and Paul McCrone

Part VI Needs of special groups

18   Mental health services for homeless people   304
      William R. Breakey, Ezra Susser and Philip Timms
19   Needs of carers   *Elizabeth Kuipers*   342
20   Mental health needs of children and young people   363
      Robert Jezzard
21   Measurement of needs in people with learning   379
      disabilities and mental health problems
      Kiriakos Xenitidis and Nick Bouras
22   Needs assessment in mental health care for older   393
      people   *Tom Reynolds and Martin Orrell*
23   Mental health needs in primary care   *Andre Tylee*   407
24   Mental health needs assessment for ethnic and   420
      cultural minorities   *Kamaldeep Bhui*
25   Needs assessment for rural mental health services   435
      Alain Gregoire
26   Needs assessment and drug misuse services   454
      John Marsden and John Strang
27   Needs assessment and eating disorders   *Janet Treasure*   472
      and Ulrike Schmidt
28   Needs assessment and alcohol   *E. Jane Marshall*   486

      Index   513

Contributors

Francesco Amaddeo, Lecturer, Dipartimento di Medicina e Sanità Pubblica, Sezione di Psichiatria, Università di Verona, Ospedale Policlinico, 37134 Verona, Italy

Bernard Audini, Senior Research Fellow, Royal College of Psychiatrists' College Research Unit, 6th Floor, 83 Victoria Street, London SW1H OHW, UK

Paul Bebbington, Professor of Social and Community Psychiatry, Department of Psychiatry and Behavioural Sciences, Holborn Union Building, Archway Campus, Whittington Hospital, Highgate Hill, London N19 5NF, UK

Jennifer Beecham, Centre for the Economics of Mental Health, Health Services Research Department, Institute of Psychiatry, De Crespigny Park, Denmark Hill, London SE5 8AF, UK; and Personal Social Services Research Unit, University of Kent at Canterbury

Marion Beeforth, Mental health service user and Chair of the Working Group on Acute Care to the External Reference Group for the National Service Framework for Mental Health

Kamaldeep Bhui, Senior Lecturer in Social and Epidemiological Psychiatry, St Bartholomew's and The Royal London, School of Medicine and Dentistry, Department of Psychiatry, Basic Medical Sciences Building, Queen Mary & Westfield College, Mile End Road, London E1 4NS, UK

Jonathan Bindman, Senior Lecturer, Health Services Research Department, Institute of Psychiatry, De Crespigny Park, Denmark Hill, London SE5 8AF, UK

Sir Douglas Black, The Old Forge, Duchess Close, Whitchurch-on-Thames, Reading RG8 7EN, UK

Nick Bouras, Professor of Psychiatry, Division of Psychiatry – GKT, Estia Centre, Guy's Hospital, London SE1 3RR, UK

William R. Breakey, Department of Psychiatry and Behavioural Sciences, Meya 4-181, John Hopkins Hospital, Baltimore, Maryland 21287-7481, USA

Chris Brewin, Professor of Clinical Psychology, Sub-department of Clinical Psychology, University College London, Gower Street, London WC1E 6BT, UK

Roy Carr-Hill, Professor of Medical and Social Statistics, Centre for Health Economics, University of York, Heslington, York YO10 5DD, UK

Richard Duffett, Consultant Psychiatrist, Goodmayes Hospital, Barley Lane, Ilford IG3 8XJ, UK

Gyles Glover, Professor of Public Mental Health, University of Durham, 15 Old Elvet, Durham DH1 3HL, UK

Howard Goldman, Professor and Co-Director, Centre for Mental Health Services Research, University of Maryland, 625 W. Redwood Street, Baltimore, Maryland 21210, USA

Alain Gregoire, Consultant Honorary Senior Lecturer in Psychiatry, Rural Mental Health Research, University of Southampton, Maples Building, Tatchbury Mount, Calmore, Southampton SO40 2RZ, UK

Rachel Jenkins, Director of WHO Collaborating Centre, Health Services Research Department, Institute of Psychiatry, De Crespigny Park, Denmark Hill, London SE5 8AF, UK

Robert Jezzard, Senior Policy Advisor, Department of Health, Wellington House, 133–155 Waterloo Road, London SE1 8UG, UK

Martin Knapp, London School of Economics and Centre for the Economics of Mental Health, Health Services Research Department, Institute of Psychiatry, De Crespigny Park, Denmark Hill, London SE5 8AF, UK

Elizabeth Kuipers, Professor of Clinical Psychology, Department of Psychology, Institute of Psychiatry, De Crespigny Park, Denmark Hill, London SE5 8AF, UK

Austin Lockwood, Research Nurse, Department of Community Psychiatry, University of Manchester, Guild Academic Centre, Royal Preston Hospital, Sharoe Green Lane, Preston, Lancashire PR2 9HT, UK

John Marsden, Senior Lecturer, National Addiction Centre, Institute of Psychiatry, De Crespigny Park, Denmark Hill, London SE5 8AF, UK

E. Jane Marshall, Senior Lecturer in the Addictions, National Addiction Centre, Institute of Psychiatry, De Crespigny Park, Denmark Hill, London SE5 8AF, UK

Max Marshall, Reader in Community Psychiatry, Department of Community Psychiatry, University of Manchester, Guild Academic Centre, Royal Preston Hospital, Sharoe Green Lane, Preston, Lancashire PR2 9HT, UK

Paul McCrone, Senior Lecturer in Health Economics, Health Services Research Department, Institute of Psychiatry, De Crespigny Park, Denmark Hill, London SE5 8AF, UK

Howard Meltzer, Principal Social Researcher, Social Survey Division (D2/03), Office for National Statistics, Pimlico, London SW1V 2QQ, UK

Richard A. Mendelsohn, Consultant in Public Health Medicine, Birmingham Health Authority, St Chad's Court, 213 Hagley Road, Birmingham B16 9RG, UK

Joseph P. Morrissey, Professor and Deputy Director, Sheps Center for Health Services Research, University of North Carolina, Chapel Hill, North Carolina 27599, USA

Elaine Murphy, East London and the City Health Authority, 81 Commercial Road, London E1 1RD, UK

Martin Orrell, Reader in Psychiatry of Ageing, Department of Psychiatry and Behavioural Sciences, University College London, Wolfson Building, 48 Riding House St, London W1N 8AA, UK

James Raftery, Professor of Health Economics, Health Services Management Centre, University of Birmingham, Birmingham B15 2TT, UK

Sian Rees, Senior manager, NHSE London Region Office; Health Services Research Department, Institute of Psychiatry, De Crespigny Park, Denmark Hill, London SE5 8AF, UK

Tom Reynolds, Consultant in Old Age Psychiatry, Our Lady's Hospital, Ennis, Ireland

M. Susan Ridgely, Senior Policy Analyst, RAND, 1700 Main Street, Santa Monica, California 90401, USA

Mirella Ruggeri, Dipartimento di Medicina e Sanità Pubblica, Sezione di Psichiatria, Università di Verona, Ospedale Policlinico, 37134 Verona, Italy

Ulrike Schmidt, Eating Disorder Unit, Institute of Psychiatry, De Crespigny park, Denmark Hill, London SE5 8AF, UK

Bruce Singh, Cato Professor of Psychiatry, University of Melbourne, Charles Connibere Building, Royal Melbourne Hospital, Melbourne, Victoria 3050, Australia

Mike Slade, MRC Clinician Scientist Fellow, Health Services Research Department, Institute of Psychiatry, De Crespigny Park, Denmark Hill, London SE5 8AF, UK

Andrew Stevens, Professor of Public Health, Department of Public Health and Epidemiology, University of Birmingham, Edgbaston, Birmingham B15 2TT, UK

John Strang, Professor of the Addictions and Director, National Addiction Centre, Institute of Psychiatry, De Crespigny Park, Denmark Hill, London SE5 8AF, UK

Geraldine Strathdee, Clinical Director, Oxleas NHS Trust, Bromley Directorate, 27 London Road, Bromley, Kent BR1 1DG, UK

Ezra Susser, Head, Division of Epidemiology, The Mailman School of Public Health, 600 West 168th Street, New York 10032, USA

Michele Tansella, Professor of Psychiatry, Director, Dipartimento di Medicina e Sanità Pubblica, Sezione di Psichiatria, Università di Verona, Ospedale Policlinico, 37134 Verona, Italy

Graham Thornicroft, Health Services Research Department, Institute of Psychiatry, De Crespigny Park, Denmark Hill, London SE5 8AF, UK

Philip Timms, Senior Lecturer in Community Psychiatry, START, Master House, 1st Floor, Dugard Way, Off Renfew Road, London SE11 4DJ, UK

Janet Treasure, Eating Disorder Unit, Institute of Psychiatry, De Crespigny Park, Denmark Hill, London SE5 8AF, UK

Andre Tylee, Professor and Head of Primary Care Mental Health Section, Health Services Research Department, Institute of Psychiatry, De Crespigny Park, Denmark Hill, London SE5 8AF, UK

John Wing, c/o Health Services Research Department, Institute of Psychiatry, De Crespigny Park, Denmark Hill, London SE5 8AF, UK

Helen Wood, Director, Greenwich Mental Health, Oxleas NHS Trust, Memorial Hospital, Shooters Hill, London SE18 3RZ, UK

Kiriakos Xenitidis, Consultant Psychiatrist, MIETS Unit, Bethlem Royal Hospital, South London & Maudsley NHS Trust, Monk's Orchard Road, Beckenham, Kent BR3 3BX, UK

Foreword

In an ideal world, demands for health care would accurately reflect health needs, and would themselves in turn be satisfied by adequate and appropriate provision of services. In the world in which we actually live, there are health needs that fail to arouse demand, being either accepted as part of life's burden, or unappreciated through simple failure to detect them or to recognise that anything can be done about them. However, demands are voiced from time to time for which it is difficult to detect or define any corresponding needs – unless perhaps the very making of a health-related demand itself constitutes a health need. This discrepancy between need and demand is important in relation to service provision, perhaps particularly because choices between alternative provisions are commonly made not as a sequel to a dispassionate appraisal and comparison of conflicting needs, but in response to the demands of pressure groups or to simple political expediency.

Such considerations make it particularly important for those qualified to do so to undertake an objective study of the constellation of needs in the field in which they are expert. Only after such an analysis is it possible to argue for what would seem to be a desirable transition, from a 'demand-led' service to a 'needs-led' service. Of course, in relation to provision of services, the weighting given to a defined need has to be modulated by considering whether in the present state of the art it can be 'cured', 'relieved', 'palliated', or in the last resort 'accepted'. The recognition and quantification of those needs that can be met is obviously of immediate importance; less obviously there is also value in the recognition and definition of needs for which there is at present no available remedy. That value consists not only in stimulating research towards a future remedy, but also in laying down the base of information for planning support services for what cannot yet be cured.

The task implicit in the title of this book is thus important; it is also distinctly difficult. Assessment of need in relation to physical illness is hard enough; when I was involved in studying the relationship between deprivation and ill health we had very largely to wield the Occam's razor of analysing the bills of mortality. Such draconian measures have fortunately little relevance to analysing needs in mental impairment and illness. However, in relation to both bodily and mental disorder, there has in recent years been considerable interest and advance in the analysis of the effects of illness on various aspects of well-being. Such analysis has to be multidimensional, comprising measures of physical and mental performance, subjective perception of well-being, fitness for work, social adaptation, and ability to participate in leisure activities. Such studies of what has been grouped under the term 'quality of life' are a necessary complement to older approaches based on diagnostic categories that may be less than clear-cut.

The editors of this book deserve warm commendation, first for tackling a difficult and important range of problems; then for assembling a group of experts capable of discussing the various aspects of a complicated and still evolving field of study; and finally for producing a work that is both scholarly and practical. As with physical disease, the provision of services for mental health is far too important to be left to the uninstructed play of market forces. I am confident that this book makes an important, and indeed necessary, contribution to the logical development of mental health services in this and other countries.

Sir Douglas Black

Preface

In the nine years since the first edition of this book was published, mental health practice and policy have undergone rapid change. In Britain, for example, most of the remaining large asylums are now empty or about to close. We have witnessed a period of unparalleled innovation with novel forms of home treatment, day care, crisis assessment, alternatives to hospital admission, increasing numbers of users and carer groups, the growth of the new paradigm of evidence-based medicine, the constant searchlight of inquiries into serious untoward incidents, and the accompanying mass media expression of public disquiet about the state of mental health services. We have seen the birth and death of supervision registers, and the first stirrings of new mental health legislation, which in future will allow clinicians to apply compulsory powers of treatment in similar fashion, whether the patient is in hospital or at home.

Even so, much of the first edition of the book remains applicable to the coming years, as much as it did to the 1990s. Our definitions of need have stood the test of time, and need can best be described as the ability to benefit from care. The importance of public health targets in the area of mental health, now manifest in *Saving Lives: Our Healthier Nation* (Department of Health, 1999*a*), is as great as it was in *The Health of the Nation* (Department of Health, 1994). The utility of survey data to inform needs assessment at the population level is even more relevant now, after the completion of the first National Psychiatric Morbidity Survey (Jenkins *et al*, 1998). But there were significant gaps in the first edition, and this second edition has been substantially extended to address these deficiencies.

During the last decade, we have seen a series of clear trends emerge. First, the role of user involvement in the planning, delivery and evaluation of treatment and care has accelerated to the point where we are beginning to see in Britain service users present on appointment committees, organisational boards, ethics committees and governmental advisory bodies. It is probable that user involvement in mental health care is now at least as well developed as in any other area of health service provision. Second, the growth and maturation of a clear research and development function within the National Health Service (NHS) has acted as a powerful lever to produce quantified assessments of the needs of populations and of individuals. Third, we have seen the role of needs assessment enter into national policy. Four of the seven standards within the National Service Framework for Mental Health (Department of Health, 1999*b*), for example, refer directly to assessing the needs of service users, or indirectly refer to needs assessments that assist in formulating an individual care plan (see Chapter 1, Table 1.2, Standards 2, 3, 4, 5). Yet the area of needs assessment in which progress has been least striking is in measuring the needs of carers. This is now set to change because Standard 6 of the National Service Framework for Mental Health – 'Caring about carers' – will require these needs to be identified and responded to:

> All individuals who provide regular and substantial care for a person on CPA [Care Programme Approach] should:
> - have an assessment of their caring, physical and mental health needs, repeated on at least an annual basis; and
> - have their own written care plan which is given to them and implemented in discussion with them.

Finally, it is sometimes helpful to step back from the detail of how to measure needs for health care and to ask *why* measure needs? In my view, an approach to health services that is fundamentally based upon need is in essence a moral choice. It is a view that attaches importance to the relief of suffering, whatever the circumstances of the person who is unwell, and which claims that a civilised society will offer services in proportion to the needs of those who may benefit from services. This sentiment was more poetically expressed by Isabel Allende (1985), when she wrote: "They also forced me to eat. They divided up the servings with the strictest sense of justice, each according to her need."

References

ALLENDE, I. (1985) *The House of the Spirits*. London: Black Swan Books.
DEPARTMENT OF HEALTH (1994) *Health of the Nation: Key Area Handbook* (2nd edn). London: HMSO.
—— (1999*a*) *Saving Lives: Our Healthier Nation*. Cm4386. London: The Stationery Office.
—— (1999*b*) *The National Service Framework for Mental Health. Modern Standards and Service Models*. London: Department of Health.
JENKINS, R., BEBBINGTON, P., BRUGHA, T., *ET AL* (1998) The British Psychiatric Morbidity Survey. *British Journal of Psychiatry*, **173**, 4–7.

Graham Thornicroft
Editor

1   Defining mental health needs

JOHN WING, CHRIS R. BREWIN
and GRAHAM THORNICROFT

This chapter sets the agenda for the book by defining the terms used in needs assessment. The topics covered include both clinical evaluation and audit, that is, analysis of face-to-face assessment of need followed by intervention and re-assessment of outcome, and the epidemiologically based equivalents required to plan and manage a geographical area rationally (Thornicroft & Tansella, 1996).

The first two chapters are therefore concerned with individual needs and Chapters 3–7 with those of an 'average' health district. The limitations of the restriction to National Health Service (NHS) services will become clearer as the book proceeds and the all-pervading overlap with other social and private services is documented. The principles of definition, however, remain constant as these boundaries are crossed and will be highly relevant as joint commissioning becomes mandatory.

A conceptual framework for planning and providing mental health services

A conceptual model can be useful to help formulate service aims and the steps necessary for their implementation. Such a conceptual model has recently been described in detail (Thornicroft & Tansella, 1999). This 'matrix' model has two dimensions: the geographical and the temporal. The first refers to three *geographical* levels: (1) country/regional, (2) local and (3) patient. The second dimension refers to three *temporal* levels: (A) inputs, (B) processes and (C) outcomes. Using these two dimensions we construct a 3×3 matrix to bring into focus critical issues for mental health service planning and provision (see Table 1.1). Practical examples of the use of the model are given in Tansella & Thornicroft (1998).

1

TABLE 1.1
The matrix model as a conceptual model for planning

Geographical dimension (C) Outcome phase	Temporal dimension		
	(A) Input phase	(B) Process phase	
(1) Country/ regional level	1A	1B	1C
(2) Local level (catchment area)	2A	2B	2C
(3) Patient level	3A	3B	3C

Source: Thornicroft & Tansella (1999).

The needs of individuals

Concepts of disability

The World Health Organization's Illness, Disability and Handicap (IDH) classification of the consequences of disease and injury works well for many straightforward medical problems (World Health Organization (WHO), 1980). The first level of the classification is concerned with a concept of 'impairment', which involves loss or abnormality of function. This concept is appropriate for the psychological impairments or dysfunctions that underlie the basic psychiatric symptoms. At a second level lie 'disabilities', which involve restrictions on personal activities that may be directly caused by impairments. At a third level, impairments and disabilities usually lead to 'handicaps', which involve disadvantages in interacting with or adapting to the individual's environment. A simple example is a violinist who develops arthritis of a finger joint (disease), which results in some loss of movement (impairment), little personal restriction (disability), but a serious occupational block (handicap).

There are two kinds of problem in adapting the IDH system for use with psychiatric disorders. First, the distinction between impairment and disability is difficult (although not impossible) to draw when the impairment is psychological. Second, the direction of cause and effect is drawn firmly from left to right. Although there is some discussion in the IDH text as to how social factors might influence disorder, impairment and disability (right to left), no criteria are suggested and the classification, in effect, ignores these possibilities.

In addition, there is a semantic problem. The terms 'disability' and 'handicap' are used interchangeably in common speech and it is very difficult to allocate separate meanings to them. For present purposes, we need to begin, rather than end, with a concept of social disablement that includes any substantial inability to perform up to personal expectation, or to the expectations of important others, and which is associated with psychiatric disorder or impairment. Someone who can perform to expectation, but chooses not to, would be excluded by definition.

In 1980, the WHO published the *International Classification of Impairments, Disabilities and Handicaps* (ICIDH). After two decades of use, it has become apparent that this classificatory system requires revision (e.g. Chamie, 1990; Badley, 1993; Brandsma *et al*, 1995; Heerkens *et al*, 1995). In accordance with this need, the WHO has started to produce a new version of the ICIDH, the ICIDH–2. It is constructed with the intention of: (a) reflecting a bio-psychosocial model in which functioning and disablement are viewed as outcomes of an interaction between the person's physical/mental conditions and the social and physical environment; (b) interpreting this interaction in a complex, bi-directional and dynamic way; (c) incorporating a universal vision of disability and functioning; and (d) using a neutral terminology.

Severity of disablement

The severity of disablement, therefore, results from: (a) the severity and duration of impairment, that is, psychological and physiological dysfunctions; (b) adverse circumstances and disadvantages, both past and present, that can affect social functioning independently; and (c) personal reactions to the first two factors, including loss of self-esteem and motivation. For convenience, (a) is measured in terms of the presence and severity of symptoms and behaviour of various kinds, (b) in terms of environmental adversity, and (c) in terms of self-attitudes.

Each component should be assessed separately so that a profile of problems is available on which judgements of need can be made. The clinical severity of symptoms, for example, can be measured in terms of intensity and persistence. Intensity tends to be equivalent to intrusiveness, which affects more general mental functioning and, in turn, affects behaviour and lowers social functioning. This is true across the whole range of symptomatology, from anxiety to auditory hallucinations. Psychotic symptoms are more likely to be intrusive and persistent, and to affect behaviour more severely, than neurotic or non-specific symptoms, but both groups of disorders can be manifested throughout the whole range of severity.

Specific features of the behaviours are often determined by symptoms. For example, over-activity associated with mania has features that differentiate it from over-activity associated with delirium, schizophrenia, agitated depression or panic. However, there are also features in common that require a similar pattern of treatment or management. People with many different disorders, or none, may harm themselves or be violent to others. Socially embarrassing behaviour can occur across all diagnoses.

Social disablement is therefore associated with an amalgam of factors that produce a pattern, level and persistence of malfunctioning that is not diagnosis-specific. It is the pattern, level and duration that principally determine need for care and services. Both in the general population (Hurry & Sturt, 1981) and in cross-sectional studies of people in contact with specialist services, the greater the number and severity of symptoms, the more severe the social disablement tends to be.

Duration carries further implications, since the other two components may be amplified if impairment persists. For example, persisting impairment may itself lead to stigma, a low standard of living and demoralisation. These, in turn, can amplify clinical manifestations such as depression and anxiety.

Case-mix

Diagnosis-related groups cannot, therefore, be used in isolation to determine needs. One diagnosis-related group, such as 'psychosis', can account for a substantial proportion of all admissions, allowing no discrimination between real needs. A multi-factorial, or 'case-mix', approach is essential (Taube *et al*, 1984). Case-mix allows the assignment of patients to recognisable groups, which reflect the problems that give rise to a need for some form of care and the cost of that care.

Targets: health gain and the prevention of disability

Thus, the target for interventions by the health and social services, in practice, should be twofold. One aim is to reduce the severity of social disablement associated with mental disorder. Any such reduction can be called a 'health gain'. The other aim is to prevent the amplification of any disablement that cannot be further reduced. Both aims require disentanglement of the three components of disablement, despite the difficulty of doing so, because each may require its own forms of intervention.

An analysis of this kind leads to setting specific targets for the provision of treatment and care, professional staff to provide it, and settings for staff and users to work in. These targets must be realistic and defined in such a way that it is possible to measure the extent to

COLLEGE LANE LRC
ITEMS CHARGED - SELF ISSUE

Date format: DD-MM-Year

16-12-2007

12:55

Salome Kiarie

DUE DATE:
11/01/2008 21:45

TITLE:Measuring mental health needs /
edited by Graham Thornicroft.

ITEM:5000296581

which they are being met, that is, measurable outcomes. Detailed examples of mental health targets are given by Jenkins in Chapter 2. A recent example of national service targets are the standards set for England within the National Service Framework for Mental Health, shown in Box 1.1.

Care and services: terminology

Care and enabling

'Care' will be defined in terms of the medical, psychological and social interventions that are considered to be 'state of the art' by well-trained mental health practitioners. It includes treatment, rehabilitation, counsel, training, supervision, resettlement and welfare. Since the term comprises reduction and further prevention of social disablement (not only the care required for symptoms and behavioural problems), it automatically includes the provision of special enabling opportunities to individuals who cannot use ordinary amenities because of temporary or persisting impairments, and therefore also includes attention to quality of life. By the same token, care also involves attention to the environment of sheltered or protected settings or activities, in order to preserve and enhance social functioning. Interventions of these kinds that are designed to prevent disablement becoming worse, rather than to reduce its severity, are included in the same way.

Services

The term 'services' includes several components. Three need to be separately specified, in terms of the agents, settings, and the organisation necessary to deliver care.

Care agents

Care is provided by formal care agents or staff, specifically trained for their functions, or by non-specific formal agents whose work often brings them into contact with mentally ill people; for example, police, fire-fighters and ambulance staff. Informal agents include relatives, friends, befrienders and voluntary workers.

Care settings

Care agents require settings to work in, including every kind from a domiciliary visit (or even a visit 'on the street') to a high-security ward.

Box 1.1
National Service Framework for Mental Health (Department of Health, 1999a)

Standard 1: Mental health promotion
Health and social services should:
- promote mental health for all, working with individuals and communities; and
- combat discrimination against individuals and groups with mental health problems, and promote their social inclusion.

Standard 2: Primary care and access to services
Any service user who contacts their primary health care team with a common mental health problem should:
- have his or her mental health needs identified and assessed; and
- be offered effective treatments, including referral to specialist services for further assessment, treatment and care if he or she requires it.

Standard 3: Primary care and access to services
Any individual with a common mental health problem should:
- be able to make contact round the clock with the local services necessary to meet his or her needs and receive adequate care; and
- be able to use NHS Direct, as it develops, for first-level advice and referral on to specialist helplines or to local services.

Standard 4: Severe mental illness
All mental health service users on the Care Programme Approach (CPA) should:
- receive care which optimises engagement, anticipates or prevents a crisis, and reduces risk;
- have a copy of a written care plan which:
  - includes the action to be taken in a crisis by the service user, their carer, and their care coordinator;
  - advises their GP how they should respond if the service user needs additional help;
  - is regularly reviewed by their care coordinator; and
- be able to access services 24 hours a day, 365 days a year.

Standard 5: Severe mental illness
Each service user who is assessed as requiring a period of care away from his or her home should have:
- timely access to an appropriate hospital bed or alternative bed or place, which is:
  - in the least restrictive environment consistent with the need to protect them and the public; and
  - as close to home as possible; and
- a copy of a written after-care plan agreed on discharge which sets out the care and rehabilitation to be provided, identifies the care coordinator and specifies the action to be taken in a crisis.

Standard 6: Caring about carers
All individuals who provide regular and substantial care for a person on CPA should:
- have an assessment of their caring, physical and mental health needs, repeated on at least an annual basis; and

- have their own written care plan which is given to them and implemented in discussion with them.

Standard 7: Preventing suicide
Local health and social care communities should prevent suicides by:
- promoting mental health for all, working with individuals and communities (Standard 1);
- delivering high-quality primary mental health care (Standard 2);
- ensuring that anyone with a mental health problem can contact local services via the primary care team, a help-line or an A & E department (Standard 3);
- ensuring that individuals with severe and mental illness have a care plan which meets their specific needs, including access to services round the clock (Standard 4);
- providing safe hospital accommodation for individuals who need it (Standard 5); and
- enabling individuals caring for someone with severe mental illness to receive the support which they need to continue to care (Standard 6).

Care coordination

Department of Health guidance introduced in 1999 revised the provisions of the Care Programme Approach (CPA) and care management to integrate these for the first time. The key link in these care arrangements is called the 'care coordinator', who will usually be a community psychiatric nurse (CPN) or a social worker, who assesses needs and who coordinates the delivery of a 'package of care' to the service user (Thornicroft, 1991*a*). This term is now used by the Department of Health to describe the roles previously called 'keyworking ' within British health services, and 'care management' within social services (Department of Health, 1999*b*).

Needs for care and services

Economical definitions of terms used in needs assessment were provided by Matthew (1971). Suitably adapted and broadened (Wing & Hailey, 1972; Brewin & Wing, 1988), they will be used throughout the rest of this chapter. More specifically, needs are defined in terms of problems for which 'state of the art' solutions exist. The following definitions are based upon a needs assessment system intended to promote comparisons between different populations, whether for clinical, research or planning purposes (Brewin *et al*, 1987; Brewin & Wing, 1988). The principles are derived from a model of day-to-day clinical practice, but they are not intended to be prescriptive.

Need

Need can be defined either in terms of the type of impairment or other factor causing social disablement or of the model of treatment or other intervention required to meet it; for example, hip replacement, insulin regime for diabetes and medication for auditory hallucinations. If an individual is socially disabled, in association with a mental disorder for which an effective and acceptable form or model of care exists, either for amelioration or prevention, the individual is in need of that intervention. There will usually be a hierarchy of methods, at the top of which may be one that produces a complete and rapid recovery with no extra ill-effects. At the bottom, there will usually be methods of amelioration, or prevention of relapse or of amplification of disablement. Perhaps the clearest and simplest definition of need is the ability to benefit from care (see Chapter 4). The fact that needs are defined does not mean that they will be met. Some may remain unmet for the immediate future because other problems must be dealt with first, or because the more effective method is not available locally, or availability is limited by rationing, or because the person in need objects, or because there are other reasons why the intervention should not be made. There are also 'potential' needs for forms of care that do not at the moment exist but which research may eventually provide. Moreover, voluntary organisations may develop services for needs that are not at present recognised or understood by most professionals (Holloway, 1994).

Two further points should be clearly understood. First, the definition does not exclude interventions that, for whatever reason, are locally unavailable. If a method of help is known, a need for it exists.

Second, the acquiescence of an individual in a situation that precludes the needed intervention does not overrule the need. Thus, many people in mental hospitals in the 1960s had grown used to their situation and a needs assessment would not have revealed problems requiring such a setting. Some who wished to stay were helped to move to less occupationally and residentially restrictive settings and, in retrospect, were pleased to have moved (Wing & Brown, 1970). A similar problem arose when a new long-stay hostel-ward was introduced as an alternative to remaining on busy acute wards (Wykes, 1981). A needs assessment is not intended to endorse the status quo. It is important not to define need in terms of the care/agent/setting already in place, thus automatically perpetuating the present allocation and priorities. At the same time, it not intended either to lead to the imposition on unwilling people of an official set of priorities. A professionally defined need may remain unmet and have to be replaced by one lower in the hierarchy, simply because the user disagrees that there is such a need.

The specification of an intervention, if available and accepted by the user following 'negotiation', leads to the choice of an agent to provide the care and a setting in which user and carer can interact (Mangen & Brewin, 1991).

Demand

A demand for care exists when individuals express a wish to receive it. Some demands are expressed in an unsophisticated form, for example, 'something needs to be done'. The user should be involved in a negotiation as to what interventions should be provided for what problems. This includes an explanation of the options. The process should not be purely top-down.

Provision

Provision includes interventions, agents and settings, whether or not used. Care coordination entails providing such a pattern of service after initial assessment and then updating the assessment regularly in order to check outcomes and to modify the pattern if needs remain unmet or change. Over-provision is provision without need. Under-provision is need without provision (unmet need).

Utilisation

Utilisation occurs when an individual actually receives care, for example, bed occupancy. Need may not be expressed as demand; demand is not necessarily followed by provision or, if it is, by utilisation; and there can be demand, provision and utilisation without real underlying need for the particular service used.

Needs assessment techniques

Methods of needs assessment can be used to extend, systematise and generalise from the principles of clinical audit, by measuring structure, process and outcome against standard guidelines, which are specified in advance. Chapters 16 and 17 describe particular techniques. The guidelines suggested can be challenged, but use of the system allows comparisons to be made, and the construction and publication of alternatives. One framework is that used by the Camberwell Assessment of Need (Slade *et al*, 1999), which includes the domains shown in Box 1.2.

Box 1.2
Areas of potential need included in the Camberwell Assessment of Need
(CAN; Slade et al, *1999)*

- accommodation
- occupation
- specific psychotic symptoms
- psychological distress
- information about condition and treatment
- non-prescribed drugs
- food and meals
- household skills
- self-care and presentation
- safety to self
- safety to others
- money
- child care
- physical health
- alcohol
- basic education
- company
- telephone
- public transport
- welfare benefits

Quality of care and quality of life

Decreasing disablement does not automatically lead to an increase in the quality of life, but it will usually increase the options available to the individual to make use of the amenities available to the generality of local people, although, clearly, the richness and variety of the social and economic opportunities available will vary. Some impairments, however, affect motivation and drive, or impose a pattern of behaviour or thought that makes it difficult for the person afflicted to use 'open' amenities. Access to public facilities may be denied or unwise. Enabling measures are then necessary in order to find other ways of realising unused potentialities.

Quality of life is therefore measurable in terms of physical necessities such as heat, light, shelter, food, security and so on, which must be provided for people who cannot procure them otherwise. A second measure should be concerned with the quality of such provisions themselves, in particular in terms of the quality of the environment and the choice available. Finally, there is the quality of personal life, the extent to which a disabled individual can maintain self-respect and autonomy, keep up interests, make a recognised contribution to society and increase his or her self-knowledge.

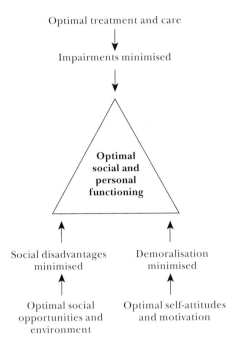

Fig. 1.1 *The components of quality assurance*

In serving these ends, quality of care and quality of life are two sides of the same coin. Fig. 1.1 shows the inter-relationships between the factors involved in decreasing social disablement and in enabling quality assurance.

The needs of groups

The epidemiology of need

The model for ordinary clinical practice has been outlined above. It is to assess an individual in order to construct a partial or complete care plan, implement it and then follow-up for re-assessment. The single-case audit cycle follows the same model. This contrasts with assessment of the needs of a diagnostic group, or of people with a particular type of clinical problem (for example, parasuicide or admission under the Mental Health Act), or of those requiring a particular form of treatment, agent or setting. In such cases, the same assessment model can be used to measure the needs of each member of the relevant group, in order to obtain a summary profile of group needs.

The needs of a defined population, such as the one for which a health authority is responsible, can be assessed most thoroughly in the same bottom-up way. The top-down information requirements of management and planning (based on national, regional and local targets and guidelines) also involve the collection of administrative and financial data.

Mental health information systems

A comprehensive mental health information system (MHIS), therefore, would cover both kinds of collection and use and the output would be available, within the limits of confidentiality, to all. Such a system would include both statistical and non-numerical information concerning: (a) local history, topography and communications; (b) socio-demographic indices and epidemiology; (c) local services (agents and settings), their functioning and efficiency; (d) clinical data about the needs of people in contact with services and how far they are being met; and (e) opinions of local users and informal carers.

Such systems would provide a data base for national and regional returns, local resource allocation and target setting, local area needs and outcome assessment, case-mix, care plans, clinical records and the audit of clinical care. To create and maintain the system, high-quality clinical information is needed that can only be obtained with the consistent collaboration of clinical teams, who have to be convinced of the practical value to them and those they are caring for (Wing, 1992).

The Körner Committee (Department of Health and Social Security (DHSS), 1982) recommended a 'minimum data-set' that should be collected across the whole of the hospital services. It was not principally concerned with the needs of people with mental disorders or with services that were community-based. The Mental Health Enquiry (MHE), which had provided a more or less continuous series of mental health statistics for decades, required only that a relatively simple manually produced set of data should be collected and sent for central processing. It was abandoned in 1986, together with the Hospital Activity Analysis.

A new set of indicators, based on the Körner data-set, was issued in 1989, but it was chiefly concerned with the needs of acute medicine and surgery. The needs of psychiatry were not well represented, the gap being particularly obvious for psychiatric services not based in hospital wards. This was not so important in the days of the MHE, when the budget for mental illness services was relatively non-competitive, in effect, 'ring-fenced', as Griffiths (1988) later recommended. However, the increasing specificity of management requirements backed by financial budgeting has changed the situation.

It therefore becomes very important to be able to judge the quality of the data collected for health service indicators (HSIs) such as CP35 (percentage total number of mental illness nurses employed in the community), or DC41 (percentage discharges to NHS hospitals outside the local area). Cooper (1989) pointed out that a system of local psychiatric case registers (PCRs) had existed for which quality of data collection had been a high priority. He recommended that the experience be utilised when setting up any alternative system to the MHE. In particular, the staff who oversee the data collection should also be concerned with the final output, and because of the fact that sequences of data about individuals have to be collected, a series of checks should be introduced to make sure that new data are consistent with the old (Wing, 1989).

A further problem arises from the multi-agency nature of psychiatric services, in which people follow complex paths from unit to unit, only some of which come under the aegis of the health authority. Domiciliary visiting has now taken a broader meaning. Some community psychiatric nurses (CPNs) work directly with general practitioners (GPs), without being part of a specialist mental health team. A MHIS has to be capable of coping with such forms of service, and provide data of value to clinical teams, purchasers and providers.

In particular, the setting of clinical as well as financial and administrative targets, demands the continuous collection of data that would serve to determine the outcome of interventions for problems, as in the classic audit and needs assessment cycles. It is as important for members of clinical teams to take part in such a monitoring process and to learn how to utilise the knowledge that it can provide as it is for administrators to understand the central requirement for planning of good-quality bottom-up information.

A medium-term aim, strongly to be welcomed, is the proposal to establish patient-based 'minimum data-set for mental health' information systems, "so that contacts with individual clients can be built into person-identified episodes of care, each with an agreed provider minimum data set" (Department of Health, 1999*b*). This principle of record linkage allows counts based on individuals as well as on events. It is most economically implemented, as demonstrated by the PCRs, by relating information to dates of contact.

Socio-demographic indices of need

The classic epidemiological studies of the early post-war years provided strong evidence that people who developed schizophrenia and people who committed suicide had often moved away from their usual area of residence before (sometimes long before) the time of clinical onset or fatality (Ödegård, 1932; Sainsbury, 1955; Hare, 1956; Dunham, 1965). The areas to which they moved were characterised by social isolation or 'anomie'. Indices of social isolation tend to be correlated with others that measure poverty, although when there are exceptions social isolation appears more important. The inclusion, for example, of marital status in the Resource Allocation Working Party (RAWP) formula for allocations to psychiatric services recognised the significance of isolation, practical as well as theoretical, for the prediction of morbidity.

More recently, administrative indices such as first and re-admission rates, and rates of accumulation beyond a year's residence in hospital, have been found empirically to be associated with a composite measure of 'deprivation', which includes marital status as one component (Thornicroft, 1991*b*; Jarman & Hirsch, 1992; Thornicroft *et al*, 1992). Such factors are shown in Table 1.2. Using data of this kind, it is possible to estimate likely psychiatric bed needs for particular areas on the basis of weighted socio-demographic indices, as shown in Table 1.3.

Setting priorities

Setting targets raises the issue of priorities in several ways. First, the targets themselves must be chosen from a wide range of possibilities. Second, once measured and found unmet, they force further selection, even when only those with roughly equivalent and affordable costs are considered. Third, the priority given to targets that are being met can be re-appraised.

The problem of priorities can be illustrated quite starkly by a consideration of the common problems of mental disorder treated in general practice (a large proportion of which are minor disorders that are not referred on) compared with those of the far fewer people with more severe disorders who are admitted to hospital. From the MHE for 1986 it can be estimated that there were 22 002 200 'in-patient days'. At £44.05 per day, this comes to £5 122 619 for an average-size local area (250 000) for that year. Croft-Jefferys & Wilkinson (1989) estimated that there were 5.79m consultations with GPs for neurosis in 1985. The average cost per visit, including home visits, medication and referrals, was £19.44, omitting indirect costs. This makes £594 913 per 250 000 per year.

Taking such figures at face value, and without examining the clinical evidence for the effectiveness and efficiency of current treatments, staff and settings, it might appear that some of the money spent on in-patients could be spared to help the much larger numbers in general practice. Indeed, there already appears to be a diversion of CPN activity in this direction in some areas (Wooff *et al*, 1986,

TABLE 1.2

Recent examples of statistically significant socio-demographic predictors of mental health services use

	Jarman, 1983	Thornicroft, 1991	Jarman & Hirsch, 1992	Thornicroft et al, 1993	Glover, 1996
Ethnic minorities	Y	Y			
Elderly living alone	Y				
Children ages <5 years	Y		Y		
Single-parent families	Y	Y			
Unskilled workers	Y				
Unemployed	Y			Y	Y
Changed address	Y	Y		Y	
Overcrowded	Y			Y	
Lack of internal amenities		Y			
No car		Y	Y		Y
Living in one room		Y			
Population density		Y		Y	
Availability of general beds		Y			
Household in single occupation			Y	Y	
Single, widowed or divorced			Y	Y	Y
Illegitimacy index			Y		
Private household with no car			Y		
Dependency ratio				Y	
Registered as permanently disabled					Y
Household not self-contained					Y
Non-permanent accommodation					Y

Y, significant association present.

TABLE 1.3

Estimated need and actual provision of general adult mental health services (for ages 15–64 years only: estimated in-patient and residential care places per 250 000 population, England 1992–1996)

Category of services	Wing, 1992[1] Expected range of places	Strathdee & Thornicroft, 1992 Expected range of places	Ramsay et al, 1997[2] Expected range of places	Actual level of provision per 250 000[3]		
				Outer London (overall)	Inner London (overall)	Range in London
Medium-secure unit	1–10	1–10	5–30	8	27	0–58
Intensive care unit/local care unit	5–15	5–10	5–20	8	16	0–41
Acute ward	50–150	50–150	50–175	73	110	48–165
24-hour nurse-staffed units/hostel wards/staff awake at night	25–175	40–150	12–50	55	35	0–164
24-hour non-nurse-staffed hostels/night staff sleep in	40–110	40–150	50–300	99	162	28–330
Day-staffed hostels	25–75	30–120	15–60	17	43	14–292
Lower-support accommodation[4]	n/a	48–100	30–120	55	95	14–272

1. All estimates given assume that each category of service exists in the given appropriate range of volume; the Wing (1992) estimates include old age assessment places, and the Strathdee & Thornicroft (1992) figures apply only to general adult services for those aged 16–65.
2. Ramsay et al (1997) estimated need levels based upon: London actual need levels based upon, for most categories of service, with a far greater variation in medium-secure beds, and NHS Executive (1996) guidance for an average of 25 places in 24-hour nurse-staffed accommodation per 250 000.
3. Actuals exclude extra-contractual referrals.
4. Includes respite beds and supported self-contained flats. As not all agencies gave information on these categories, these estimates should be regarded as conservative.
Source: Ramsay et al, 1997.

1988). But, without a proper MHIS, it is impossible to have a clear idea of what such shifts might mean in terms of priorities, targets and outcomes for the two groups.

A second illustration of problems arising from the allocation of priorities arises from the rule enunciated earlier in this chapter, to the effect that preventing the amplification of social disablement is as important as demonstrating a diminution. Targets have to be set in such a way that the effects of preventive care can be measured positively, even though the degree of impairment is no longer expected to be much reduced. One way to do this is to ensure, as part of the regular needs assessments, that interventions previously not found to be successful may be offered again from time to time, without pressure.

These considerations raise the issue of priority starkly, and illustrate why it is necessary for an MHIS to generate data that accurately reflect the needs for caring, enabling and prophylactic services. Based on the clinical and social characteristics of all those known to all the responsible authorities, The Audit Commission (1992) calculated that public expenditure on community-based care in England (including that provided by primary care services) cost more than in-hospital care, whereas 10 years previously, at equivalent prices, the expenditures were more or less equal. The report points out that:

> "[n]o authority visited had any information systems that could tell managers in either authority the range of services deployed to a particular individual from health and social services – let alone from the independent sector or from relatives and friends. There was very little available on unit costs of services, and there was only occasional systematic information available to managers (let alone users and carers) on the range of services available throughout an area. Such information systems as exist are nearly always service orientated. There is a particular need to strengthen the information available to users and carers outlining their entitlement and services available to them."

A more detailed account of ways of determining priorities for mental health care within localities is given by Murphy in Chapter 8, and within sectors by Strathdee & Thornicroft in Chapter 10, while the closely related issues of costing care and services are considered by Beecham & Knapp in Chapter 12.

The way in which an MHIS, based on a combination for good-quality bottom-up clinical information and top-down administrative data, can underpin both clinical care and resource management is summarised in Fig. 1.2.

Top-down information

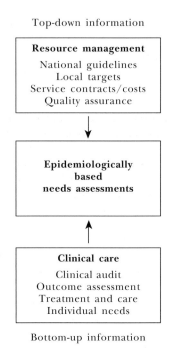

Fig. 1.2 Use of a mental health information system for high-quality local planning

Conclusions

Up until now, the assessment of needs for mental health care and services has proceeded in a relatively haphazard and informal way, particularly in areas not served by a PCR. Little attention has been paid to basic questions about what needs are and how to measure them. Assessment of individual needs has relied on the expertise and implicit models of care held by individual clinicians, on informal audit procedures and, in cases where patients have been compulsorily detained, on Mental Health Act commissioners. The trend is now clearly evident for the evaluation of clinical practice to become more systematic and routine. At the individual level, models of good practice are being specified, along with increased recognition of the needs of others in patients' social networks, such as relatives (see Chapter 19 by Kuipers). The technical challenge of computerising information collection and deployment in such a way that it can aid routine decision-making is being addressed. Assessment tools are now available for comparing patients' needs across time and across settings. And, at the service level, comprehensive assessments are now being developed that examine not only patient outcomes but aspects of organisation, funding, and structure (see, for example, Chapter 13 by Ridgely *et al*).

In attempting to cover the many disparate topics that are relevant to needs assessment, we have organised the book in an approximate sequence, beginning with the most general considerations and ending with the most specific techniques and issues. The first two chapters deals with basic definitions of need as they can be applied to mental health, differentiating them from associated concepts such as demand, utilisation and quality of life. Needs assessments are put into a general context of audit, evaluation and planning. The setting of general targets for the assessment of need is discussed from a national perspective.

In Chapters 3–7, the focus is on the needs of populations and the information requirements of districts. Sources of information, both local and national, are discussed, with the aims of purchasing authorities and provider units in mind. Chapters 8–12 deal with the issues involved in choosing between the competing needs of a population, that is, setting priorities and costing services.

The emphasis then shifts in Chapters 13 and 14 to evaluating the ability of services to meet needs, starting with an example of a heavily researched and coordinated evaluation of new arrangements for the delivery of community care services, and concluding with an example of a local audit of admissions to a particular hospital provider unit.

Chapters 15–17, by contrast, deal with the needs of individuals. Chapter 15 by Lockwood & Marshall gives an account of the methods that have been used to assess the needs of individual patients, and of the differing levels of detail required for community surveys, the long-term mentally ill, and so on. Chapter 16 by Brewin is concerned with how the collection of data required for assessing individual needs can be routinised, and describes a number of patient information systems. This is followed by a description of the advantages and disadvantages of new techniques for computerising patient assessment.

Becoming yet more specific, Chapters 18–28 describe the needs of special groups such as the homeless and relatives of the mentally ill.

References

Audit Commission (1992) *Community Care: Managing the Cascade of Change.* London: HMSO.

Badley, E. M. (1993) An introduction to the concepts and classifications of the International Classification of Impairments, Disabilities, and Handicaps. *Disability Rehabilitation*, **15**, 161–178.

Brandsma, J. W., Lakerveld-Heyl, K., Van Ravensberg, C. D., *et al* (1995) Reflection on the definition of impairment and disability as defined by the World Health Organization. *Disability Rehabilitation*, **17**, 119–270.

Brewin, C. R. & Wing, J. K. (1988) *The MRC Needs for Care Assessment Manual.* London: MRC Social Psychiatry Unit, Institute of Psychiatry.

—, —, MANGEN, S., *ET AL* (1987) Principles and practice of measuring needs in the long term mentally ill. The MRC Needs for Care Assessment. *Psychological Medicine,* **17**, 971–981.

CHAMIE, M. (1990) *The Status and Use of the International Classification of Impairments, Disabilities, and Handicaps (ICIDH).* World Health Status Q, 43. Geneva: WHO.

COOPER, J. (1989) Information for planning. Case registers and Körner. In: *Contributions to Health Services Planning and Research* (ed. J. K.Wing), pp, 115–120. London: Gaskell.

CROFT-JEFFERYS, C. & WILKINSON, G. (1989) Estimated costs of neurotic disorder in UK general practice. *Psychological Medicine,* **19**, 549–558.

DEPARTMENT OF HEALTH (1989) *Working for Patients.* Cm 555. Working Paper 6, Medical Audit. London: HMSO.

— (1999*a*) *The National Service Framework for Mental Health. Modern Standards and Service Models.* London: Department of Health.

— (1999*b*) *Effective Care Co-ordination in Mental Health Services. Modernising the Care Programme Approach.* London: Department of Health.

DEPARTMENT OF HEALTH AND SOCIAL SECURITY (1982) *A Report on the Collection and Use of Information about Hospital Clinical Activity in the NHS.* London: HMSO.

DUNHAM, H. W. (1965) *Community and Schizophrenia. An Epidemiological Analysis.* Detroit: Wayne State University Press.

GLOVER, G. (1996) Health service indictors for mental health. In: *Commissioning Mental Health Services* (ed. G. Thornicroft & G. Strathdee), pp. 311–318. London: HMSO.

GRIFFITHS, R. (1988) *Community Care. Agenda for Action.* London: HMSO.

HARE, E. H. (1956) Mental illness and social conditions in Bristol. *Journal of Mental Science,* **102**, 349–357.

HEERKENS, Y. F., VAN RAVENSBERG, C. D. & BRANDSMA, J. W. (1995) The need for revision of the ICIDH: an example of problems in gait. *Disability Rehabilitation,* **17**, 184–194.

HOLLOWAY, F. (1994) Need in community psychiatry: a consensus is required. *Psychiatric Bulletin,* **18**, 321–323.

HOUSE OF COMMONS (1990) *National Health Service and Community Care Act.* London: HMSO.

HURRY, J. & STURT, E. (1981) Social performance in a population sample. Relation to psychiatric symptoms. In: *What is a Case? The Problem of Definition in Psychiatric Community Surveys* (eds J. K. Wing, P. Bebbington & L. N. Robins), pp. 202–213. London: Grant McIntyre.

JARMAN, B. (1983) Identification of underprivileged areas. *British Medical Journal,* **286**, 1705–1709.

— & HIRSCH, S. (1992) Statistical models to predict district psychiatric morbidity. In: *Measuring Mental Health Needs* (eds G. Thornicroft, C. R. Brewin & J. Wing), pp. 62–80. London: Gaskell.

MANGEN, S. & BREWIN, C. R. (1991) The measurement of need. In: *Social Psychiatry. Theory, Methodology and Practice* (ed. P. Bebbington), pp. 162–182. London: Transaction Publishers.

MATTHEW, G. K. (1971) Measuring need and evaluating services. In: *Problems and Progress in Medical Care* (ed. G. McLachlan). Sixth series. London: Oxford University Press.

NHS MANAGEMENT EXECUTIVE (1991) *Health Service Indicators. New Perspectives.* Consultation draft. London: Department of Health.

ÖDEGÅRD, Ö. (1932) Emigration and insanity. A study of mental diseases among Norwegian-born population in Minnesota. *Acta Psychiatrica et Neurologica Scandinavica,* Supplement 4.

RAMSAY, R., THORNICROFT, G., JOHNSON, S., *ET AL* (1997) Levels of in-patient and residential provision throughout London. In: *London's Mental Health* (eds S. Johnson, R. Ramsay, G. Thornicroft, *et al*), pp.193–219. London: King's Fund.

SAINSBURY, P. (1955) *Suicide in London.* London: Chapman and Hall.

SLADE, M., THORNICROFT, G., PHELAN, M., *ET AL* (1999) *Camberwell Assessment of Need (CAN).* London: Gaskell.

STRATHDEE, G. & THORNICROFT, G. (1992) Community sectors for needs-led mental health services. In: *Measuring Mental Health Needs* (eds G. Thornicroft, C. R. Brewin & J. Wing), pp. 140–162. London: Gaskell.

TANSELLA, M. & THORNICROFT, G. (1998) A conceptual framework for mental health services: the Matrix model. *Psychological Medicine*, **28**, 503–508.

TAUBE, C., LEE, E. S. & FORTHOFER, R. N. (1984) Diagnosis-related groups for mental disorders, alcoholism and drug abuse. Evaluation and alternatives. *Hospital and Community Psychiatry*, **35**, 452–455.

THORNICROFT, G. (1991*a*) The concept of case management for long-term mental illness. *International Review of Psychiatry*, **3**, 125–132.

—— (1991*b*) Social deprivation and rates of treated mental disorder: developing statistical models to predict psychiatric service utilisation. *British Journal of Psychiatry*, **158**, 475–484.

—— & TANSELLA, M. (1996) *Mental Health Outcome Measures*. Heidelberg: Springer-Verlag.

—— & —— (1999) *The Mental Health Matrix*. Cambridge: Cambridge University Press.

——, MARGOLIUS, O. & JONES, D. (1992) The TAPS Project .(6): New long-stay psychiatric patients and social deprivation. *British Journal of Psychiatry*, **161**, 621–624.

——, DE SALVIA, G. & TANSELLA, M. (1993) Urban-rural differences in the associations between social deprivation and psychiatric service utilisation in schizophrenia and all diagnoses: a case-register study in Northern Italy. *Psychological Medicine*, **23**, 487–489.

WING, J. K. (ed.) (1989) *Health Services Planning and Research. Contributions from Psychiatric Case Registers*. London: Gaskell.

—— (1992) *Epidemiologically Based Needs Assessment. Report 6. Mental Illness*. London: NHS Management Executive, Leeds.

—— & BROWN, G. W. (1970) *Institutionalism and Schizophrenia*. Cambridge: Cambridge University Press.

—— & HAILEY, A. M. (eds) (1972) *Evaluating a Community Psychiatric Service. The Camberwell Register, 1964–1971*. London: Oxford University Press.

WOOFF, K., GOLDBERG, D. & FRYERS, T. (1986) Patients in receipt of community psychiatric nursing care in Salford 1976–82. *Psychological Medicine*, **16**, 407–414.

——, —— & FRYERS, T. (1988) The practice of community psychiatric nursing and mental health social work in Salford. Some implications for community care. *British Journal of Psychiatry*, **152**, 783–792.

WORLD HEALTH ORGANIZATION (1980) *International Classification of Impairments, Disabilities and Handicaps*. Geneva: WHO.

WYKES, T. (1981) A hostel-ward for 'new' long-stay patients. An evaluative study of 'a ward in a house'. In: *Long-term Community Care. Experience in a London Borough. Psychological Medicine Monograph Supplement No. 2* (ed. J. K. Wing), pp. 57–97. Cambridge: Cambridge University Press.

2   Health targets

RACHEL JENKINS and BRUCE SINGH

Management by objectives is a tool well known in business for identifying the individual steps and targets necessary to achieve common goals. Defining measurements makes it possible to organise feedback from results and to review and revise objectives, roles, priorities and reallocation of resources systematically in a business environment (Drucker, 1981). Of the broad range of government responsibilities in public health, none is more fundamental than the obligation to provide goals and direction to guide health programmes along a productive course.

Some general prerequisites pertain to the successful application of the process of setting objectives; they include the ability to define a problem clearly, the availability of effective intervention, the social acceptability of the interventions and the means to track progress. Three basic types of objectives can be developed: outcome objectives, process objectives and input objectives.

International context

Establishing targets in public health as a national effort has been undertaken by many countries, in particular the USA (American Public Health Association, 1991), the UK (Department of Health, 1992) and Australia (Commonwealth Department of Human Services and Health, 1994), as research has unveiled more opportunities, population growth and industrialisation have created more problems and economic pressures have offered more constraints. In this environment, many governments have felt the need to clarify national directions in health. An additional force driving such exercises has been the realisation that efforts to improve health must be linked to other efforts aimed at improving social and economic conditions. The complexity of the task requires careful integration and planning. A motivating force for many of these international efforts has been the World Health Organization (WHO) project 'Health for All by the Year 2000'. As part of this initiative, the

WHO prepared a document setting out global aspirations towards health for all by the year 2000 and suggested a number of targets, including two on mental health. These were published (WHO, 1981) and have since been revised. This stimulated member nations to agree to take specific steps to improve the health prospects of their citizens. An integral part of the WHO project was a commitment by member nations to establish a national health strategy and monitor and evaluate that strategy for effectiveness and appropriateness. Every three years, participating nations report on their progress to WHO. There is a wide variety in both the structure and focus of various national goal-setting efforts, this reflecting the fact every country has different needs and different uses to which the goal-setting process can be put. Some countries provide only broad indicators of national problems and priorities. In fact, these are often couched more as national hopes and aspirations than as attainable goals. For others, they reflect more the process of consensus building than predicting an achievable outcome. However, the process in the UK, Australia and the USA has been more specific, utilising a national goal and objective-driven plan (Commonwealth Department of Human Services and Health, 1992, 1998; Human Rights and Equal Opportunity Commission, 1993).

The UK experience

In the late 1980s, there was a gradual rise in interest in the theoretical and practical development of outcome indicators to measure progress in achieving real health gain and their value to clinicians, planners and policy makers alike.

In 1990, Jenkins reviewed theoretical issues concerning outcome indicators and proposed a framework for a system of mental health care outcome indicators, based on the traditional public health model of prevention (Jenkins, 1990). These issues received further discussion in a series of collaborative workshops between the Royal College of Psychiatrists and the Faculty of Public Health Medicine (Jenkins & Griffiths, 1991; Griffiths *et al*, 1992). This work laid the foundations for the inclusion of mental illness as a key area in England's Health of the Nation strategy in 1992 (Department of Health, 1992, 1994).

Overall objectives for mental illness in England were summarised in 1991 as follows (Department of Health, 1994):

(a) to reduce the incidence and prevalence of mental disorders;
(b) to reduce the mortality associated with mental disorders;
(c) to reduce the extent and severity of other problems associated with mental disorders, for example:
(i) poor physical health
(ii) impaired social functioning

  (iii) poor social circumstances

  (iv) family burden;

(d) to ensure appropriate services and interventions are provided;

(e) to reverse the public's negative perception of mental illness, for example:

  (i) counter fear, ignorance and stigma

  (ii) create a more positive social climate in which to seek help

  (iii) improve quality of life for people with mental health problems; and

(f) to research causes, consequences and the care of specific mental disorders.

Within these overall objectives, England's Health of the Nation strategy, recognising the importance of affective disorders (Department of Health, 1992), set three specific targets for reducing morbidity and suicide:

(a) to significantly improve the health and social functioning of people with mental illness;

(b) to reduce the overall suicide rate by at least 15% by the year 2000 from 1990 levels of 11 per 100 000; and

(c) to reduce the lifetime suicide rate of severely mentally ill people by at least 33% by the year 2000.

The White Paper laid out a tripartite framework for action: improving information and understanding about mental illness, developing comprehensive local services, and developing good practice. To assist in implementing the strategies outlined in *Health of the Nation*, the *Mental Illness Key Area Handbook* was produced (Department of Health, 1994), which set out more detail for the tripartite framework for national and local action to achieve the targets. It is important to note that all the Health of the Nation targets were set out as goals for all agencies and sectors to work to achieve rather than the health sector alone; and so an important part of the overall Health of the Nation strategy was the construction of 'healthy alliances' working together to achieve the national goals.

Improving information and understanding about mental illness

National epidemiology

Large-scale epidemiological surveys are useful to assess the scope for public health interventions, the requirements for primary care and the use of existing specialist services. They can obtain representative information for a large geographical area, valid information on prevalence and disability, and information on associated factors of possible causal importance. By repeating community surveys, it is possible to monitor the health of the population, trends in disorders, and changes in potential risk factors.

Therefore, as part of the agenda to improve information and understanding about mental illness, including affective disorders, the Department of Health for England, together with the Welsh Office and the Scottish Home and Health Department, commissioned the Office of Population Censuses and Surveys (OPCS) (now the Office of National Statistics) to survey the psychiatric morbidity of the country in collaboration with an advisory group of psychiatric epidemiologists (OPCS, 1995; Jenkins *et al*, 1998). The survey programme aimed to obtain a national picture of the prevalence, severity and duration of mental disorders and their accompanying disability and associated risk factors, and the extent to which health and social care needs are met by services. This was the first national survey in any country to collect data on prevalence, risk factors and associated disability simultaneously in household, institutional and homeless samples by use of standardised assessment techniques. The survey covered affective disorders as well as other psychotic and neurotic disorders, and alcohol and drug misuse.

The household survey found that one in six adults aged 16–64 years who live in private households had suffered from some type of neurotic disorder in the week before the survey interview, half of which was mixed anxiety–depression.

All types of common mental disorder, especially depression and mixed anxiety–depression, were more frequent in women than in men. Other key associated demographic risk factors for the neurotic disorders included marital status, where rates were substantially higher in separated, divorced and widowed individuals of both genders, and among cohabiting women. Unemployment was the strongest risk factor, with unemployed people twice as likely to suffer from a neurotic disorder as people in work. Common mental disorders were also associated with physical complaints, and about half of those with depression or anxiety also suffered from long-standing physical complaints.

Common mental disorders were associated with increased rates of general practitioner (GP) consultation. Subjects with significant depressive symptoms were asked about suicidal ideation. Just under 1% of the total sample in the household survey reported suicidal thoughts in the previous week, two-thirds of them women.

The overall prevalence of psychosis was 4 per 1000, with rates for urban dwellers being twice that for those living in the country. Of people with psychosis, two-thirds were in touch with specialist services, 18% had only seen their GP and a further 18% had not sought professional help at all. There is therefore significant unmet need. The levels of social disability were high for neurosis as well as for psychosis.

The results of the Great Britain survey programme – particularly the high prevalence of affective disorders, the high levels of social disability, the high rates of suicidal thoughts, the high levels of morbidity in the homeless, the surprising regional variations in the levels of psychosis, and the socio-demographic associations – have had a number of implications for strategies to support the implementation of the targets.

First, the high prevalence of neurosis, particularly depression and anxiety, means that it is imperative to ensure appropriate education and training of primary care teams, and to develop good practice guidelines for use by primary care teams, with locally agreed criteria for referral, and shared care if appropriate. Primary care provides many opportunities for prevention and early detection that could be used more systematically. Schools and workplaces are also important settings for prevention, early detection and prompt management of affective disorders.

The high levels of social disability found in depression and anxiety as well as in psychosis mean that all assessments should include social needs as well as mental and physical health needs, and that care plans must address social disability as well as health issues in an integrated way.

The high rates of suicidal thoughts emphasise the importance of teaching good suicide assessment and management techniques to health and social care professionals, and of developing national and local action to minimise environmental risk factors for suicide, including controlling access to the means of suicide and supporting high-risk groups.

The high levels of morbidity in the homeless mean that every locality needs to commission services for the homeless to ensure they receive adequate primary and secondary care, and to tackle the root cause of homelessness.

The regional variations in rates of psychosis should be taken into account when assessing needs for specialist services, as should the association of mental disorders with other demographic factors such as unemployment and living conditions when assessing health needs and allocating financial resources to geographical areas.

Public information strategy to improve information and understanding about mental disorders including affective illness

A public information strategy launched in 1993 to increase understanding and reduce stigma involved the dissemination of a series of booklets to primary care, including, for example: *Mental Illness: What does it Mean?*, which explained terms in clear and concise ways; *A Guide to Mental Health in the Workplace*, which encouraged employers to adopt health policies that address mental as well as physical health; and *Sometimes I Think I Can't Go On Any More*, which sought to raise public awareness on the nature of suicide and to offer advice to those trying to help friends and relatives who may be at risk (Department of Health, 1993).

The government has organised a variety of national conferences to assist dissemination of information and understanding about affective disorders. These include the following aspects: suicide prevention (e.g. Jenkins *et al*, 1994); mental health promotion and prevention in primary care (e.g. Jenkins & Üstün, 1998); and mental health in the workplace where occupational doctors have a primary care role (e.g. Jenkins & Coney, 1992; Jenkins & Warman, 1993).

Outcome measurement

The Department of Health commissioned the Royal College of Psychiatrists Research Unit in 1992 to develop a brief standardised assessment procedure to enable the first mental illness target to be measured in a routine clinical setting at each Care Programme Approach (CPA) review. This was developed, piloted, launched and is now relatively widely used in this country and in Australia. In extensive field trials, the scale has been shown to have excellent interrater reliability and to indicate changes over time that closely reflect the clinical impression of the patient's progress (Wing *et al*, 1998).

Developing comprehensive local services

Specialist care

The 1993 Health of the Nation *Mental Illness Key Area Handbook*, revised in 1994 (Department of Health, 1994), was the first comprehensive document on mental illness for managers since the 1975 White Paper, *Better Services for the Mentally Ill* (Department of Health and Social Security, 1975). It gave detailed guidance to both purchaser and provider health and social service managers on the range of services needed for people with mental illness.

Two of the top priorities for the National Health Service (NHS) agenda of the 1990s were the continuing implementation of community care policies and the development of the 'internal market', which, under both Conservative and Labour governments, emphasises different forms of 'primary care-led commissioning of services'.

In August 1995, the Secretary of State for Health asked NHS regional directors to review the progress made in their region towards the delivery of modern and effective mental health services. The results of that review were published in 1996, when the government committed itself to delivering the full 'Spectrum of Care' (Department of Health, 1996*a*) required for a comprehensive local mental health service, where people are looked after as close to home as is compatible with the health and safety of themselves and the public.

A small number of people with the most complex and challenging problems require 24-hour nursed care; in the absence of such provision, individuals either take up acute beds for prolonged periods of time or get into serious difficulties in the community (Department of Health, 1996*b*).

As the large, long-term mental hospitals have closed, considerable efforts have been made to ensure that the money freed up by their closure remains allocated to mental health services and that the community services put in place are comprehensive and provide the complete 'spectrum of care' of a range of types of treatment in a range of different settings and including social care, employment and housing, as well as medical treatment. Effort has gone into defining the number and types of beds required within a community-based service.

The government paper *Modernising Mental Health Services: Safe, Sound and Supportive* (Department of Health, 1998) continued this policy, announcing the development of a National Service Framework (Department of Health, 1999*c*) and set out the range and type of services to be provided for working age adults in all areas of England and Wales. The Framework covers all mental health and social care services, including primary care, mental health promotion and mental ill health prevention. Particular emphasis is laid on establishing assertive outreach services and 24-hour services, including 24-hour nursed beds and crisis services. It also announces a major review of the Mental Health Act to allow treatment to be administered compulsorily in the community.

Continuing development of good practice

Care Programme Approach

As in the USA, community workers and community mental health teams (CMHTs) have formed the backbone of the community service and they have shown the same tendency to drift into treating people with 'less severe illness' (most often people with affective disorders) and to neglect the care of people with chronic schizophrenia (Audit Commission, 1994).

Central strategies to deal with this problem and achieve good health outcomes are the CPA (Department of Health, 1995) and guidance on criteria to be used to prioritise the use of the scarce resources of secondary care mental health professionals. The key elements of the CPA are that every patient in touch with secondary care services should receive a health and social care needs assessment, a package of care to meet those needs, a keyworker and a regular review as appropriate. The CPA is tiered so that patients with the greatest needs receive the most complex multi-disciplinary package of care. The Department of Health definitions of 'severe mental illness' used to define which patients are given priority access to secondary mental health services include bipolar depression and severe affective disorders but exclude 'milder' affective disorders, which are considered to be the province of primary care.

Primary care

GPs come into contact with and are responsible for treating the majority of psychiatric disorders in the population. Particular attention has been paid to continuing medical education and updating GPs and practice teams in the recognition, detection and management of common mental disorders, such as anxiety and depression . The Defeat Depression campaign (Rix *et al*, 1999) was run jointly by the Royal College of Psychiatrists and the Royal College of General Practitioners, supported by the Department of Health.

The Department of Health, in collaboration with the Mental Health Foundation and the Gatsby Trusts, funded a senior mental health fellow in general practice for four years to cascade knowledge and skills about affective disorders through GP tutors and course organisers. This scheme has now evolved into a Royal College of General Practitioners' Unit for Mental Health Education in Primary Care, largely focused on the affective disorders. Primary care in the UK is delivered by multi-disciplinary, usually GP-led teams that always include nurses and may sometimes include a counsellor. The Unit has therefore developed a 'train the trainers' course, which trains pairs of teachers (usually a GP and a community psychiatric nurse (CPN)), who then offer flexible, multi-disciplinary, practice-based training in their localities (Armstrong, 1997).

The Department of Health also funded a national primary care facilitator to take a national lead in mental health education for primary care facilitation. This has now developed into a national training centre for primary care nurses in depression.

The Department of Health commissioned a critical review of psychotherapy research (Roth *et al*, 1996), which emphasised the value of psychological interventions in other medical problems such as heart disease and asthma. In 1992, the Department of Health took up the new step of funding a national primary care nurse facilitator to take a lead in mental health education for primary care nurses and facilitators (Armstrong, 1995). This has now evolved into two ongoing initiatives: one, a self-financing national education centre for primary care nurses that works in close partnership with the educational centre for general practice; the other, a mental health facilitator, who, working with the national primary care facilitation programme continues to provide support and education to the network of facilitators.

The Department of Health also funded a number of developmental projects in primary care (Jenkins, 1992; Jenkins & Üstün, 1998). The experience gained in these pilots was made widely available through the Department of Health publication, *The Primary Mental Health Care Toolkit*, which contains tools designed by the project teams for the assessment and management of common disorders. An example is a protocol specially developed for use by practice nurses during the course of existing 'well person clinics' to identify and support people at high risk of developing an affective disorder (Armstrong, 1993).

Another approach tried during this period was to encourage grassroots primary care practitioners to share their ideas and projects with each other. The Department of Health funded three 'innovations in primary care mental health' conferences. A continuing data base and network of innovations has now been developed, sited at the Sainsbury Centre for Mental Health.

The workplace

The principal issues in the workplace are similar to those in primary care, that is, there is a high prevalence of morbidity, a substantial proportion of which is undetected, hidden morbidity; and that which is recognised is not always managed optimally and is one of the top three causes of sickness absence and the second most common cause of absences longer than 21 days. This is almost certainly an underestimate because of the stigma that still attaches to mental health problems. This untreated and poorly managed morbidity has major public health consequences for the economy, as well as for individuals and their families. For a number of years, therefore, the Department of Health convened an inter-agency group to coordinate activities in the workplace. Representatives from the trade union council, employers' bodies, the Health and Safety Executive, the Institute of Personnel Management and other relevant organisations discussed what each separate organisation could do and also developed a joint programme of work. An example of the joint work was the production of a resource pack for management training and development, *Mental Well Being in the Workplace* (Doherty & Tyson, 1998).

Co-sponsored conferences on the issue of mental health in the workplace took place in 1992 and 1993, and both conferences led to major publications (Jenkins & Coney, 1992; Jenkins & Warman, 1993), the first of which was sent to all NHS managers. Work to increase employers' awareness of the issues and to encourage them to take appropriate action included publication of an information leaflet *A Guide to Mental Health in the Workplace*, a resource pack *ABC of Mental Health in the Workplace* (Department of Health, 1996*c*) and providing information stands at large conferences for employers, including a stand on rural stress (affecting farmers and agricultural workers).

Employers have been encouraged to develop workplace health policies to address the mental as well as physical needs, to value mental health of the workforce, to promote understanding of mental health problems and reduce stigma, to reduce workplace stress, to improve detection and management of illness, including suicidal risk, and to improve rehabilitation back to work.

A part-time fellow in occupational mental health, funded by the Department of Health and the independent sector, worked to improve the knowledge and understanding of occupational physicians about mental health issues. Mental health topics were included for the first time in the professional examinations for occupational physicians.

During this period, the Health and Safety Executive (another government agency) greatly expanded the part of its work dealing with work-induced stress. They produced materials for employers giving advice on reducing workplace stressors and improving support to employees. The first prosecution under the Health and Safety Act (1974) for stress-related ill health provided added impetus to the campaign.

The Department of Health produced its own policy on mental health for its civil servants early in 1994. Initiatives within the NHS included Department of Health support for a stress fellowship in general practice, regular presentations to NHS audiences on issues relating to mental health at work, and production for NHS employers of an organisational stress audit package, produced by the health educational authority. Mental health and the NHS workforce was also one of the priorities for the research and development programme. Two of the studies commissioned focused on the prevalence of mental illness in the workplace: a study of factors influencing mental illness in this setting (Wall *et al*, 1997) and a longitudinal study of 224 medical students over a 10-year period to consider the long-term predictors of stress and depression in this group (Firth-Cozens & Morrison, 1989).

The first study found that there is considerably more mental ill health in terms of stress and depression, both overall and in many of the professional groups, within the NHS than in the rest of the working population. There are particularly large proportions of high scorers in women managers and women hospital doctors. Both studies found good evidence that the following factors are strongly related to high stress levels and minor affective disorder:

    (a) management issues such as poor communication and low participation;

    (b) interrupted or inadequate sleep patterns;

    (c) high work demands/poor support;

    (d) difficult relationships with colleagues and patients;

    (e) alcohol use, particularly in young women doctors;

    (f) high self-criticism; and

    (g) avoidance coping styles.

Prisons

One of the series of surveys of psychiatric morbidity commissioned by the Department of Health was carried out among male and female remand and sentenced prisoners (Singleton *et al*, 1998). This showed very high rates of all forms of mental illness, personality disorders and substance misuse. Neurotic disorders were found in 58% and 75% of male and female remand prisoners respectively and in 39% and 62% of male and female sentenced prisoners. The Department of Health has now provided funding to adapt the WHO ICD–10–PHC guidelines for prisons.

Prevention

This recognises the fact that affective disorders are influenced by such factors as early childhood experiences, genetic contributions, physical health, stressful life events and chronic social difficulties. These influences may be moderated by intervening factors such as social supports and individual coping skills. The opportunities for primary and secondary prevention in primary care are very great since it is here that recognition of patient risk factors and detection of illness usually occurs. The common element in major life events, whether anticipated or catastrophic, is the threat to the individual's security and social integration. Empirical evidence shows that elevated rates of threatening life events precede the onset of severe depressions (Paykel & Cooper, 1991). However, the statistical associations between stressful events and illness are modest and most people remain well under conditions of high stress (Hinkle, 1987).

Considerable research effort has been applied to identifying factors that contribute to individual vulnerability.

Some universal prevention strategies in place in Great Britain include government legislation and initiatives on car seat-belts and safe driving to reduce the risk of injury, and an emphasis on good nutrition and exercise. In addition, there have been two campaigns run by the Royal College of Psychiatrists, the first on improving public awareness of depression and the second on tackling stigma. Broad policy initiatives of the New Labour government are also aimed at preventing mental ill health. The 'new deal' is an initiative to help the longer-term unemployed to obtain jobs, the minimum wage provides a 'floor' to low pay and the social exclusion unit is focusing on reducing rough sleeping, truancy and school exclusion.

Some selective prevention measures appropriate for specific subgroups of the population with increased risk of illness include school- and work-based preventive activities, and health interventions in young unsupported teenage mothers. Newpin is one such voluntary scheme.

Indicated prevention measures are for people at high risk of illness, for example people with strong genetic loading for psychosis, and for people who have experienced severe emotional stress, and for providing support to older people, especially those with physical and sensory disability.

Suicide prevention

Following the publication of the Health of the Nation strategy, many commentators were sceptical about the potential to influence suicide rates. However, experience over the course of the strategy 1992–1996 was encouraging; and the overall suicide rate has fallen by 11.7% in five years (see Fig. 2.1).

Most people who kill themselves are suffering from a mental illness at the time. The strategy included education of health and social care professionals about suicide risk, supporting high-risk groups (people with severe mental illness, those committing deliberate self-harm, certain occupational groups such as doctors, vets, farmers, pharmacists and nurses), consideration of methods of reducing access to the means of suicide, development of primary and secondary care services, research and audit so we learn the lessons for prevention, and working with the media to encourage responsible reporting that does not glamorise and does not report the method of suicide.

The National Confidential Inquiry into suicides and homicides by people with a mental illness was established and began to collect information on suicide in 1993. It provided valuable insights into

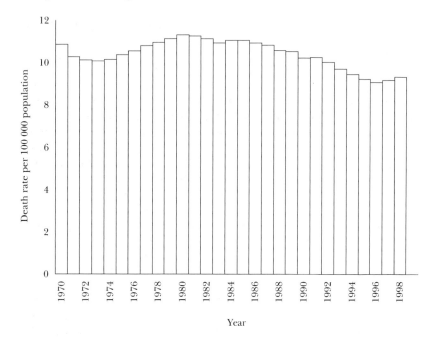

Rates are calculated using the European Standard Population to take account of differences in age structure.
These are three-year average rates: deaths for 1993 and 1994 have been re-coded by ONS so that death rates for all years should now be broadly comparable.

Fig 2.1. Death rates for suicide and undetermined injury, all age groups, England 1970–1998 (Source: ONS)

suicide and the recent report (Department of Health, 1999*a*) stresses the need for clarity of responsibilities, multi-disciplinary cooperation and communication, treatment compliance, risk assessment skills, adequate staff numbers, audit programmes to maintain clinical skills, quality of patients' living environment, integration between the voluntary and statutory services, and risk associated with change in care regimens.

In 1997, England had a change of government and the Health of the Nation Strategy was succeeded by *Saving Lives: Our Healthier Nation Strategy* (Department of Health, 1999*b*), which has set a single target to reduce overall suicide rates by a further 20% between 1997 and 2010. The White Paper has put forward an extremely comprehensive framework of activity to attain the target, including primary, secondary and tertiary prevention, and has suggested many examples of action for national government, for local partnerships between agencies, and for individuals themselves. Action for national government includes publishing the Mental Health National Service Framework, investing more resources in mental health services, improving employment opportunities, reducing homelessness, prompting pre-school education and educational achievement, and considering the mental as well as physical health impact when developing wider government policies. Suggested action for local partnerships includes implementing the National Service Framework, encouraging development of healthy schools and workplaces, developing local support networks – culture-, age- and gender-sensitive – which meet the needs of high-risk groups, improving community safety, developing effective housing strategies, encouraging open and green space for children and families, and other leisure facilities, and identifying local resources and services for mental health, and helping them to work in partnership. Suggestions for individual action include: supporting others at times of stress; using educational and training opportunities; using opportunities for relaxation and physical exercise; drinking sensibly and avoiding illegal drugs; increasing understanding of good mental health; contacting help quickly when difficulties start; and getting involved with service planning (Department of Health, 1999*c*).

The Australian experience

The Australian health ministers endorsed the concept of setting national goals and targets as a means of making significant improvement in the health status of Australians at a National Health Summit in 1993 and agreed that this concept should be embedded within the broader framework of a national health policy. They saw that such a process would provide a way of focusing the health system on improving health outcomes rather than on focusing on activity levels and throughputs. They believed that this could achieve more equitable outcomes in health by addressing some of the underlying determinants of ill health. They expected that these goals and targets would specify priority population groups for specific targets, particularly those that have the greatest gap in health status. In addition, they would provide a way of monitoring and reviewing progress towards improved health outcomes, assessing the effectiveness of a range of preventive measures, and provide a means of involving sectors other than health in health policy and planning. Four areas were initially chosen as foci for action (Commonwealth Department of Human

Services and Health, 1994) on the basis that the conditions were of major concern to the health of Australians, that effective interventions to improve outcomes were possible and that methods of measuring progress in achieving these goals were available. They were cardio-vascular disease, cancer, injury and mental health.

The national mental health goals for Australia

The public health impact of mental health disorders was categorised into two areas: morbidity, which contributed to reduced health, well-being and social functioning, and mortality, the deaths associated with mental disorders. Two overarching goals address these areas.

(a) to reduce the loss of health, well-being and social functioning associated with mental health problems and mental disorders;
(b) to reduce the rate of suicide among people with mental disorders.

Two underlying principles of key importance in achieving the goals were also specified. One was that the government should ensure that services and legislation protect the human rights of people with mental disorder in accordance with the United Nations Resolution on the Protection of Rights of People with Mental Illness and the Australian Health Minister's national mental health statement of rights and responsibilities. Second was that the government should implement strategies to improve community attitudes and under-standing in order to reduce stigma and discrimination. These areas were highlighted because an enquiry by the Human Rights and Equal Opportunity Commission of Australia (Human Rights and Equal Opportunity Commission, 1993) into those with mental illness suggested that Australia had fallen short of being able to comply with the United Nations declaration. The report emphasised the frequent discrimination against, and denial of rights and services to, people with mental disorders. In addition, a survey conducted by a public relations company as part of the national mental health strategy had found considerable confusion and ignorance in the community about what qualifies as a mental disorder and extreme pessimism regarding outcomes for people who seek assistance with mental health problems.

Reduction of health, well-being and social functioning
owing to mental disorder

In addressing the first goal, as in the UK, targets were defined for two groups of disorders, namely depression and related disorders (so-called high-prevalence disorders) and schizophrenia and other psychoses (low-prevalence disorders).

The targets for depression and related disorders. These were to reduce the prevalence following trauma or bereavement by 20% by the year 2000, to improve the quality of life for those affected by reducing the duration of disabling symptoms by 20%, to reduce the likelihood of relapse following a first episode of depression by the year 2000 and to develop appropriate outcome measures by the end of 1997. Priority populations specified were children and young people under 25 years, people aged 65 years and over, those in post-trauma or bereaved situations, post-partum women, carers of those affected by mental disorder, and siblings and children of those with mental disorders. Strategies were developed into primary, secondary and tertiary preventive.

Under *primary prevention* were the following:

(a) the establishment of school-based mental health promotion programmes at all levels of the education system;

(b) support for the national strategy for the prevention of child abuse and neglect;

(c) ensuring that early identification of disruptive behaviour disorders in children and adolescents and the development of effective intervention strategies were encouraged;

(d) ensuring the training of health and educational professionals involved in antenatal and early childhood centre care in the identification of mothers at risk of depression;

(e) the establishment of early post-vention outreach services for critical incident and stress debriefing following specific traumatic events and disaster situations;

(f) ensuring the provision of information support and respite on a national basis to carers, relatives and friends of those affected by mental disorders; and

(g) enhancing access to community services to minimise the social and economic disadvantage commonly experienced among specific groups, e.g. those from non-English speaking back-grounds.

Under *secondary prevention*, the following strategies were highlighted:

(a) increasing the number of school-based assessment and coun-selling services, so that early detection could be introduced into in-service programmes and basic training for teachers, particularly secondary teachers;

(b) the development of comprehensive school-based programmes to support and assist children experiencing grief, trauma, parental and marital discord and separation; and

(c) the development in conjunction with the relevant professional groups of specific programmes for GPs in the recognition of affective management and relapse prevention of new cases of depression and related disorders.

Tertiary prevention strategies proposed were:

(a) the development and implementation of best practice clinical guidelines for the primary care sector for the management of depression;
(b) collaboration of goals with professional groups and the National Community Attitude Strategy to enhance understanding and awareness of depression and related disorders in the general community.

Targets for schizophrenia and other psychoses. These were to improve the quality of life, independence and subjective well-being of those affected by schizophrenia and other psychoses, by reducing the duration of disabling symptoms from an episode of these disorders by 20% by the year 2000 and significantly reducing the likelihood of relapse following a first episode of disorder, as well as developing appropriate outcome measures by the end of 1997. The priority populations were young people aged 14–30 years and those with long-standing disability resulting from these disorders.

In terms of specific strategies under *primary prevention*, only one was advocated, namely the promotion of research into the causes of schizophrenia and other psychoses. Under the *secondary prevention* rubric, the following strategies were proposed:

(a) enhancing the ability of community and primary health care providers and the recognition of the early manifestation of schizophrenia and other psychoses;
(b) in collaboration with relevant professional groups, facilitation of the early treatment of schizophrenia through best practice guidelines for recognition and management;
(c) providing incentives for continuing education of mental health staff or the assessment and management of the early manifestation of schizophrenia;
(d) providing easy access to care at an earlier stage of illness; and
(e) the establishment of measures to increase the treated prevalence of schizophrenia and other psychoses.

Under *tertiary prevention* it was proposed that:

(a) Governments should attempt to enhance community understanding and awareness of schizophrenia and other psychoses in order to reduce stigma and discrimination.

(b) Governments in collaboration with key consumer and professional groups should enhance knowledge and positive attitudes to those with mental disorders among mental health professionals and other health professionals.

(c) Teams should ensure early intervention in relapsing cases and should extend the quality and deployment of known effective interventions with particular emphasis on partnership between the consumer and service providers.

Reduction of suicide

Targets for suicide reduction. In the goal on suicide, the targets were to reduce by 15% the expected Australian suicide rates over the next 10 years, to reduce by 25% the suicide rate in people suffering from schizophrenia and other psychoses over 10 years, and to develop appropriate outcome measures by the end of 1995. The priority populations were males aged 15–34 years and males aged 65 years and over, because of the high levels of suicide in these groups in the Australian context.

Under *primary prevention* the strategies were:

(a) the encouragement of further community debate on legislation to restrict the use of firearms for non-essential purposes; and

(b) the implementation of protocols for specialist mental health intervention and other strategies, such as peer support in schools, where a high-risk situation is perceived to exist, for example, where a suicide has occurred.

Under *secondary prevention* the strategies were:

(a) the improved recognition and treatment of depression, a major precursor to suicide in general practice, by providing incentives for GPs to participate in continuing education;

(b) the better management of suicide attempts through improved access to health services and specific management protocols for those presenting to emergency departments;

(c) the fostering of enhanced community recognition of depression and related disorders through the further development of depression awareness campaigns; and

(d) in conjunction with professional groups, the development of strategies to improve the management of suicide attempters and to deal with suicidal ideation with patients with schizophrenia and other psychoses.

The Australian guidelines were published in 1994 and responsibility for implementing them fell to both Commonwealth and State governments. Much progress has been made in their implementation, although systematic evaluation of this has not been achieved. Many of the strategies suggested were implemented as part of the first national mental health strategy that focused on the care of people with schizophrenia and related disorders 1992–1997 (Commonwealth Department of Human Services and Health, 1992) (for example, the development of the Australian clinical guidelines for the management of early psychosis (Commonwealth Department of Human Services and Health, 1998). Additional focus on the depression targets and strategies is now part of the Second National Mental Health Plan released by the Australian Governments (e.g. depression awareness campaign, which extends the established guidelines for recognition and management of depression in primary care). The process of setting the goals and targets, however, was an extremely powerful one for highlighting the need to focus on outcomes rather than process measures in mental health. It is the expectation that Australia will report to the WHO on its national health policy by a focus on its progress in meeting a comprehensive range of targets that have been specified.

Conclusions

The process of setting national health targets is a powerful way of engendering commitment at government, national, regional, local and individual level to achieve measurable health outcomes. It influences distribution of resources in terms of finance, time and training. It encourages examination and implementation of interventions with proven effect that have not hitherto been widely disseminated.

References

American Public Health Association (1991) *Healthy Communities 2000 Model Standards and Guidelines for Community Attainment of the Year 2000 National Health Objectives.* Washington, DC: APHA.
Armstrong, E. (1993) Mental health check. *Nursing Times*, **89**, 40–42.
—— (1995) *Mental Health Issues in Primary Care*, p. 92. London: Macmillan.
—— (1997) *The Primary Mental Health Care Toolkit.* London: Department of Health.
Audit Commission (1994) *Finding a Place: A Review of Mental Health Services for Adults.* London: HMSO.
Commonwealth Department of Human Services and Health (1992) *National Mental Health Plan.* Canberra: Australian Government Printing Service.
—— (1994) *Better Health Outcomes for Australians. National Goals, Targets and Strategies. Better Health Outcomes into the Next Century.* Canberra: Commonwealth Department of Health.
—— (1998) *Second National Mental Health Plan.* Canberra: Australian Government Printing Service.

DEPARTMENT OF HEALTH (1992) *The Health of the Nation: A Strategy for Health in England.* Cm. 1986. London: HMSO.

—— (1993) *Mental Illness: What Does it Mean?, A Guide to Mental Health in the Workplace* and *Sometimes I Think I Can't Go on Anymore.* A series. London: Department of Health.

—— (1994) *The Mental Illness Key Area Handbook,* 2nd edition. London: HMSO.

—— (1995) *Building Bridges: A Guide to Arrangements for Inter-agency Working for the Care and Protection of Severely Mentally Ill People.* London: Department of Health.

—— (1996*a*) *The Spectrum of Care: Local Services for People with Mental Health Problems.* London: Department of Health.

—— (1996*b*) *Commissioning 24 Hour Nursed Care for People with Severe and Enduring Mental Illness.* London: Department of Health.

—— (1996*c*) *ABC of Mental Health in the Workplace.* London: HMSO.

—— (1998) *Modernising Mental Health Services: Safe, Sound and Supportive.* London: Department of Health.

—— (1999*a*) *Safer Services: National Confidential Inquiry into Suicide and Homicide by People with Mental Illness.* London: Department of Health.

—— (1999*b*) *Saving Lives: Our Healthier Nation.* Cm. 4386. London: The Stationery Office.

—— (1999*c*) *National Service Framework for Mental Health: Modern Standards and Service Models.* London: Department of Health.

DEPARTMENT OF HEALTH AND SOCIAL SECURITY (1975) *Better Services for Mentally Ill.* Cmnd 6233. London: HMSO.

DOHERTY, N. & TYSON, S. (1998) *Mental Well Being in the Workplace: A Resource Pack for Management Training and Development.* London: Health and Safety Executive Books.

DRUCKER, P. F. (1981) *Toward the Next Economics and Other Essays.* New York. Harper and Row.

FIRTH-COZENS, J. & MORRISON, L. A. (1989) Sources of Stress and Ways of Coping in Junior House Officers. *Stress Medicine,* **5**, 121–126.

GRIFFITHS, S., WYLIE, I. & JENKINS, R. (1992) *Creating a Common Profile for Mental Health.* London: HMSO.

HEALTH AND SAFETY ACT (1974) London: HMSO.

HINKLE, L. E. (1987) Stress and disease: the concept after 50 years. *Social Science and Medicine,* **25**, 561–566.

HUMAN RIGHTS AND EQUAL OPPORTUNITY COMMISSION (1993*)* *Human Rights – Mental Illness.* Canberra: Australian Government Printing Service.

JENKINS, R. (1990) Towards a system of outcome indicators for mental health care. *British Journal of Psychiatry,* **157**, 500–514.

—— (1992*)* Developments in the primary care of mental illness – a forward look. *International Review of Psychiatry,* **4**, 237–242.

—— & CONEY, N. (1992) *Prevention of Mental Ill-health at Work.* London: HMSO.

—— & GRIFFITHS, S. (1991) *Indicators for Mental Health in the Population.* London: HMSO.

—— & ÜSTÜN, T. B. (eds) (1998) *Preventing Mental Illness: Mental Health Promotion in Primary Care.* Chichester: Wiley.

—— & WARMAN, D. (1993*)* *Promoting Mental Health Policies in the Workplace.* London: HMSO.

——, GRIFFITHS, S., WYLIE, I., *ET AL* (1994) *The Prevention of Suicide.* London. HMSO.

——, BEBBINGTON, P., BRUGHA, T., *ET AL* (1998) The British Psychiatric Morbidity Survey. *British Journal of Psychiatry,* **173**, 4–7.

OFFICE OF POPULATION CENSUS AND SURVEYS (OPCS) (1995) *OPCS Surveys of Psychiatric Morbidity in Great Britain.* Reports 1–8. London: HMSO.

PAYKEL, E. C. & COOPER, Z. (1991) Recent life events and psychiatric illness. In: *The European Handbook of Psychiatric and Mental Health* (ed. A. Seva), pp. 350–363. Barcelona: Editorial Anthropos.

RIX, S., PAYKEL, E. S., LELLIOTT, P., *ET AL* (1999) Impact of a national campaign on GP education: an evaluation of the defeat depression campaign. *British Journal of General Practice,* **49**, 99–102.

ROTH, A., FONAGY, P., PARRY, G., *ET AL* (1996) *What Works for Whom? A Critical Review of Psychotherapy Research.* New York: Guilford Press.

SINGLETON, N., MELTZER, H. & GATWARD, R. (1998) *Psychiatric Morbidity among Prisoners in England and Wales.* London: Office for National Statistics.

WALL, T. D., BOLDEN, R. I., BORRILL, C. S., *ET AL* (1997) Minor psychiatric disorder in NHS trust staff: occupational and gender differences. *British Journal of Psychiatry*, **171**, 519–523.

WING, J. K., BEEVOR, A. S., CURTIS, R. H., *ET AL* (1998) Health of the Nation Outcome Scales (HoNOS). Research and development. *British Journal of Psychiatry*, **172**, 11–18.

WORLD HEALTH ORGANIZATION (1981) *Development Indicators for Monitoring Progress Towards Health for All by the Year 2000.* Geneva: WHO.

WORLD HEALTH ORGANIZATION COLLABORATING CENTRE (2000) *WHO Guide to Mental Health in Primary Care* (adapted for the UK from ICD–10, Chapter 5, Primary Care version). London: Royal Society of Medicine Press.

3   Population surveys of morbidity and need

RACHEL JENKINS and HOWARD MELTZER

The heavy burden posed by mental disorders in all regions of the world makes it imperative that countries develop explicit policies and implementation strategies to tackle this burden (Murray & Lopez, 1996; Jenkins, 1997). Such policies will need to include action to improve information and understanding about mental illness, action to develop services and improve practice in order to promote mental health and reduce morbidity and disability, and action to reduce mortality from mental illness.

The information available to those concerned with mental health policy has generally been limited in scope and geographical coverage. Routine statistics (e.g. on hospital admissions) and small local surveys cannot provide nationally representative information on need and may be misleading if used as the basis for mental health policy. There are therefore a number of reasons for carrying out large-scale community studies of psychiatric morbidity.

Effective policy needs to be based on epidemiology and the social and economic consequences of psychiatric morbidity. Representative information in a geographical area is a desirable prerequisite for planning health and social services. In addition to estimating prevalence, severity, duration and accompanying social disability, community surveys can document the use of existing services and can estimate the extent of unmet needs and the services required to meet them.

Information on prevalence and associated factors of presumed causal importance allows aetiological hypotheses to be generated and tested, albeit with the limitations inherent in cross-sectional studies. It also allows assessment of the potential scope for public health interventions. By repeating community surveys, it is possible to monitor the health of the population and trends in disease, together with changes in potential risk factors.

As well as mental health surveys of the general household adult population, there are also policy-driven reasons to carry out mental health surveys of the prison population, people who are homeless and people in institutional care. Although these groups represent a relatively small percentage of the total population, they are likely to be extensive users of mental health services and pose particular challenges to mental health service providers. Surveys on the development and well-being of children and adolescents also have a key role to play in completing the epidemiological picture of the nation's mental health.

This chapter explores the role of such surveys in health planning and research, drawing on the UK experience, with particular emphasis on the implications not just for specialist care, but also for primary care, schools, workplaces and the interface between health and social care.

Rationale of the survey programme

The survey programme was announced in 1992 as part of England's Health of the Nation strategy, which, while setting specific targets for reducing morbidity and mortality, laid out a tripartite framework for action: improving information and understanding about mental illness, developing local comprehensive services, and developing good practice (Department of Health, 1992, 1994). The survey programme was an integral part of the agenda to improve information and understanding about mental illness. The Department of Health commissioned the Office of Population Censuses and Surveys (OPCS) (now the Office for National Statistics (ONS)) to survey the psychiatric morbidity of the country in collaboration with an advisory group of psychiatric epidemiologists (see Appendix 3.1). This chapter provides an overview of the survey programme to date as a whole, and the reader is also referred to Chapter 2 of this volume for further details.

The survey programme initially consisted of four surveys, commissioned in 1992, and a series of subsequent surveys covering additional population groups (Jenkins *et al*, 1997a, 1997b, 1998). The surveys were commissioned by the Department of Health for England, together with the Welsh Office and the Scottish Home and Health Department, to give a national picture of the prevalence, severity and duration of mental health problems and their accompanying disability, associated risk factors, and the extent to which health and social care needs are met by services. The survey data aimed to provide a baseline measure of the health of the nation target to improve the health and social functioning of people with mental illness.

TABLE 3.1
Research programme of psychiatric morbidity surveys in Great Britain

Survey	Sample size	Fieldwork
Adults living in private households	10 108	April–September 1993
Adults with psychosis living in the community	300	October–December 1993
Residents of institutions catering for people with mental disorders	1191	April–July 1994
Homeless people	1166	July–August 1994
Male and female remand and sentenced prisoners*	3142	September–December 1997
Children and adolescents aged 5–15 years in private households	10 438	January–May 1999

* In England and Wales.
Source: Thornicroft & Tansella (1999).

The four initial surveys consisted of a private household survey of 10 000 adults aged 16–64 years, an institutional survey, a survey of a supplementary sample of people with known psychosis living in households, and a survey of homeless and roofless people. The subsequent surveys included a survey of people in custody (with a subsample followed up 12 months later) and a survey of children and adolescents aged 5–15 years. Two new surveys will shortly be reported: a repeat household survey that will include adults aged 16–74 years and a survey of young people looked after by local authorities (see Table 3.1).

Methods of the survey programme

Sampling strategy

The private household survey used the small users 'Postcode Address Files' as the sampling frame, with 90 delivery points randomly selected in each of 200 postal sectors. It was stratified by regional health authority and social class (giving 18 000 delivery points in order to yield 10 000 subjects; see Fig. 3.1).

18 000 addresses in great Britain selected from the Postcode Address Files
15 765 private households found at these addresses
12 730 adults aged 16–64 years selected for interview 10 108 adults cooperated

Fig. 3.1 Summary of the sampling procedure

The supplementary sample of people with known psychosis living in households was carried out in order to provide additional information on service use. It was obtained by random samples from a listing of everyone with known psychosis compiled by general pracitioners (GPs) and community mental health teams (CMHTs) in the same 200 postal sectors as were sampled in the private household survey. Overall, about 300 adults were interviewed. This survey was carried out in order to provide additional information on service use of people with psychosis, owing to the relatively low prevalence of psychosis among the private household population.

The institutional survey was carried out in hospitals and residential homes randomly selected from Department of Health data-bases, and in hostels and group homes selected from lists obtained from health and local authorities, stratified by institutional size. Overall, information was collected on 1180 residents in 208 establishments.

The sample for the survey of homeless and roofless people was randomly selected from lists of homeless people in temporary housing in private-sector-leased accommodation and from hostels for the homeless, night shelters and people sleeping rough who were in contact with day centres. Five hundred and thirty residents were interviewed from a sample of 92 hostels; 268 were interviewed in private-sector-leased accommodation; 187 were interviewed in 29 night shelters; and 181 were interviewed in 30 day centres.

For the prison survey, in order to provide separate prevalence estimates for male and female remand and sentenced prisoners, the aim was to achieve interviews with over 1200 male remand, 1200 male sentenced and 800 female prisoners.

To avoid the possibility of over- or under-sampling any possible clusters of prisoners with mental problems, all prisons in England and Wales were included in the survey and a sample of inmates drawn from a list of inmates in all locations within each prison using a fixed sampling fraction. The sampling fractions used were 1 in 34 male sentenced prisoners, 1 in 8 male remand prisoners and 1 in 3 women prisoners (whether remand or sentenced). All 131 prison establishments open at the time fieldwork commenced agreed to participate in the survey. Interviews were obtained for 1250 male remand, 1121 male sentenced, 187 female remand and 584 female prisoners.

This was the first overall national survey programme in any country to collect data on prevalence, risk factors and associated disability simultaneously in household, institutional and homeless samples by the use of standardised assessment techniques.

Interviewing procedures and questionnaire content

Although the survey research programme on psychiatric morbidity was split up into separate surveys, the aim was to get comparative data, as far as possible, across all the surveyed populations.

All responders in the household survey were interviewed by Office of Population Censuses and Surveys social survey interviewers using: the Revised Clinical Interview Schedule (CIS–R; Lewis *et al*, 1992) leading to ICD–10 diagnostic categories (World Health Organization (WHO), 1992); the Psychosis Screening Questionnaire (Bebbington & Nayani, 1995), specifically developed for the survey; questions about alcohol and drug misuse and dependence using quality/ frequency questions from the regular national surveys of alcohol and tobacco consumption; questions about stressful life events, social support, social disability, activities of daily living (ADLs), education and employment; and questions about long-standing illness and medication. Those subjects scoring over 12 on the CIS–R and/or positive on the Psychosis Screening Questionnaire were asked further detailed questions on use of health, social and voluntary care services and informal care, and had a follow-up interview administered by psychiatrists, Schedules for Clinical Assessment in Neuropsychiatry (SCAN; Wing *et al*, 1990), to provide a one-year prevalence of functional psychosis. In the supplementary sample, all were approached for a SCAN interview.

In the institutional survey, the same procedure was carried out, except that proxy information was sought for those who were unable to cooperate with the interview. In the hostels and private-sector-leased accommodation, a similar procedure to that in the household survey was followed, with the addition of the 12-item

General Health Questionnaire (GHQ; Goldberg, 1972). Pilot studies indicated that a shorter questionnaire was needed for the sample from night shelters and day centres. Therefore, for these two samples, the 12-item GHQ replaced the CIS–R, and fewer questions were included on the social environment and use of services.

Results

Household survey

Neurosis

The household survey achieved a response rate of 80%. One in six adults aged 16–64 years who lived in private households had suffered from some type of neurotic (non-psychotic) disorder in the week before the survey interview, half of which was mixed anxiety–depression. All types of neurotic disorders were more common among women than men (see Table 3.2).

TABLE 3.2
Prevalence of psychiatric disorders per 1000 population in adults aged 16–64 years in Great Britain in 1993

	Rate per thousand in past week (s.e.)		
	Women	Men	All adults
Mixed anxiety and depressive disorders	94(5)	54(4)	77(3)
Generalised anxiety disorder	34(3)	28(2)	31(2)
Depressive episode	25(2)	17(2)	21(1)
Phobias	14(2)	7(1)	11(1)
Obsessive–compulsive disorder	15(2)	9(2)	12(1)
Panic disorder	9(1)	8(2)	8(1)
Any neurotic disorder	195(7)	123(5)	160(5)

	Rate per thousand in past 12 months (s.e.)		
	Women	Men	All adults
Functional psychosis	4(1)	4(1)	4(1)
Alcohol dependence	21(2)	75(5)	47(3)
Drug dependence	14(2)	29(3)	22(2)

s.e., standard error.
Source: Thornicroft & Tansella (1999).

Marital status was strongly associated with neurotic disorder: rates were substantially higher in separated, divorced and widowed individuals of both genders and among cohabiting women. Table 3.3 shows the socio-demographic associations of a raised total CIS–R score based on multiple logistic regression analysis. Unemployed people (see Table 3.4) were about twice as likely to suffer from neurotic

TABLE 3.3
Odds ratio of socio-demographic correlates of the Revised Clinical Interview Schedule (CIS–R; Lewis et al, 1992) score

CIS–R score of 12 or more	Adjusted odds ratio	Confidence interval
Gender		
Male	1.00	–
Female	1.56**	1.37–1.78
Age (years)		
16–24	1.00	–
25–34	1.07	0.87–1.32
35–44	1.23	0.99–1.53
45–54	1.24	0.99–1.55
55–64	0.72**	0.56–0.91
Family unit type		
Couple, no children	1.00	–
Couple, 1 or more children	1.03	0.87–1.21
Lone parent + child	1.56**	1.26–1.93
One person only	1.48**	1.25–1.76
Adult with parents	0.76	0.54–1.05
Adult with one parent	0.80	0.54–1.19
Employment status		
Working full-time	1.00	–
Working part-time	1.19	1.00–1.42
Unemployed	2.26**	1.87–2.72
Economically inactive	1.71**	1.47–2.00
Accommodation		
Detached	1.00	–
Semi-detached	0.96	0.80–1.15
Terrace	1.19	1.00–1.43
Flat/maisonette	1.15	0.93–1.43
Tenure		
Owner/occupier	1.00	–
Renter	1.33**	1.16–1.53
Locality		
Semi-rural/rural	1.00	–
Urban	1.21**	1.06–1.38

**$P<0.01$.

TABLE 3.4
Prevalence of psychiatric disorders by economic activity

	Working full-time	Working part-time	Unemployed	Economically inactive
Neurosis rate per 1000 in past week	118 (6)	160 (10)	259 (17)	212 (10)
Psychosis rate per 1000 in past 12 months	2 (1)	5 (2)	7 (2)	9 (2)
Alcohol dependence rate per 1000 in past 12 months	54 (4)	42 (6)	89 (13)	29 (4)
Drug dependence rate per 1000 in past 12 months	13 (2)	17 (4)	83 (12)	23 (3)

disorders compared with people in work, and those living in urban settings were 1.5 times as likely to suffer them than rural dwellers. Employment status is even more strongly associated with neurotic disorder.

About half of individuals identified as having a neurotic disorder also suffered from long-standing physical complaints, compared with only 30% of people without a neurotic disorder. This differential was seen across all ages and both genders.

Subjects with significant depressive symptoms were asked about suicidal ideas. Just under 1% of the total sample in the household survey reported suicidal thoughts in the preceding week, two-thirds of them women. However, only one-fifth of those reporting suicidal ideas were receiving antidepressant medication and only one-sixth were receiving counselling or psychotherapy.

Alcohol and drug use

One adult in 20 had experienced symptoms of alcohol dependence in the preceding year and one in 40 dependence on drugs. Men were over three times as likely as women to be dependent on alcohol and twice as likely to be dependent on drugs (see Table 3.2). Alcohol dependence was nearly twice as common among those who were unemployed as in those who were working; drug dependence was over five times more frequent among unemployed people (see Table 3.4).

Use of mental health services

Individuals with neuroses were twice as likely as those without to have consulted their GP in the fortnight before interview. Three-quarters of people with neurosis had consulted their GP only in the past year, and a further 8% had had contact with a mental health service in the last year as well as consulting their GP. However, 16% of those with a neurotic disorder had not consulted any professional about their mental health, usually because they thought no one could help (see Table 3.5).

Psychosis

The overall prevalence of psychosis in the household survey was four per 1000, with that for urban dwellers being twice that for those living in the country. There is therefore significant unmet need for specialist support for people with psychosis (see Table 3.6). Table 3.6 shows the extensive use of GPs in managing patients with psychosis, with just over a third also being in contact with specialist mental health services.

Social disability

The levels of social disability found in the household survey, not only in people with psychosis but also in those with neurosis and in those who were experiencing suicidal thoughts, is astonishingly high

TABLE 3.5

Use of services in the past year by gender: adults with a neurotic disorder (%)

	Women	*Men*	*All*
Consulted GP and had contact with mental health services[1]	9	6	8
Contact with mental health services only	0	2	1
Consulted GP only	77	71	75
Neither consulted GP nor had contact with mental health services	13	21	16
Base[2]	865	535	1390

1. Includes psychiatrist, psychotherapist, community psychiatric nurse, psychiatric social worker or counsellor.
2. Base excludes 167 people for whom mental health services data were missing.

TABLE 3.6
Use of services in past year by gender: adults with a psychotic disorder (%)

	Women[2]	Men[2]	All
Consulted GP and had contact with mental health services[1]	[9]	[7]	36
Contact with mental health services only	[–]	[1]	1
Consulted GP only	[12]	[12]	55
Neither consulted GP nor had contact with mental health services	[1]	[1]	7
Base		44	

1. Includes psychiatrist, psychotherapist, community psychiatric nurse, psychiatric social worker or counsellor.
2. Bases for men and women are too small to show percentages; actual fugures are presented in square brackets. The final column shows percentages.

(see Table 3.7) and emphasise the need for integrated assessment and management of health and social care needs.

Institutional survey

The survey of adults living in institutions covered those aged 16–64 years who were permanently resident in institutions catering for people with mental health problems in Great Britain. Residents

TABLE 3.7
Difficulties in activities of daily living (ADLs) in household samples

Subject group	*% with any ADL difficulties*	*Base*
Suicidal thoughts in past week	50	80
Psychosis in past year	40	44
Neurosis in past week	32	1557
None of the above	12	8184

were defined as permanently resident if they had been living in the sampled establishment for six months or more, or had no other permanent address, or were likely to stay in the establishment for the foreseeable future. In 1994, approximately 33 200 adults aged 16–64 years were permanently resident in accommodation of this type.

Seventy per cent of residents for whom diagnoses were obtained suffered from schizophrenia, delusional and schizoaffective disorders, 8% from neuroses or non-psychotic disorders, and 8% from affective psychoses. Of the remaining 10%, 8% had other disorders, and for 80% there was insufficient information for a diagnostic classification. The distribution of disorders varied according to whether the setting was a hospital or residential accommodation. The prevalence of schizophrenia and related disorders was higher in hospitals (74% compared with 67% in residential accommodation), while neurotic disorders were more prevalent among those in residential accommodation (12% compared with 4% in hospitals). The majority of residents with schizophrenia and related disorders had a length of stay of two years or more, with a median length of stay of 2.5 years. Residents with affective psychosis showed similar lengths of stay. Conversely, most residents with neurotic disorders had a length of stay of less than two years with a median length of stay of 1.5 years.

Psychiatric morbidity among homeless people

The survey of psychiatric morbidity among homeless people covered a broad range of people who did not have adequate shelter. They were defined according to their accommodation circumstances: residents of hostels, of private-sector-leased accommodation or of night shelters, or as homeless people sleeping rough and using day centres.

The prevalence of neurosis was 38% among hostel residents, 35% among private-sector-leased accommodation residents, 60% among night shelter residents, and 57% among homeless people sleeping rough (compared with 14% in private households). The prevalence of psychosis was 8% among hostel residents, 2% among private-sector-leased accommodation residents and was not estimated in night shelter residents and people sleeping rough (compared with 0.4% in private households).

The prevalence of alcohol dependence was 16% among hostel residents, 3% among private-sector-leased accommodation residents, 44% among night shelter residents and 50% among homeless people sleeping rough (compared with 5% of private household residents).

The prevalence of drug dependence on non-cannabinoid drugs was 6% in hostel residents, with a further 5% dependent on cannabis only. Twenty-two per cent of night shelter residents were dependent on non-cannabinoid drugs, rising to 39% when cannabis was included. In people sleeping rough, 12% were dependent on non-cannabinoid drugs, rising to 24% when cannabis was included.

The supplementary sample of people with known psychosis

Subjects for the supplementary survey were obtained from GPs or mental health teams (following Local Research Ethics Committee approval). Doctors and other health professionals were asked to approach their clients who were suffering from a psychotic disorder and ask them to participate in the OPCS survey. Therefore, if the subjects screened positive on any of the five sift criteria, they were confirmed as having a psychotic disorder.

The analysis in this section brings together people with a psychotic disorder from the private household survey (44 adults), people with psychosis living in private households who were known to their GP or mental health team (244 adults), and adults with a psychotic disorder identified in the institutional sample who would be regarded as living in residential households, that is, those living in supported accommodation such as recognised lodgings or small-group homes. Adults with psychosis identified by the survey of homeless people were not included in this analysis because only a very small number were considered to be living in private households, for example those living in private-sector-leased accommodation.

This sample is not representative of all people with psychotic disorders because individuals in the different subsamples had different probabilities of selection, and the results have not been re-weighted to compensate for this, partly because of the complexity involved and partly because of the likelihood of some duplication of addresses in the various sampling frames used.

Three-fifths of this sample of people with psychosis had consulted a GP in the past year about a mental, nervous or emotional problem. One-half of the sample had been an out-patient during the previous year for a mental, nervous or emotional problem. Almost one-half of this sample had received a domiciliary visit from a community psychiatric nurse (CPN), one-quarter had been visited by a social worker, and one in six had received visits from a home care worker. One-fifth had been an in-patient for a mental problem in the past year.

More than three-fifths of the sample reported difficulties with at least one of the ADLs covered by the surveys, the commonest problem being difficulty in dealing with paperwork. At least two-thirds of the people with psychosis said they needed help and most of them received it.

Only one in five of the sample of people with psychosis was in employment, half were unable to work and one in eight was un-employed. Nine-tenths of the sample controlled their own finances, and about one-half of those who did received a state benefit relating to invalidity or disability.

About one-quarter of this sample were identified as having a small primary support group, and one-third had a severe lack of perceived social support.

Around three-fifths of this sample of people with psychosis were regular smokers, and two-fifths smoked 20 or more cigarettes a day. A smaller proportion of this sample were heavier drinkers than in the general population living in private households. However, one in 10 of this sample reported illicit use of drugs, compared with around one in 20 in the household survey.

The prison survey

The ONS survey of psychiatric morbidity among prisoners in England and Wales was commissioned by the Department of Health in 1997. The main aim of the survey was to collect baseline data on the mental health of male and female remand and sentenced prisoners in order to inform general policy decisions.

These baseline data were compared with corresponding data from previous ONS surveys of individuals resident in private households and institutions catering for people with mental health problems and homeless people. In addition, the survey aimed to examine the varying use of services and the receipt of care in relation to mental disorder, and to establish key, current and lifetime factors that may be associated with mental disorders of prisoners. The survey included assessment of personality disorder, neurosis, psychosis, alcohol and drug dependence, deliberate self-harm, post-traumatic stress and intellectual functioning, and the comorbidity of these disorders. All prisons in England and Wales were included in the survey. All prisoners aged 16–64 years were eligible for selection in the sample. Women prisoners and men on remand are a comparatively small proportion of the total prison population. Therefore, these groups were over-sampled to provide adequate numbers to allow separate analysis of the data for these groups.

Seventy-eight per cent of male remand prisoners, 64% of male sentenced and 50% of female prisoners had a personality disorder. Ten per cent of male remand, 7% of male sentenced, and 14% of female prisoners had a functional psychosis. Fifty-nine per cent of remand and 40% of sentenced male prisoners had a neurotic illness, while the corresponding figures for women were 76% and 63%.

The proportion of prisoners who had thought of committing suicide at some time was very high. For example, 46% of male remand prisoners had thought of suicide in their lifetime, 35% in the past year and 12% in the week prior to interview. The rates for female remand prisoners were even higher. The rates of suicide attempts were also very high – 27% of male remand prisoners said they had attempted suicide at some time in their life, 15% in the preceding year and 2% in the previous week.

Implications

The surveys have greatly enhanced the national data available to the government for planning purposes by adding data on population epidemiology (morbidity, disability, associated risk factors and linked service use) to the existing routine collection of data on service use.

The surveys demonstrated a number of significant findings, which need to be taken into account in the planning and delivery of mental health services in Great Britain. The very high prevalence of neurosis, some of which is extremely severe and associated with suicidal risk, means proper attention must be given to the education and training of primary care teams about mental health (Jenkins, 1992, 1998), to the primary/secondary care interface (Strathdee & Jenkins, 1996), and to supporting primary care teams with good practice guidelines (Armstrong, 1997; World Health Organization & Royal Society of Medicine, 2000), agreed criteria for referral, and with shared care where appropriate. It is also clear that the prevention and early detection and amelioration of the more common and less severe forms of neurosis will need to be addressed more widely in schools, workplaces and in other communities (Jenkins & Üstün, 1998). This will require systematic effort by developers and evaluators of preventive interventions. The regional variation in psychosis and the association of mental disorders with socio-demographic factors such as unemployment and living conditions mean that these variables must be taken into account when assessing health needs and when allocating financial resources.

The high levels of social disability associated not only with psychosis but also with neurosis mean that individuals must receive proper integrated assessment of their social needs as well as their health needs, and that care plans must address social disability as well as health issues in an integrated way.

The high rates in the household survey of suicidal thoughts in people with depression mean that teaching good suicidal assessment and management techniques to health and social care professionals must be a priority (Jenkins *et al*, 1994), as should the national and local action to minimise environmental risk factors for suicide and to reduce access to the means for suicide.

The high levels of morbidity in the homeless must be addressed by purchasing of services for homeless people in every locality to ensure adequate primary and secondary care.

The extremely high levels of morbidity in the prison population mean that it is essential to ensure access to high-quality primary and secondary mental health care. The government is now commissioning prison health care from the NHS and has funded the adaptation of the ICD–10 mental health guidelines for prisons.

Conclusion

The survey programme has achieved a representative baseline framework of information on the mental health of our nation and the associated health care response to this, as described by users of the NHS in Great Britain. By repeating the survey programme in future years, it will be possible to monitor and estimate the extent to which the objectives for mental health prevention and treatment services can be more accurately based. By doing so, attention can be given both to common mental disorders and to severe mental illness by means of specific, well-informed mental health policies.

Appendix 3.1

Advisory Group of Psychiatric Epidemiologists

Professor Rachel Jenkins (Chair)
Professor Paul Bebbington
Professor Glyn Lewis
Dr Terry Brugha
Dr Michael Farrell
Dr Jacqueline Alarçon
Dr Jeremy Coid

References

ARMSTRONG, E. (1997) *The Primary Mental Health Care Toolkit.* London: Department of Health.

BEBBINGTON, P. E. & NAYANI, T. (1995) The Psychosis Screening Questionnaire. *International Journal of Methods in Psychiatric Research,* **5**, 11–20.

—, DUNN, G., JENKINS, R., *ET AL* (1998) The influence of age and sex on the prevalence of depressive conditions: report from the National Survey of Psychiatric Morbidity. *Psychological Medicine,* **28**, 9–19.

DEPARTMENT OF HEALTH (1992*a*) *The Health of the Nation: A Strategy for Health in England.* Cm. 1986. London: The Stationery Office.

— (1993) *The Public Health Information Strategy – Improving Information on Mental Health.* London: Department of Health.

— (1994) *Mental Health Area Handbook.* London: The Stationery Office.

GOLDBERG, D. P. (1972) *The Detection of Psychiatric Illness by Questionnaire (GHQ).* Maudsley Monograph 21. London: Oxford University Press.

JENKINS, R. (1992) Developments in the primary care of mental illness – a forward look. *International Review of Psychiatry,* **4**, 237–242.

— (1997) Reducing the burden of mental illness. *Lancet,* **349**, 1340.

— (1998) Mental health and primary care – implications for policy. *International Review of Psychiatry,* **10**, 158–160.

— & ÜSTÜN, T. B. (eds) (1998) *Preventing Mental Illness – Mental Health Promotion in Primary Care.* Chichester: Wiley.

—, GRIFFITHS, S.,WYLIE, I., *ET AL* (eds) (1994) *The Prevention of Suicide.* London: The Stationery Office.

—, BEBBINGTON, P., BRUGHA, T., *ET AL* (1997*a*) The National Psychiatric Morbidity Surveys of Great Britain – strategy and methods. *Psychological Medicine,* **27**, 765–774.

—, —, —, *ET AL* (1997*b*) The National Psychiatric Morbidity Surveys of Great Britain – initial findings from the Household Survey. *Psychological Medicine,* **27**, 775–790.

—, —, —, *ET AL* (1998) British Psychiatric Morbidity Survey. *British Journal of Psychiatry,* **173**, 4–7.

LEWIS, G., PELOSI, A., ARAYA, R., *ET AL* (1992) Measuring psychiatric disorders in the community: a standardised assessment for use by lay interviewers. *Psychological Medicine,* **22**, 465–486.

MURRAY, J. L. & LOPEZ, A. D. (eds) (1996) *The Global Burden of Disease.* Harvard: Harvard School of Public Health/Harvard University Press.

STRATHDEE, G. & JENKINS, R. (1996) Purchasing mental health care for primary care. In: *Commissioning Mental Health Services* (eds G. Thornicroft & G. Strathdee). London: The Stationery Office.

WING, J. K., BABOR, T., BRUGHA, T., *ET AL* (1990) SCAN: Schedules for clinical assessment in psychiatry. *Archives of General Psychiatry,* **47**, 589–593.

WORLD HEALTH ORGANIZATION (1992) *International Classification of Diseases and Related Health Problems. Tenth revision (ICD–10).* Geneva: WHO.

— & ROYAL SOCIETY OF MEDICINE (2000) *WHO Guide to Mental Health in Primary Care.* London: Royal Society of Medicine.

4 Commissioners' information requirements on mental health needs and commissioning for mental health services

ANDREW STEVENS, JAMES RAFTERY and RICHARD A. MENDELSOHN

The commissioning of mental health services continues to be influenced by the rapid development of mental health policy nationally (Department of Health, 1998*a*, 1999*b*) and the desire to replace the internal market of the NHS with a more collaborative, coordinated approach that seeks to maximise quality and health improvement (Secretary of State for Health, 1997). In keeping with the health service reforms of the early 1990s (House of Commons, 1990), the purchaser/provider split has been retained in the most recent reorganisation, but somewhat de-formalised with 'commissioning' rather than 'purchasing' and with primary care groups and primary care trusts (PCG/Ts) taking on part of the role of district health authorities (DHAs). Like the old purchasers, these commissioning agencies are now responsible for spending the resources available, to improve the health of their 'responsible' population. The commissioning agencies must set the pattern of spend between different services and base this pattern on an assessment of the needs of the population so as to maximise health improvement.

There is a new local collaborative approach in the commissioning of mental health services that applies to all relevant stakeholders. Such stakeholders include local authorities, which also, therefore, have an interest in needs assessment – specifically of the social care requirement for individuals with mental health problems. Indeed, joint health and social service needs assessment is now a formal requirement (Department of Health, 1998*a*). Local authorities have also been subject to reorganisation (Secretary of State for Health, 1998) and for the first time are subject to joint health and social services planning and priorities guidance (Department of Health, 1998*b*), which may make closer working a reality. Allowing the development of alternative models of either the commissioning or the provision of mental health and social services may also assist closer collaboration (Department of Health, 1998*c*). In particular, the possibility of the creation of mental health care trusts across both types of organisation has been signalled (Department of Health, 2000). Such collaboration between health and social services has to date been hampered by the overlap of responsibilities, tightening local authority finance, the different geographical boundaries of different authorities and the differing nature of the assessment of the individual needs and the population needs.

This chapter looks at the information requirements of commissioners of specialist mental health and social care services. It considers the developing policy context, that is, the modernisation programme in the National Health Service (NHS) and the drive to increase partnership working. It then examines the main areas of information required: population needs assessment, service description and specification, and service monitoring. It concludes with an overview of future information developments and recommends the need for commissioners to develop wide-ranging support in order to cope with the pace of change.

The term 'commissioners' refers principally to those who have to assess need and plan mental health services, and the term 'commissioning' refers to activities that include contracting, purchasing and action to achieve mental health improvement.

The National Health Service re-reorganisation

The *New NHS: Modern, Dependable* (Secretary of State for Health, 1997) signalled a new approach in the NHS, replacing the internal market with a system (in theory) more based on partnership and driven by performance. While retaining the separation between the planning and procurement of health care and its provision, there is a renewed emphasis on public sector planning and quality assurance, as well as an enhanced role for primary care.

The planning and procurement of health care is meant to take place within an overarching Health Improvement Programme (HImP), a local action plan to improve health and health care led by health authorities, but inclusive of all elements of the local 'NHS family' and social care providers. By definition, it sets strategy locally as well providing a development and accountability framework (see Fig. 4.1). Such a local strategy should include mental health, as it is one of the government's four priority areas to improve health and tackle health inequality in England (Department of Health, 1999*a*), and be informed by the national mental health strategy (Department of Health, 1998*a*).

Quality assurance within the NHS is delivered by new mechanisms that set standards and measure performance. Thus, nationally, standards in mental health, as in other services, are specified through a National Service Framework (NSF) (Department of Health, 1999*b*)

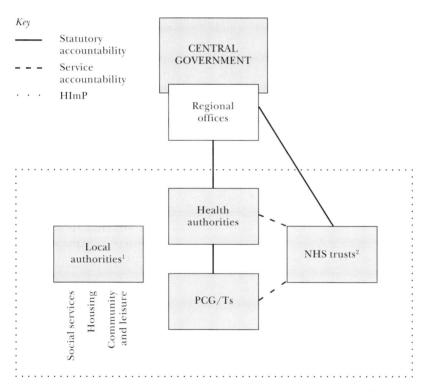

1. May combine to form mental health care trusts in some places from 2002.
2. Only those statutory functions most closely associated with mental health services shown.

NB At the time of writing, the reduction of the number of health authorities to create a few strategic health authorities, and the passing on of many of their functions to PCTs, is underway.

Fig. 4.1 Accountability framework of the statutory agencies in mental health and social care provision and their relationship to the local Health Improvement Programme

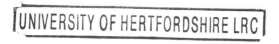

and guidelines are issued by a new statutory body, the National Institute for Clinical Excellence (NICE). Locally, delivery should be ensured by 'clinical governance' (a new corporate responsibility at all levels to ensure clinical quality) underpinned by 'professional self-regulation' and 'lifelong learning' (Department of Health, 1998*d*). Performance is monitored at the trust level by the Commission for Health Improvement, at the health authority level by the Performance Assessment Framework and at the user level by the NHS Patient Survey. However, unless these processes are adequately resourced, the aspirations to improve quality, manage risk and measure performance will by stymied by lack of clinical time, inadequate investment in information systems and slow accumulation of the evidence base.

In an attempt to improve equity of primary care development and provision, realise the potential of a primary care-led NHS and increase local accountability and responsiveness, PCG/Ts have been created in England, local health groups in Wales and local health care cooperatives/trusts in Scotland. In England, PCGs can operate in a purely advisory role for the health authority or take on responsibility for some or all of a unified (a combination of hospital and community health services, cash-limited general medical services and prescribing) health care budget. Progression to primary care trusts (PCTs) is expected, replacing the health authority role in many ways, and also such that they might provide community health services, including specialised mental health services.

Thus, the old functional relationships of unitary health authorities (which combined and replaced family health services authorities (FHSAs) and DHAs), local authorities, primary care and the specialised mental health and social care services are no longer as fixed as they once were. The division of commissioner and provider functions is shown in Table 4.1 and their statutory and service accountability is shown in Fig. 4.1. Such de-formalisation in the functions of commissioning and providing of mental health and social services is not without its dangers, for example the temptation to divert resources from severe and enduring mental illness to less severe forms (Burd *et al*, 1999) and de-prioritisation in comparison to physical health and illness such as cardiovascular disease.

The commissioner's role

If the commissioner's aim is to respond to the population's health needs to optimise mental health improvement, they need to know what those needs are and what services are already provided. The most significant constraints on commissioning are the current pattern

TABLE 4.1

Commissioners and providers of care (simplified)

Service	Commissioners	Providers
Mental health provision in primary care	PCG/Ts responsible to health authorities	Primary health care team with social services, voluntary sector and independent sector
Secondary and specialised community care	PCG/Ts in collaboration with health authority commissioning teams	Community mental health trusts and a range of voluntary and independent providers*
Social care	PCG/Ts and trust in collaboration with local authority and commissioing teams of health authorities	Local authority services, housing associations and private and voluntary sector*

* These may combine to form mental health care trusts from 2002.

of services and the overall finance. The total budget is outside the commissioner's control. It is allocated by Parliament, the Department of Health (NHS Executive, 1998*a*) and health authorities and PCG/Ts in turn. Commissioning agencies, in theory, may move money between services (e.g. from surgery to mental health) and between providers, but in practice such changes are usually at the margin.

Five stages of commissioning activity have been identified as follows (NHS Management Executive, 1991*a*):

(a) assessment of health and (possibly) social needs of the local population, including a perspective that includes users and carers and other 'stakeholders' with reference to national and local strategies: e.g. *Safe, Sound and Supportive* (Department of Health, 1998*a*); *Saving Lives* (Department of Health, 1999*a*); *National Service Framework for Mental Health* (Department of Health, 1999*b*); and *A Plan for Investment. A Plan for Reform* (Department of Health, 2000);

(b) appraisal of service options for meeting those needs, in the light of the existing services and including an examination of the evidence base for any particular model of care;

(c) specification of the preferred pattern of service development;

(d) developing, with providers' models which reflect the preferred pattern of service development compatible with funding limits;

(e) monitoring the provision of the procured services and the health of the population.

These rational and methodical stages will often be blurred and will usually be iterative in the real world. In practice, there are three main activities for which information is required:

(a) an assessment of need;
(b) service description, specification and associated costs; and
(c) monitoring through the collection of routine data and audit.

These activities demand a number of skills within commissioning agencies. For example, in a PCG/T, the chief officer is responsible for the overall performance of the group/trust via an accountability agreement with the responsible health authority. He or she is assisted by a number of fellow executive and non-executive board members (the latter bringing a range of interests from the local community). High-quality commissioning requires public health (needs assessment, evaluation of evidence and interpretation of the service) finance and contract management skills. Practising each set of skills depends upon the generation of separate but related sets of information from the epidemiology and effectiveness literature and from various sources on service utilisation. The roles of needs assessment and contract management are closely related and should work in parallel, but with a respective bias towards the content of the commissioned care and the process of achieving it (Fig. 4.2).

'Need' from a health commissioner's viewpoint

The assessment of health needs is considered from a variety of angles in this book; however, 'need' as a concept can mean different things to professionals from different disciplines (Stevens & Gabbay, 1991).

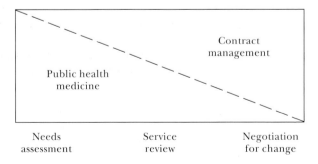

Fig. 4.2 Roles of public health medicine and contract management in purchasing care

Indeed, often, the terms 'need', 'want', 'demand' and even 'supply' are used loosely and sometimes synonymously. From a commissioner's point of view, the appropriate definition of 'need' is one that is based on "the population's ability to benefit from care" (NHS Management Executive, 1991*b*). 'Want' refers to what users would like but may not act upon, 'demand' refers to expressed want and 'supply' to services/care that are actually available. In the provision of mental health services, a reasonable goal of those who commission care (including those specifying service requirements at the national level) would be to increase the overlap between need, demand and supply (Stevens & Gabbay, 1991; Stevens & Raftery, 1994). Fig. 4.3 shows the relationship between need, demand and supply in mental health care and gives examples of each.

Each component of the commissioner's definition of need is important. First, the *population's* ability to benefit is the aggregate of the individuals' ability to benefit along with the benefit to the wider population, for example, reduction of fear of danger. At the population level, this will depend on the epidemiology, that is, the incidence and prevalence (of different degrees of severity) of the condition and its effects and complications. Second, the *ability* to benefit does not mean that every outcome is guaranteed to be favourable, but it does mean that there is only a need where the intervention and/or the care setting is effective (meets the objectives of that intervention). This is crucial because the ability to benefit differentiates need from demand and want, and limits the call on providers, so that in terms of health care we can talk about health care requirements. Third, the benefit measured should include not only the clinical status and well-being compared with that without the intervention, but also reassurance, both to the individual and to the professional, that avenues of potential benefit have been explored, for example confirming the diagnosis, supportive care and relief of pressure on other carers. Finally, care should include health care whose components comprise health prevention and promotion, diagnosis, treatment, continuing care, rehabilitation and terminal care, as well as components of social care and general care.

Since need has now been defined as the ability to benefit, it is also worth distinguishing it from efficacy, effectiveness and outcome.

Need	Population's *ability to benefit*
Efficacy	Intervention's/care setting's *potential to benefit* in ideal (experimental) conditions
Effectiveness	Intervention's/care setting's *potential to benefit* in everyday conditions
Outcome	*Achieved benefit* in the local setting

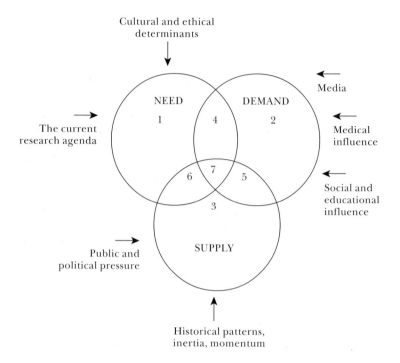

Examples include:
1. Compliance theory for schizophrenia.
2. Complementary therapies for severe mental illness (SMI).
3. Behavioural modification in eating disorders.
4 Useful daytime occupation.
5. Non-directive counselling in primary care.
6. Detention under Mental Health Act.
7. Assertive Community Treatment for SMI.

Fig. 4.3 The relationship between need, demand and supply in mental health care and their determinants

Need defined in this way has formed the basis for the *epidemiological assessment* of need, which in conjunction with the *comparative* and *corporate* approaches can guide the commissioning of mental health care. Indeed, a whole literature based on the epidemiological assessment of health care needs has now arisen, which includes mental health topics such as adult mental health services (Wing, 1994), child and adolescent mental health (Wallace *et al*, 1997), and alcohol misuse (Edwards & Unnithal, 1994).

Main methods of assessing need

The epidemiological assessment of need

Measuring the population's ability to benefit form health care generates two very specific information requirements:

(a) the local prevalence and incidence of disease, ranged by severity (prevalence – the number of cases per unit population at a point in time, or over a period – is usually the appropriate measure for chronic disease; and incidence – the number of new cases per unit time – is usually appropriate for measuring acute disease); and

(b) the effectiveness of the care and care settings available or potentially available to cope with it.

Together these measurements form the basis of the epidemiological approach to needs assessment. Both incidence/prevalence and effectiveness present challenging information problems. *Local* data on the occurrence of health problems are rarely available with the exception of where, on rare occasions, the local area has been the site of an epidemiological survey or study (Sashidharan *et al*, 1995), and those instances where diseases are so definite and so certain to present to hospital services that they are fully recorded in the hospital data systems, for example, appendicitis.

The way round this problem is to apply the results of national estimates to the local population, adjusting for factors that might account for local variation to generate indicative incidences and or prevalences. National sources of data for occurrence of mental health problems include the National Psychiatric Morbidity Survey (Meltzer *et al*, 1995) and the results of the GP morbidity surveys (Office of Population Censuses and Surveys (OPCS), 1995).

The collection of these and similarly secondary sources of ad hoc data suggests the need for commissioning agencies to have access to either a virtual or actual repository of expertise and literature.

Information on the effectiveness of health care and health care settings is growing exponentially. Some of the existing effectiveness literature has already been summarised (Conway *et al*, 1996; Department of Health, 1999*b*) in addition to the protocols and reviews of mental health interventions available in the Cochrane library, for example 'Assertive Community Treatment for people with severe mental disorders' (Marshall & Lockwood, 1998).

There are also databases of systematic reviews and other collections of both systematic and non-systematic reviews which can be found via the internet (see Booth, 1998). Evidence has also been actively disseminated by the NHS Centre of Reviews and Dissemination at the University of York, for example on mental health promotion in high-risk groups (NHS Centre for Reviews and Dissemination, 1997). Finally, primary sources of evidence on effectiveness are still invaluable (Thornicroft *et al*, 1998).

The epidemiological approach to needs assessment, although the theoretical ideal for commissioners, is not the only approach. In reality, the commissioning policy of the commissioning agencies is likely to be influenced just as much by the two other approaches: comparative assessments and the corporate approach. Strictly, neither measures the ability to benefit from health care, and both certainly include elements of demand (what actually presents to professionals) and supply (services already in existence elsewhere), but each can give clear pointers to priorities for change.

The comparative assessment of need

The comparative approach involves making comparisons between health authorities or localities. With the drive to reduce inequalities and increase social equity, such an approach is likely to become significant in analysing differences between PCG/Ts. However, such comparisons are limited by the available sources of data. Examples include:

(a) Morbidity and mortality: suicide rates as in *Our Healthier Nation* indicator for mental illness (Department of Health, 1999*a*; NHS Executive, 2000), rates of death mentioned as associated with schizophrenic psychoses – *Public Health Common Data Set* (Department of Health, 1998*e*) – and variations in morbidity in primary care (OPCS, 1995).

(b) Service utilisation and provision: mental health unit costs, emergency psychiatric re-admission percentage rates (NHS Executive, 2000), rates of detention under the 1983 Mental Health Act and use of prescribing analysis and cost (PACT) data for prescribing in primary care either within or between health authorities (Department of Medicines Management, 1996).

(c) Costs and outcomes: usually available only through local data and measurement, for example specific service reviews at either the health authority or regional office level (e.g. NHS Executive, West Midlands, 1999).

The comparative approach gives insights into possible priorities for change by exploring differences both within and between health authorities. Morbidity and mortality data may reveal local 'outliers' of either need or performance. To the degree that they are responsive to health service performance, these indicators serve as proxy outcome measures of local health services, although it is accepted that there are concerns about the use of suicide as an overall indicator of mental health.

Data on service utilisation and provision compared between districts, expose the relative differences in supply across the country. High levels do not necessarily mean 'overmet' need, nor low levels 'unmet need', but both can trigger scrutiny on whether the levels of provision might be adjusted. The health service indicators (HSIs), which used to contain 72 indicators in mental health services, have been replaced by the less comprehensive indicators in the public health common data-set, in reality making comparative needs assessment more difficult.

Good-quality comparative cost data are elusive because of the variety of methods used to calculate costs. Crude measures such as cost per in-patient day or per clinic attendance, which might be available, are very limited as they are usually derived 'top-down' (by dividing all units of activity by all relevant expenditure). To be meaningful, costs must relate to defined activities 'bottom-up' (the sum of identified resources tied up in the delivery of a particular service). For example, commissioners will probably have access to, for contractual reasons, the entire spend for a trust's service or even client group across trusts (if there is more than one provider), for, say, elderly mentally ill costs. However, they also need to know the *unit cost* of the range of services, such as for a residential place, an in-patient episode for acute care and assessment, or a year's community care, which could then be compared with published unit costs (see Netten *et al*, 1998).

Of course, value for money implies a measure of value – hence the need for outcome measurements. In theory, it is only when outcomes are included that comparisons of cost-effectiveness are valid. Despite the development of validated measures of outcome (Wing *et al*, 1998), they are not yet available routinely. In practice, comparative cost data provide clear prompts for commissioners, both to question the value of services commissioned and to decide when not to do so because the cost is trivial. Arguments put forward by providers to justify greater than average or expected cost not explained by restructuring costs, for example, must put the onus on the provider to demonstrate that the additional cost is justified, that is, by getting down to the collection of adequate outcome data.

The corporate approach to needs assessment

The 'corporate' approach to needs assessment involves the com-missioning agency systematically synthesising the views of interested and informed parties in local mental health care. This is an extremely important part of needs assessment, especially within the process of the HImP and the increasing breadth of involvement of other parties. These will typically include:

(a) the mental health commissioning team (if any), experts and advisers;

(b) users and carers;

(c) PCG/Ts, members of the primary health care team (PHCT) and social services;

(d) providers and their clinical staff and those involved in linking in to the development process of the local HImP;

(e) other local agencies, e.g. the voluntary sector, independent sector and local authority; and

(f) the regional office of the NHS Executive.

Inevitably, some of these will reveal as much about demand (users, carers and PHCT members) and about supply bias (providers and other local agencies) as they do about need. But, many of these sources, particularly providers, that is, the local psychiatrists and GPs, are in a position to alert purchasers to major crises and reflect unmet needs much more quickly than a formal needs assessment, as well to provide feedback on the quality of services. The establishment of PCGs as sub-committees of the health authority will help to consolidate this process.

Service description

Quantity

Irrespective of whether needs are assessed epidemiologically, comparatively or corporately (and preferably in combination), a baseline service description is vital. Ideally, a full service description would include details of costs and expected performance, that is, expected outcomes. The routine measurement of outcomes is some way off and therefore current service specifications rely on descriptions of facilities and levels of activity.

The level of service description required is not of a universal standard and may include staff, equipment, estate, accreditation standards, rules and protocols. 'Estate' ranges from beds and places through to wards, community settings or entire service systems. Commissioners need to have an intelligible description of a service, but often the level of detail is restricted because providers may be allowed to organise services as they see fit (provided desired outcomes can be guaranteed) and also because of the cost of collecting and interpreting the detailed data.

A variety of levels of description can be outlined from crude to fine:

(a) *Total cost and capacity of a health authority's specialist mental health service.* Such a description will have developed from the 1991 starting level for the block contract used by purchasers of mental health care. Quality may be based on provider reassurances of satisfactory services and the degree of fulfilment of national (patient charter) and local standards.

(b) *Cost and capacity of subsections of a specialist mental health service within and across trusts.* Such subsections might include: adult general specialist services; elderly mental health; child and adolescent services; substance misuse; forensic; and learning disabilities. This refinement of (a) marks the first step in recognising the heterogeneity of the service. Value for money, however, remains impossible to judge without more detail on the type of settings in which clients are cared for.

(c) *Cost, capacity, activity and staffing of services might be further disaggregated to more specific services* (as shown in Table 4.2). Such a specification would include the unit costs for components of the service, defined as the largest homogenous service unit feasible; locations, types of wards, community mental health teams, functional mental health teams, etc. Since staffing levels are currently measured reasonably well, they can measure the scale of a service and hence check the accuracy of costing.

The level of information referred to in (c) should be the minimum that commissioners should aim for, as it is the crudest level at which any meaningful judgement of service effectiveness and efficiency can be made.

While greater levels of detail than in Table 4.2 are possible, they are not recommended for the reasons given above (provider prerogative and expense considerations). The function column could be expanded, for example, to show the use of agreed protocols, admission thresholds, etc., but the basic format is probably sufficient for commissioners to understand the services specified. The information recorded in such a table also forms the basis for service monitoring (Table 4.2).

Agreement about priorities requires negotiation and an understanding of the relative costs and benefits of various options. Other changes in services will rely on marginal year-to-year change and will focus on areas where there are the best opportunities for relatively painless shifts in the balance of care. The key information set that will need to be shared between commissioners and providers will be a clear description of local mental health and social care services contracted and paid for.

TABLE 4.2
Detailed service specification

Location or non-locational service	Function	Capacity	Activity level	Staffing	Cost	Unit cost[1]
In-patient ward	Acute assessment	X beds	X consultant episodes	X WTE[2]	£XK	£XK per bed
CMHT	Assertive outreach	X open cases	X contacts	X WTE	£XK	£XK per open case
24-hour staffed crisis centre	Crisis management	X clients	X consultant episodes	X WTE	£XK	£XK per placement

1. Including pro rata proportion of overheads.
2. WTE, whole time equivalent.

A range of contract types have been developed since the inception of the internal market in 1991. Such contracts now form part of the annual Services and Financial Framework (SaFF) agreement between commissioners and providers and include block, cost and volume, and cost per case contracts. The extra-contractual referral system which operated on a cost per case basis and dealt with 'one-off' high-cost, low-volume cases and out-of-district referrals is being replaced by the out-of-area treatment system (NHS Executive, 1998*b*), except for referrals to independent providers. It is likely that there will need to be annual reviews based on block contracts even within the new long-term service agreements (Department of Health, 1998*f*).

Quality

Quality can be divided into broad fields, clinical and non-clinical, each of which can be assessed according to its structure, processes and procedures, and outcome. Some quality criteria will fulfil national concerns, such as the patients charter and *Our Healthier Nation* (Department of Health, 1999*a*), while others will have been generated locally according to local priorities. Although specific examples may differ between commissioning agencies, it is possible to describe a quality matrix that captures the current approach to quality specification within contracts (see Table 4.3). Very few of these are obligatory and they will be superseded by the need to develop measures within the context of the national performance assessment framework (NHS Executive, 1999*a*), and the need to fill Clinical Governance requirements.

Service monitoring – quantity and quality

Theoretical framework

In monitoring services, the commissioner's interest in a service can be illustrated as in Chart 1. This extends beyond ensuring that services meet need to a clear picture of value for money. There is, therefore, an interest in both sides of the chart:

Chart 1:

Resources   · · · · · ➤   Health care (quality and quantity)

Partly because commissioning agencies have a responsibility to the whole resident population, and partly because the relevance of health care depends on to whom the care is given, Chart 1 can be made slightly more elaborate:

TABLE 4.3
Quality matrix

	National	Local
Generic	Clinical Governance action plan and annual reports Waiting times Confidential enquiry reports Minimum data-set requirements	Critical incidence reports Patient profiling Caseload audits
Specific	National Service Framework requirements NHS Plan requirements Adherence to Children Act	Care Plan Approach implementation audit User participation programmes Mental health promotion initiatives

Chart 2:

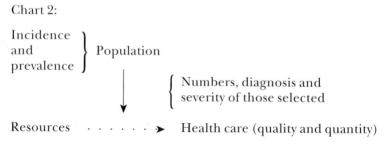

It is necessary to measure the characteristics of the population treated vis à vis the population at large to take into account issues of equity and appropriateness, that is, to ensure that care given was to the people with the greatest need. The information needed for Chart 2 will be substantially satisfied by informing services, as illustrated in Table 4.2 (setting the baseline from which to measure need).

In an ideal world, commissioners would go further. This real interest should not be confined to the health care received but include the health gain achieved (for the resources put in):

Chart 3:

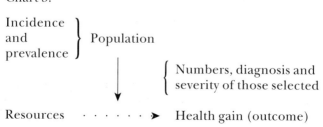

Thus, the key information required pertains to outcome accompanied by severity measurement (on the same scale) of users as they enter the service.

Practical considerations

While such key information has yet to be incorporated routinely, in practice commissioners will have to rely on structure, process, proxy outcome measures or ad hoc clinical audit projects which can examine aspects of service delivery. Measuring structure means maintaining knowledge of the provider's services as described above (Table 4.2). As regards the monitoring process, this may sometimes be a close substitute for monitoring outcome, where research has demonstrated a close relationship between process measures and outcomes (the analogy in physical ill health is 'door to needle' time for thrombolytic therapy in acute myocardial infarction), for example measurement of the time interval between addiction and the first treatment in opiate services (Strang, 1991) or the proportion of people with schizophrenia whose cases have been reviewed according to the Care Programme Approach (CPA), emergency readmission rates in schizophrenia or periodic rating scores with depression, etc.

Thus, although Chart 3 summarises the commissioner's idealised interest, in reality a wider range of items is actually monitored. Thus, the measurements are as outlined below:

Chart 4:

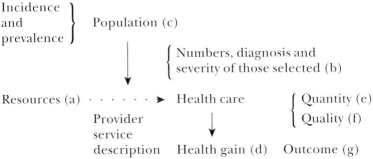

(a)   Resources, i.e. cost

Resource utilisation can be examined by comparing expenditure over a given period of time (out-turn) against that allocated for a particular service, although this is not necessarily monitored routinely. The annual service level agreement, if specified carefully, can allocate all the risk of overspends to the provider at the beginning of a contractual period. In practice, the risk tends to be shared between commissioners and providers by means of clauses within service level agreements, which are triggered by activity and cost deviations from planned levels.

(b)   Number and characteristics of patients treated

Both the number of people treated (which is what is usually, albeit crudely, contracted for), and their medical characteristics, require measuring. Ideally, outcome might be measured as the difference between the patient's starting condition (or rather expected untreated end condition) and the actual end condition. In the field of mental health, this is difficult since the prediction of the natural history of a particular case or set of cases is more problematic because of the interaction with many variables that influence outcome (as opposed to just treatment). In practice, the best that is currently recorded for in-patient care is dependent on the contract minimum data-set with items such as diagnosis (without severity), episode length and patient details.

Another potential approach is the measurement of case-mix related to resource utilisation. Indeed, for other sectors in the NHS, health care resource groups are now measured routinely, but have not been derived for mental health. Yet another approach, albeit only at the development stage, is to use health benefit groups (HBGs) – relatively homogenous groups of conditions that require a similar intervention; for example, short-term depression and anxiety and psychosis with and without risk.

(c)   Population not treated

Commissioners will wish to know about those who might be treated, but who in fact have not been. In other areas of commissioning, for example orthopaedics, estimates of unmet need could be made by measuring the difference between prevalence, incidence and activity. In psychiatry, this is probably insufficient because the risk is that the most severely ill, and not the mildest, may fail to receive treatment. Such a position would be extremely rare in general medicine or surgery, because the most severe are the most likely to seek care and to be considered the most rewarding to treat. Neither of these conditions is met by people with severe schizophrenia and people with challenging behaviour. Commissioners must insist on the monitoring of the most severely psychiatrically ill.

(d)   Provider service description

The provider service description provides the framework for monitoring the service. The commissioner's understanding of what is monitored depends on separating out the measurements of the service into relatively homogeneous units, such as acute in-patient beds, elderly long-stay places, community contacts, etc. (see Table 4.2).

(e)   Activity levels

Activity levels in the specialist mental health services have traditionally been mainly measured in terms of consultant finished episodes and out-patient contacts. In all specialities, this is at best a very crude measure of quantity and fails to measure quality at all. In mental health, the poverty of this measure is exacerbated by a number of features:

- In-patient care is a small and diminishing part of mental health care.
- In many respects, in-patient care actually represents an alternative model of care to that practised (i.e. community care) for certain patients.
- The chronicity and episodic nature of mental illness means that episodes are often part of a larger sequence and vary in length and intensity.
- There is a diversity of health professional contacts – psychiatrists, psychologists, CPNs, occupational therapists, etc.

A number of other routine process measures also give information of doubtful value on the service to be purchased. The CPN contact rate says nothing about what happened, how long for, or to what end; nor does the day hospital attendance rate.

The present minimum contract data-set became operational in 1993–1994. It provided data on the main types of activity rather than needs and associated prices. Acute psychiatry admissions were dealt with as one medical speciality among many, with an annual census to cover those in long-stay institutions. A new minimum data-set (Glover *et al*, 1997) is being developed and should help support the monitoring of long-term service agreements in terms of capacity and number of patients and case-mix cared for.

The different secondary care settings to be measured need to cover different settings:

- acute in-patient care
- longer-term in-patient care
- crisis houses
- out-patients
- day care

- community contacts
- residential care.

As there is a tendency for these to be alternatives to each other in many situations (i.e. intensive community care may keep someone out of hospital), they need to be measured comparably. Therefore, the three-way measurement of capacity (e.g. number of open cases a community team can manage), activity level (total admissions in the case of in-patients or contacts elsewhere) and new cases seen should apply to each. Furthermore, in the case of out-patients or community care, they should be recorded irrespective of whether contact is with a psychiatrist or with another member of the team.

(f)   Health care – quality

A list of list of clinical and non-clinical quality items is given in Table 4.3. Some of these are open to routine monitoring at different intervals, for example GP communication and waiting times. Other quality measures can be constructed for particular parts of the service, and the items suggested, for example patient satisfaction, can be tailored to the service. Whatever measures are preferred locally, monitoring is essential if they are to mean anything.

(g)   Health care – clinical, quality and outcome

Outcome measurement will be fragmentary for some time to come, although we now have the tools to measure outcomes in both adult and child and adolescent mental health service, for example the Health of the Nation Outcome Scale (HoNOS; Wing *et al*, 1998). Until such measures are accepted by mental health professionals and information systems support their routine use, local clinical audit may be the most useful way to make progress.

Developments in and support for commissioning

Future requirements in commissioning

The NSF (Department of Health, 1999*b*) and the NHS Plan (Department of Health, 2000) have set the agenda for change. However, achieving change will require protracted negotiation and information exchange, and will have to take place within the SaFF of the local HImP of the health authority (Department of Health, 1998*h*). New funding was originally made available through the NHS Modernisation Fund (NHS Executive, 1999*b*) to support the national strategy (Department of Health, 1998*a*). Such funding was to be targeted at specific schemes to modernise mental health services, for example increasing the use of atypical antipsychotics, and increasing access to 24-hour nursed beds and assertive outreach services. Such national priorities remain, but without ring-fenced funding.

There is also the requirement to develop 'long-term service agreements' (Department of Health, 1998*f*). These agreements are meant to reflect ongoing dialogue between clinicians, users and carers, as well as managers. Ideally, they should: engage with those who contribute to the 'pathway of care' based on HBGs; include measurable targets for improvement; incorporate incentives for improving quality and cost-effectiveness with clear responsibility for financial risk management; and form the basis for a continuing, open and cooperative relationship between commissioners and providers.

Our Healthier Nation (Department of Health, 1999*a*) reiterated the need to address inequalities, and this applies equally to mental health as to cardiovascular disease, cancers and accidents. Such inequalities in mental health are well recognised (Bunting, 1997), and action must be taken locally to address them by considering barriers to service uptake, local resource allocation, and the impact of social and demographic factors on case recognition and referral (Henderson *et al*, 1998).

Developing support for commissioning

High-quality commissioning requires robust routine information on activity and high-quality intelligence.

Developing current routine information

The development of information management and technology has finally been put on a firmer footing in the NHS with the publication of a strategy (Department of Health, 1998*i*). This strategy sets out how information can be used to support quality within the NHS. A variety of initiatives will be developed which include: electronic patient records and electronic health records; remote on-line services for patients and professionals to access; access for NHS users of accredited independent multimedia background information; and on-line access for professionals to local and national evidenced-based guidelines.

Potentially, such developments provide the opportunity for better routine data collection to support commissioning, as the inadequacies of the current Körner-based mental health data have been highlighted by Glover (1995). These inadequacies are that the activity data are episodic and hospital-based and do not reflect the rhythm of clinical activity. This rhythm is often community-based, occurs over a long time-frame and includes many different players. Consequently, much effort has gone into the development of a new minimum data-set for specialist mental health care. Such a data-set has to meet a variety of needs for those providing care, for those managing services and for those commissioning services.

So far, one incarnation of a new *prototype* minimum data-set has been piloted and was well received, where the records formed part of a computerised system (Glover *et al*, 1997). This prototype comprised data items on: patient registration; personal and socio-demographic details; referral details; status at review; details of the CPA; diagnosis and HoNOS scores; care delivered since last review; and care planned. However, this initiative failed and the Mental Health Minimum Data Set (MHMDS) project was re-established in 1997 (Department of Health, 1997). Again, it has been piloted and has shown that although much of the data already exists within operational systems, drawing together the 'mental health care spell' has proven difficult.

The latest MHMDS (Department of Health, 1997) contains items that match the prototype but include details of the mental health care package (in-patient days, NHS community bed days, sheltered work and others) and the mental health care spell (speciality code, spell days in period, days of minimal CPA and complex CPA and others). It is clear, however, that trusts are not all in a position to provide such data-sets; indeed, at the time of a recent telephone survey, 22% were not able to produce MHMDS and 34% did not use HoNOS (NHS Executive, 1998*c*). Such lack of progress is regrettable, as the lack of high-quality routine data has seriously hampered the development of sophisticated mental health commissioning processes.

Commissioner's intelligence network

The need for intelligence – interpreted as anything that helps to throw light on the local population's health and social care needs and the services they receive – is likely to increase. This will be true where skills and knowledge built up within health authority commissioning teams are disseminated out into other organisations and therefore become diluted. This intelligence is not only numerical but also contextual, not only local but also national, and not only routine but also ad hoc. These dimensions and the types of information are illustrated in Table 4.4.

Some information needs will be met locally via professional and lay networks, and some will be met nationally and systematically by bodies such as NICE. Access to and ability to use sources of evidence will be critical, whether it is via a local postgraduate or in-house library or by developing systematic searching skills.

There is also a need to develop tools to help to assess needs, building on the approach of the mental illness needs index methodology (Glover *et al*, 1998). Such a tool kit should take into account all the

TABLE 4.4
Broad categories of intelligence for purchasing, with examples

	Local		National	
	Routine	*Ad hoc*	*Routine*	*Ad hoc*
Numerical	Contract data-sets, population registers	Local surveys, use of primary care morbidity data	Public health common data-set, general household survey	Epidemiological study data
Textual	Service agreements	Local reports	High-level government circulars Cochrane Library	Royal College reports, NSF and NHS Plan

relevant socio-demographic factors, including age/gender structure and ethnicity, as well as housing and employment rates of the population, and use evidence-based normative levels of services that take into account the range of community services available. It also needs to be robust enough to operate at the locality level. Inevitably, such a model has elements of need, demand and supply, but might provide some indicators against which local service provision can be measured. Development of the York psychiatrist index of needs to locality is also needed (Carr-Hill *et al*, 1994).

Conclusion

The next few years will see the further development of policy around mental health and the provision of services. Initiatives that will impact on commissioners and the need for information will include the review of the Mental Health Act, changes to the CPA, developments around personality disorder, high-security service changes, the development and implementation of a mental health information strategy, and changes to the configuration of mental health services.

Such an array of initiatives, added to those referred to in the introduction, presents opportunities for commissioners in collaboration with providers, both statutory and voluntary, and users to shape services to local needs while maintaining effectiveness and efficiency. Such developments, however, must be supported by information at all stages, including the planning, implementation and monitoring of service changes.

References

BOOTH, A. (1998) The Internet: quantity not quality. *Student British Medical Journal*, **6**, 49.

BUNTING, J. (1997) Morbidity and health-related behaviours of adults – a review. In: *Health Inequalities* (eds F. Drever & M. Whitehead). Office for National Statistics Decennial Supplement No.15. London: The Stationery Office.

BURD, M., CHAMBERS, R., COHEN, A., *ET AL* (1999) Mental health services – primary concerns for the future. *British Journal of General Practice*, **49**, 399.

CARR-HILL, R. A., HARDMAN, G., MARTIN, S., *ET AL* (1994) *A Formula for Distributing NHS Revenues Based on Small Area Use of Hospital Beds.* York: Centre for Health Economics, University of York.

CONWAY, M., SHEPHERD, G. & MELTZER, D. (1996) Effectiveness of interventions for mental illness and implications for commissioning. In: *Commissioning Mental Health Services* (eds G. Thornicroft & G. Strathdee), pp. 247–264. London: HMSO.

DEPARTMENT OF HEALTH (1997) *Report on the Review of Patient Identifiable Information.* Appendix 12. Caldicott report. London: Department of Health.

—— (1998*a*) *Modernising Mental Health Services: Safe, Sound and Supportive* (incorporating emerging findings of the National Service Framework External Reference Group). Health Service Circular HSC 1998/233; Local Authority Circular (98)25. London: Department of Health.

—— (1998*b*) *Modernising Health and Social Services: National Priorities Guidance 1999/2000–2001/2002.* London: NHS Executive.

—— (1998*c*) *Partnerships in Action (New Opportunities for Joint Working between Health and Social Services.* London: Department of Health.

—— (1998*d*) *A First Class Service-Quality in the New NHS.* London: The Stationery Office.

—— (1998*e*) *Public Health Common Data Set.* London: Department of Health.

—— (1998*f*) *Commissioning Services 1999–2000.* Health Services Circular 1998/074 Appendix A. London: Department of Health.

—— (1998*g*) *National Service Frameworks.* Health Service Circular: HSC 1998/074. London: Department of Health.

—— (1998*h*) *Health Improvement Programmes; Planning for Better Health and Better Health Care.* Health Services Circular 1998/167, Local Authority Circular (98)23. London: Department of Health.

—— (1998*i*) *Information for Health: An Information Strategy for the Modern NHS 1998–2005.* London: Department of Health.

—— (1999*a*) *Saving Lives: Our Healthier Nation.* Cm. 4386. London: The Stationery Office.

—— (1999*b*) *A National Service Framework for Mental Health.* London: Department of Health.

—— (2000) *A Plan for Investment. A Plan for Reform.* London: The Stationery Office.

DEPARTMENT OF MEDICINES MANAGEMENT (1996) *Typical and Atypical Antipsychotics – Medicine Management Report, No. 31.* Keele: Keele University.

EDWARDS, G. & UNNITHAL, S. (1994) Alcohol misuse. In: *Health Care Needs Assessment, The Epidemiologically Based Needs Assessment Reviews* (eds A. Stevens & J. Raftery), Chapter 17. Oxford: Radcliffe Medical Press.

GLOVER, G. (1995) Mental health informatics and the rhythm of community care. *British Medical Journal*, **311**, 1038–1039.

——, KNIGHT, S., MELZER, D., *ET AL* (1997) The development of a new minimum data set for specialist mental health care. *Health Trends*, **29**, 48–51.

——, ROBIN, E. & EMAMI JAND ARABSCHEIBANI, G. R. (1998) A needs index for mental health care. *Social Psychiatry and Psychiatric Epidemiology*, **33**, 89–96.

HENDERSON, C., THORNICROFT, G. & GLOVER, G. (1998) Inequalities in mental health. *British Journal of Psychiatry*, **173**, 105–109.

HOUSE OF COMMONS (1990) *National Health Service and Community Care Act.* London: HMSO.

MARSHALL, M. & LOCKWOOD, A. (1998) Assertive Community Treatment for people with severe mental disorders (Cochrane Review). In: *Cochrane Library,* Issue 3. Oxford: Update Software.

MELTZER, H., GILL, B., PETTIGREW, M., *ET AL* (1995) *OPCS Surveys of Psychiatric Morbidity in Great Britain. Report 1. The Prevalence of Psychiatric Morbidity among Adults Living in Private Households.* London: HMSO.

NETTEN, A., DENNETT, J. & KNIGHT, J. (1998) *Unit Costs of Health and Social Care.* Kent: Personal Social Services Research Unit, University of Kent at Canterbury.

NHS CENTRE FOR REVIEWS AND DISSEMINATION (1997) *Effective Health Care – Mental Health Promotion in High Risk Groups.* York: University of York.

NHS EXECUTIVE (1998*a*) *Health Authority Revenue Allocations Exposition Book.* Leeds: Department of Health.

—— (1998*b*) *The New NHS Guidance on Out of Area Treatment.* Consultation Paper. Leeds: NHS Executive.

—— (1998*c*) *Mental Health Minimum Data Set Project: Summary Results of a Telephone Survey of Mental Health Service Providers.* London: NHS Executive.

—— (1999*a*) *The NHS Performance Assessment Framework.* Leeds: NHS Executive.

—— (1999*b*) *Health and Personal Social Services Modernisation Fund.* Leeds: Department of Health.

—— (2000) *Quality and Performance Management in the NHS: NHS Performance Indicators.* Leeds: NHS Executive.

NHS EXECUTIVE, WEST MIDLANDS (1999) *West Midlands Review of Specialist National Health Services to Meet Health Needs of Children and Young People.* West Midlands: Department of Health.

NHS MANAGEMENT EXECUTIVE (1991*a*) *Role of District Health Authorities – Analysis of Issues.* London: Department of Health.

—— (1991*b*) *Assessing Health Care Needs.* London: Department of Health.

OPCS (1995) *Morbidity Statistics from General Practice. Fourth National Study 1991–1992.* MB5 No. 3. London: HMSO

SASHIDHARAN, S. P., COMMANDER, M. J., ODELL, S. M., *ET AL* (1995) *The West Birmingham Psychiatric Epidemiology Research Project. Report 1: Use of Specialist Mental Health Services.* Birmingham: The University of Birmingham.

SECRETARY OF STATE FOR HEALTH (1997) *The New NHS: Modern, Dependable.* London: The Stationery Office.

—— (1998) *Modernising Social Services.* Cm. 4169. London: The Stationery Office.

STRANG, J. (1991) Injecting drug misuse. *British Medical Journal,* **303**, 1043–1046.

STEVENS, A. & GABBAY, J. (1991) Needs assessment, needs assessment. *Health Trends,* **23**, 22.

—— & RAFTERY, J. (1994) Introduction to epidemiological needs assessment. In: *Health Care Needs Assessment, The Epidemiologically Based Needs Assessment Reviews* (eds A. Stevens & J. Raftery), vol. 1, pp. 11–30. Oxford: Radcliffe Medical Press.

THORNICROFT, G., STRATHDEE, G., PHELAN, F., *ET AL* (1998) Rationale and design. PriSM psychosis study I. *British Journal of Psychiatry,* **173**, 363–370.

WALLACE, S. A., CROWN, J. M., BERGER, M., *ET AL* (1997) Child and adolescent mental health. In: *Health Care Needs Assessment, The Epidemiologically Based Needs Assessment Reviews* (2nd series) (eds A. Stevens & J. Raftery), pp. 55–128. Oxford: Radcliffe Medical Press.

WING, J. K. (1994) Mental illness. In: *Health Care Needs Assessment, The Epidemiologically Based Needs Assessment Reviews* (eds A. Stevens & J. Raftery), vol. 2, pp. 202–304. Oxford: Radcliffe Medical Press.

——, BEEVOR, A. S., CURTIS, R. H., *ET AL* (1998) Health of the Nation Outcome Scales (HoNOS). Research and development. *British Journal of Psychiatry,* **172**, 11–18.

5 Measuring (relative) need for mental health care services

ROY CARR-HILL

Predictive models of morbidity and resource allocation

In the British National Health Service (NHS), at every level from sector team to the Department of Health, mental health care needs must be met from finite resources. Achieving this efficiently depends on effective targeting both in individual and area terms. Assessing the relative need of individuals is probably even more complicated for mental illness than for general medicine, because of difficulties with diagnoses. Here, however, the focus is on the prior question of how resources should be distributed between areas. This requires a method of quantifying how need for mental health services is distributed at an area level.

In this chapter, we will explore the extent to which it is possible to predict the need for mental health services and to use this as a basis for allocating health services resources. Other work in this area is briefly and critically reviewed, but the main focus of this chapter is the approach adopted by the team who developed the most recent resource allocation formulae, which have been used since April 1996. The main features of the approach and the results are presented here; full details are given in Car-Hill *et al* (1994) for readers interested in a more detailed account of this highly technical area.

The Original Resource Allocation Working Party (RAWP) approach

Initially, in 1976, the RAWP opted for standard mortality ratio[1] (SMR) using the following terms:

(a) morbidity measures need;
(b) mortality is a good proxy for morbidity; and, therefore,
(c) mortality is a good proxy measure for need.

One can agree with the first statement, but might want to take issue with the current appropriateness of the second assumption, and to ask what level of association counts as 'good'?

The assessment that the level of association is 'good' depends on how accurate you want to be. If the allocations are treated only as indicative targets around which the recipients can negotiate, then clearly the requirement for accuracy is much less. If the allocations are to a large group, then biases/errors will, with luck, cancel each other out, so that a crude approximation to morbidity will be sufficient. However, neither of these pertains here: allocations are treated as definitive targets towards which budgets are moved; and, at least relative to the original RAWP exercise, the boards cover much smaller populations.

Moreover, several analyses with area data[2] have shown that socio-demographic factors are related to morbidity over and above the statistical associations of mortality with morbidity. However, reliance on area data runs the risk of committing the 'ecological fallacy', in that associations observed on an area level may not be reflecting associations at an individual level. This is especially a problem when only one pair of variables is being considered, because there may well be other cognate variables that are associated with both mortality and morbidity and which provide at least a partial explanation of their joint association.

Changing patterns of mortality

When RAWP was writing, the majority of early deaths were the result of (an accumulation of) socio-economic disadvantages (over the century) that, it was reasonable to presume, also reflected the pattern of real morbidity and therefore the need for health care. Moreover, there were substantial numbers of deaths under 65 years (or 75 years). But the pattern was already shifting, so that now the majority of deaths are the result of a combination of chronic, degenerative diseases; and because most live longer than 65 years (or 75 years), the numbers of deaths under 65 years (or under 75 years) and the implications for

---

[1] Although of course, the original RAWP was not wedded to SMRs; they examined the evidence. In the particular case of psychiatric services, their preferred choice was marital status.

[2] The argument is rather silly with individual data. Of course, most (except accident victims) are ill before they die; but, assuming one could accurately measure levels of morbidity, who dies for a given level of morbidity is almost entirely socially determined.

health care are prone to random disturbance (for example, accidents are not health care-intensive deaths).

Most agree that the emphasis should be on being as up to date as possible. But it has to be recognised that, inasmuch as death/ mortality does reflect morbidity and socio-economic conditions, this is more correctly seen as a consequence of the accumulation of socio-economic disadvantage over the previous 70 years, rather than a reflection of current conditions.

Evidence-based resource allocation

There have been several approaches to resource allocation:

(a) *historical*: increments on historical budgets
(b) *normative*: pontification as to the variables that should be included
(c) *regression*: examining evidence in a purely statistical sense
(d) *modelling*: attempting to understand how need is translated into resource utilisation.

The argument here is that any formula should be based on the best empirical evidence about the distribution of need. Basing allocations on increments to previous (historical) budgets, or on regression of a series of historical budgets over a number of years, is inadequate because that simply rewards those who have, for whatever reasons, done well in the past. One alternative is to use normative judgements about what the allocation of resources should be; that is, presumptions that the need for mental health care services should be proportional, for example, to the extent of broken families, marital disharmony or even mortality. The remaining alternative is to attempt to understand how need for mental health care need *is* and *should be* translated into resource use, taking into account variations in supply. Our position is that the latter is preferable at least in the first instance.[3]

In order to carry out this kind of analysis, we need comprehensive data on need and utilisation. The first step, therefore, is to understand the epidemiology of the utilisation of mental health care services.[4]

Epidemiological evidence

There is strong evidence linking psychiatric service utilisation rates with lower social class, male gender, single marital status and some domiciliary aspects, such as living alone, in overcrowded accommodation

---

[3] Although this is not agreed in all parts of the UK.
[4] Note that this is not the same as the epidemiology of mental illness. Some utilisation is inappropriate; and some need for service is unmet.

or in highly transitory neighbourhoods. In addition, reasonable evidence links residential mobility and living in inner cities with higher service utilisation rates; however, the association between population density and mental health services and poverty is more tenuous.

In principle, if one makes an assumption about the average costs and average efficiency of the appropriate treatment protocols, one could extrapolate from these epidemiological data to an assessment of the need for mental health care services (Bevan, 1998).

Previous studies at an area level

For this reason, many or most of the studies – including many of those above and the study discussed in this chapter – have been at an area level. Jarman *et al* (1992) have shown the association between admission rates to psychiatric hospitals in England, but UPA–8 scores (Jarman, 1984) accounted for only 23% of the variation between districts. In particular, two of the components (elderly living alone and children under five years) had very poor predictive capacity. Other variables such as ethnic origin are ambiguous; for example, ethnic origin groups together Caribbeans who use mental health services frequently and those from the Indian subcontinent who use those services relatively little.

Within districts, the Royal College of Psychiatrists (1988) found a reasonably high correlation between the Jarman UPA–8 index and ward admission rates in Hammersmith; Kammerling & O'Connor (1993) found a similar association in Bristol, but noted that unemployment rate and ethnicity produced better predictions; and Cotgrove *et al* (1992) found no correlation in Bloomsbury and Islington.

Glover *et al* (1997) argue that, because admissions and discharges may be influenced by clinical style, the period prevalence admission rate (the number of people per unit of population) is preferable, as it is likely to reduce distortion both from this and from coding errors. They analysed data from 558 wards in North East Thames Region after excluding the City of London wards and the 14 wards in north Essex, which are served by a provider unit in an adjacent region.

Of the 9610 admissions in these wards during the calendar year 1991 appearing in the hospital episode statistics (HES), repeated admissions were identified by birth date, gender and electoral ward of residence. Regression equations were developed among wards within each catchment area, relating the standardised period prevalence admission ratio to variables drawn from census local-based statistics. In half the areas, this produced an adjusted r^2 value greater than 0.5; only two areas showed values below 0.25. However, they found that models based on Essex wards predicted higher than observed numbers of people admitted in both outer and inner London, while a model based on outer-London wards predicted lower than observed numbers in both Essex and inner London. This probably suggests that Essex providers have more generous bed provision relative to need and thus lower admission thresholds.

Kisely (1998) reviewed the Kings Fund report on mental health needs in London (Johnson *et al*, 1997), demonstrating graphically the selective use of routine data on prevalence of psychoses and schizophrenia and health services activity measured in terms of bed occupancy and finished consultant eipsodes. He showed that only for detection under the Mental Health Act is London truly higher (Strathdee & Thornicroft, 1996). He goes on to argue that epidemiological data based on measures of social deprivation in the community for which services are purchased are a better basis. We extend this to argue that the best way to estimate the correct response to need is to examine how local services respond to those epidemiological data.

Developing a model

The difficulty with all these analyses is that they are 'empiricist' in the sense that they simply report correlations between different variables. These correlations could arise in a variety of ways; and, in particular, correlations between one index or one indicator and resource use at an area level may mask a more fundamental relationship at the individual level. Indeed, there is in general a danger in drawing inferences from area data. The most famous example of this is Durkheim's *Suicide*, in which he showed that rates of (male) suicide were higher in northern Germany, although there was no information on *who* had committed suicide. Seventy years later, Selvin (1958) emphasised that this did not mean that it was the Protestants who committed suicide. It is for these reasons that we argue that we have to develop a model of the process.

Rationale for our procedure

In order to explain our approach, we have to set down a (simplified) model of how we see the process from the needs for mental health care services to utilisation.

Individual-level analysis

The starting point is an individual who, whether or not they feel ill, needs mental health care services. The presumption is that the assessment of need for a given level of underlying morbidity would be uniform across the intended domain of application of the formula. We realise that there is a vast literature on the disjunction between underlying morbidity (whatever that is) and need for health care. These are dealt with elsewhere (see Thornicroft, 1991). We start here with a distribution of (unmeasured or imperfectly measured) need. This pattern of needs is translated into utilisation through a variety of filters (and sometimes processes of amplification) as in Fig. 5.1. Note that care can be inappropriately given in response to the presentation of 'illegitimate' needs, just as there may be needs that are entirely unmet because they never pass the first hurdle.

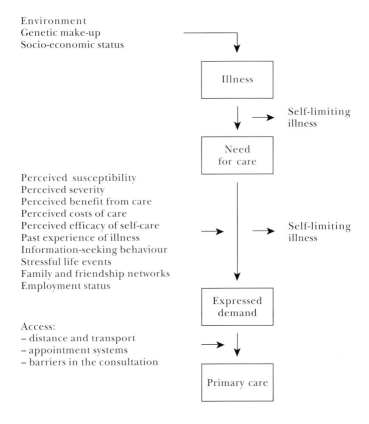

Note: Socio-economic status variables may affect not only health status but also 'objective' need, the rate of expression in the form of demand, levels of accessibility and availability, and GP decision-making. The feedback loop may be either positive or negative.

Fig. 5.1. Factors influencing demand for primary medical care

The experience of utilisation itself leads to an increase (or decrease) in future utilisation and, at a group level, to a particular pattern of supply of services, which themselves modify the process of filtering, as shown in Fig. 5.1. There is, therefore, a cycle of feedback processes alternatively reinforcing or dampening down utilisation.

The problem, therefore, is to identify the extent to which different-ial needs lead to differential utilisation, after controlling for all these extraneous factors. Note that if there were not these various filters, then we could simply evaluate the power of the association between self-reported morbidity (supposed to be a reflection of true morbidity with random noise) and the resource consequences of utilisation (at either an individual or group level), without any of the fancy statistical footwork.

We have described these processes as operating on an individual level. However, in order to estimate such a model, we would need to have data not only on self-reported morbidity, but also on each of the filters indicated in Fig. 5.1 (which is unrealistic), or an agreed way of estimating morbidity uncontaminated by these various filters (which is the focus of some of our current research). Moreover, the requirement for individual data raises all the problem of obtaining a 100% coverage for a population survey (it is a lot easier to collect data for those have passed through institutional records).

It is for this reason that we have moved to estimating the relation-ship between 'needs' and utilisation on an area level. And while in many respects this is just a repeat, writ large of the individual argument because of the dangers of the ecological fallacy (see above), we have to make explicit the assumed processes underlying the demand for health care.

Area-level analysis

The underlying socio-economic and demographic characteristics of the population generate a specific distribution of health care needs, in terms of mental illness morbidity that is treatable. These needs give rise to a certain level of demand for mental health care, although some needs will be unmet and some services will be provided inappropriately. The determinants of this demand considered here are, however, now just the health characteristics of the population. Social characteristics may also influence demand independently of health status. According to this model, therefore, social needs and expectations of the population may have influ-ences on demand over and above any health care needs measured simply through morbidity.

In the same way, the availability of health and related welfare services can affect expectations, and therefore demand for health care. More specifically, in the analysis to develop the formula, we argued that it was likely that the *perceived* availability of local services would be a major determinant of local demand. For example, when a general practitioner (GP) decides whether or not to refer a patient to a consultant, he or she may be influenced by the time the patient will have to wait for treatment. And what matters in the referral process is the GP's perception of the expected waiting time, and not necessarily any objective measure of waiting time. This emphasis on perceived accessibility – which is of course unobservable – is important because it draws attention to the potential for very local variations in effective supply, even though the physical supply of beds available to GPs may be constant across a district.

Supply can influence utilisation in other ways. For example, the level of supply will influence the extent to which demand for health care can be met in situations where there is excess demand for health care. In addition, there is a body of research that suggests that 'supplier-induced demand' – that is, the level of demand that might be influenced by (GP) provider behaviour – might be an important consideration (Cromwell & Mitchell, 1986).

In short, an underlying need for health care in the population is augmented by social circumstances and expectations to generate demand for health care. In the light of this demand and the local political process, NHS services are provided. The adequacy of the supply response will then affect future expectations, and therefore future demand. Further, the level of utilisation over time affects the physical availability of services, which in turn affects perceived availability, and so the process continues. Moreover, the activities of the NHS might have an effect on the underlying health status of the community, and hence a feedback from supply to demand. The actual use of NHS facilities is therefore a dynamic process, with many of the links in Fig. 5.2 containing time lags.

Modelling this process with real data

Modelling such a dynamic process is clearly complex, and calibrating a satisfactory empirical model impossible, given the current limited availability of data. In particular, there is a lack of adequate time series data, and many of the existing measures of utilisation and supply are very crude.

At best, we can obtain cross-sectional data on utilisation, supply and, often for a different date, proxies for need. In this situation, our measures of supply and utilisation are jointly determined (see

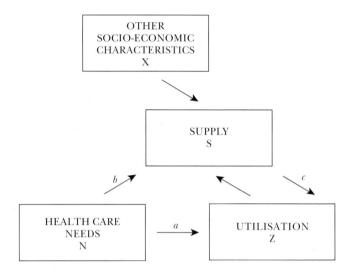

Fig. 5.2 Interrelationship between need, supply and utilisation

Appendix 5.1). That is, they are both affected by the same processes, either at the same time or with lags. In the terminology of econometrics, the variables are endogenous.

The extent to which supply variables are correctly treated as endogenous has been discussed in the literature (Cromwell & Mitchell, 1986; Sheldon & Carr-Hill, 1992). Much depends on the level of analysis being adopted. Thus, given historical administrative arrangements in England, the supply of beds made available at the district level may indeed have been influenced by historical aggregate needs within districts. However, it is not necessarily the case that physical supply of beds is endogenous at the ward level. Nevertheless, what affects utilisation is perceived supply, and this will vary according to the characteristics of the local area (electoral ward) and the GPs acting as agents within it. Therefore, there is every reason to suppose that endogeneity exists even at the small area level.

Because of the assumptions we have had to make, the model developed in the Appendix is almost certainly a simplification of reality, in the sense that it fails to capture the subtle interaction of needs, supply and utilisation over time. Yet, even if the model specified in equations (1) and (2) were theoretically sound, the narrow availability of data and limitations of statistical methods might constrain the ability to build a meaningful empirical model of the demand for health care. In particular, given that the relationship (2) exists, it is almost certainly inappropriate to seek to estimate the utilisation equation (1) by means of ordinary least squares (OLS) regression, as was attempted in the review of RAWP, because the simultaneous determination of U and S would lead to biased estimates of regression coefficients. As a result, it is necessary to examine the possibility of endogeneity, and if it exists to use more advanced statistical estimation techniques, such as two-stage least squares.

Given the simultaneity represented by the pair of arrows between supply and utilisation and in the above equations, there is 'endogeneity', and estimation using OLS will leads to biased coefficients and, of course, distortions in terms of which variables are identified as statistically significant. The problem arises because in the equation for utilisation, the supply variables are correlated with the error term, which violates one of the basic estimating assumptions of OLS. We therefore have to estimate using two-stage least squares or some other econometric technique to take account of these correlations. The argument is based on Fig. 5.2. On this basis, we develop a system of equations:

$$U_i = g_1(N_i, S_i)$$

and

$$S_i = g_2(N_i, U_i, X_i)$$

On that level, the processes described above can be summarised schematically as in Fig. 5.2 (without pretending that this is anything other than a schematic presentation). Note that:

(a) Socio-economic factors that generate illegitimate needs are bundled together with those that inhibit the expression of 'real' needs. We take it that, while the care given may be inappropriate or ineffective, the presumption is that the level of expression of illegitimate needs at secondary care level is small,[5] although this does sometimes pose problems of interpretation (see below); and we ignore the problem that care might be inappropriate or ineffective by presuming average levels of efficiency.

(b) Patterns of supply may have arisen in response to the distribution of real need for health care, but they are also affected by historical patterns of provision. Given that we are concerned with identifying the impact of the distribution of real need on utilisation, we have to separate the former 'legitimate' from the latter 'illegitimate' supply.

---

[5] This may be much more of a problem when we are considering discretionary care and interventions or 'needed' prevention.

This latter problem of separating 'legitimate' from 'illegitimate' supply was considered at length by Carr-Hill *et al* (1994). They showed how, under reasonable assumptions, the correct approach was to estimate the *total* effect of 'true' needs variables on utilisation, that is, not controlling for supply. But in order to do that we have to identify the 'true' needs variables in the first place. The procedure followed by the group who developed the so-called York formulae for England was to identify a set of 'pure' needs variables from a two-stage least squares estimation and then to estimate the fixed coefficients on those variables within a multi-level model (or to estimate the coefficients in a standard OLS with dummy variables) for each English district health authority (DHA) (as was), in order to control for the potential differences in policies and practices between areas. The full argument is given in Appendix 5.2. The major difficulty is the identification of a set of 'pure' needs variables, purged of the effects of 'extra' supply.

Second stage

As explained, the units of analysis were small geographical areas. Although this was the most practical method of examining the relationship between needs and utilisation using routinely collected data, as explained above, it suffers from a further complicating factor (the 'ecological fallacy'). It might reasonably be assumed that medical and administrative policies (as adopted, say, by hospitals, DHAs or family health service authorities) have an influence over a geographical area that is wider than the small area unit of analysis. This is particularly likely in districts outside the metropolitan areas, which are primarily supplied by one hospital. In these circumstances, it is quite plausible to suggest that there are systematic 'district' effects that influence utilisation across a number of observational units.

The reasons for this are also associated with the 'ecological fallacy'. This can be illustrated with reference to a diagram (Fig. 5.3). In this example, there are three health authorities. The numbers in the diagram refer to small areas (wards) within each health authority. Needs are measured using census or similar data. The expenditure responses of each health authority to variations in needs are roughly similar, as shown by the slopes of the regression lines for each health authority. However, authority HA1 devotes a higher level of resources to the services than HA2, which in turn devotes more than HA3. The average needs and costs of each health authority are indicated by the black circles. If these are used in a regression, the thick regression line SS may result. This line bears no relation to actual responses to needs within health authorities, and is mainly determined by variations in expenditure policy between health authorities.

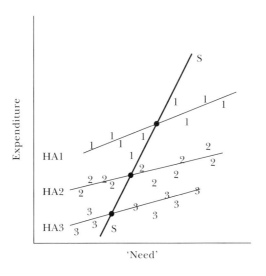

Fig. 5.3 Ward-based and authority-based relationships compared

If phenomena of this sort exist, the use of aggregate health authority expenditure data in a regression analysis, as is the practice in calculating the Standard Spending Assessment for local authorities, may be principally capturing historical spending variations between health authorities, rather than genuine responses to needs. If we are searching for some 'standard' response to needs, we should be seeking to identify the individual slopes of the sort HA1, HA2 and HA3. The government then has to select a particular slope as the 'standard'. Implicit in its methods is the assumption that the national average of individual authority slopes should be favoured. As shown above, this is most emphatically *not* achieved by using aggregate data. Instead, it is necessary to identify the average of the slopes found *within* health authorities.

This poses a problem for statistical estimation, because the fundamental assumption of randomly distributed error terms may be violated. Therefore, we use multi-level modelling techniques to identify and abstract from higher-level supply effects (Paterson & Goldstein, 1991). In effect, multi-level modelling adds a further set of supply variables into the model: the policy effects of administrative areas. An alternative to this procedure is to use dummy variables for each authority (Blundell & Windemeijer, 1997); the choice depends on whether or not one believes that the data from one year should be treated as *sui generis* or whether they are better seen as a sample of possible years. On the whole, we prefer the latter assumption (also we would need to introduce nearly 200 dummy variables if we were to use the Blundell's blunderbuss approach). In addition, the multi-level analysis enables us to explore the robustness of the models using regression techniques, and can be used to investigate the extent and causes of inter-authority variation, which is much more difficult with the dummy variable procedure.

Data used to develop a model

Collection of data

The units of analysis used in the study were 4985 'synthetic wards', small areas with an average population of 9643 covering the whole of England. These synthetic wards were electoral wards, aggregated with contiguous wards where necessary so that none had a population of less than 5000. For each synthetic ward, data were assembled relating to socio-economic conditions, the supply of health services and the use of in-patient services.

The socio-economic variables comprised detailed demographic data prepared by the Office of Population Censuses and Surveys, health status variables and broader social and economic variables derived from the 1991 census. The demographic data were used to standardise all variables for which age was thought to be an important determinant, as follows. The national rates M_{jk} for the variable for age group j and gender k were applied to local population sizes P_{ijk}. This gave the equation:

$$EN_i = \sum_{j=k}^{18} \sum_{k-l}^{2} M_{jk} P_{ijk}$$

where EN is the expected number of observations of the phenomenon of interest in area i. The indirectly standardised rate is then the ratio of the actual number of observations to this expected number. We found little difference between values and rankings of wards using a direct standardisation method and indirect standardisation.

The health status variables included a variety of age-specific standard-ised mortality ratios, standardised ratios of self-reported limiting long-standing illness (derived from the 1991 census) and low birth weight data. We abstracted data from the census on 37 socio-economic variables that could possibly influence demand for health care. In summary, the census variables covered the following aspects of social and economic circumstances: housing tenure; housing amenities; car ownership; overcrowding; ethnicity; country of origin; elderly living alone; lone parents; students; migrants; unemployment; educational qualifications; social class; and non-earning households. Clearly, several measures could be added to these. But we believe that for the purposes of this study the range of issues covered is sufficient to capture the important social causes of the need for health care.

We created four supply variables to capture the effect of varying availability of health services to the wards' populations. These sought to measure the accessibility of NHS in-patient facilities, GP services, the provision of residential and nursing homes, and the accessibility of private inpatient facilities. When deriving measures of accessibility, it is necessary simultaneously to reconcile the supply of facilities, their proximity to the ward of interest, and the impact of competing populations and competing supply. This was done by using the methods of spatial interaction modelling (Appendix 5.2).

To develop measures of accessibility, we used the following indicators of the size of service provision: the number of available beds for NHS in-patient facilities; the number of GPs for GP services; and the number of patients present on census night for private hospitals. Hospitals and GP surgeries were located using grid reference, and we calculated distances to populations on the basis of straight line distances to ward centroids. The proportion of those aged 75 years or over living in nursing or residential homes was the remaining health care supply variable. Limitations of data and the timescale of the project precluded development of more refined variables.

Rates of use standardised for age and gender were calculated from the HES, which cover all finished in-patient and day care hospital episodes. There were 566 887 valid records for the financial year 1990–1991 and 9 042 169 records for 1991–1992. The data available contained the following information: district of treatment; method of admission; source of admission; category of patient (public/private); waiting time for elective admission; age group; speciality group; operation group (×4); order number of episode; duration of episode; discharge destination; patient classification (day/ordinary); and synthetic ward of residence.

Ideally, the analysis would have taken into account the variability of use of hospital care by patients with specific diagnoses or for specific procedures. However, all diagnostic and procedure data were deleted from the HES before they were sent to us. Instead, we assigned each episode to one of 12 speciality groups.

Two types of cost were calculated for each episode: the standard cost, which is the national average cost for a particular age, gender and speciality group; and the estimated cost, which is the speciality-specific cost for the length of stay of that particular episode – that is, speciality fixed cost + speciality variable cost × length of stay. Standard costs seek

TABLE 5.1

In-patient cost curves 1991–1992 according to current Department of Health and revised York formula (relative costs per head of population; overall average = 1)

Age (years)	Non-acute	
	Department of Health	York
0–4	0.00	0.27
5–14	0.01	0.61
15–44	0.18	0.55
45–64	0.56	0.35
65–74	1.53	0.76
75–84	3.76	2.47
≥85+	9.39	4.96

to remove local variations in policy and practice from the measures of use, but do not capture variations in length of stay brought about by variations in need. For this reason, the Department of Health technical advisory groups recommended using estimated costs as the basis for the analysis of acute episodes. The fixed cost per psychiatric episode was estimated (average over speciality groups nos 700–715) as £1031.30 and the cost per bed day as £86.50. These cost data also facilitated the construction of age–cost curves for in-patients, defined as the national average costs per head of population within age bands (Table 5.1). Figure 5.4 shows the links between the various data sources and the master database.

Statistical modelling

The model presented here is for psychiatry[6] and was derived from analysis of 1991–1992 data in England. To develop a model with reasonable statistical specification with these data, we found it necessary to use standard costs as the dependent variable (that is a

---

[6] Admission in the specialities of geriatrics, psychiatry and learning disability were modelled separately from those in the acute sector because of the higher proportion of admissions with long lengths of stay. These groups were modelled separately and in combination and are legitimately aggregated, because they have in common the need for continuing long-term care. It proved impossible to derive a satisfactory model for learning disability.

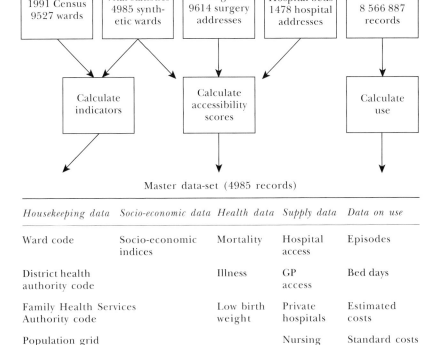

Fig. 5.4 Links between the various data sources and the master data-set

standard value for the costs for a given age–gender group) as some episodes had very long lengths of stay and therefore very high estimated costs. The most 'parsimonious' two-stage least squares model (i.e. the model with the smallest number of statistically significant variables without using explanatory power) is shown in Table 5.2. There is some evidence of mis-specification ($x^2(32) = 67.5$; critical value – 61.1), but this must be expected with so many observations. Age–gender standard-isation appears to have been satisfactory.

It is important to understand the significance of the fact that the supply variables are confirmed as endogenous. In purely statistical terms, this means that any attempt to estimate the equations without taking into account the inter-relationships identified in the diagrams and discussions above will lead to erroneous results. In substantive terms, some of the results are 'obvious' in that a small area's utilisation of in-patient mental illness services tends to increase when there are

TABLE 5.2
Mental illness model, England, 1991–1992

Variable	Coefficient	Standard error	β value
Access to non-acute NHS beds	−0.333	0.128	−0.175
Access to GP	0.323	0.081	0.136
Proportion of population aged 75+ not in nursing/residential home	−0.767	0.167	−0.091
Access to private hospitals	0.158	0.101	0.158
Proportion of households headed by lone parent	0.145**	0.026	0.136
Proportion of dependants with no carer	0.119**	0.033	0.070
Proportion with head born in New Commonwealth	0.058**	0.012	0.113
Proportion of pensionable age living alone	0.205**	0.075	0.057
SMR for ages 0–74	0.254**	0.061	0.097
Proportion of adult population permanently sick	0.212**	0.032	0.179
Percentage of population in urban enumeration districts	−0.109**	0.040	−0.042
Proportion of 17-year-olds who are students	−0.069**	0.033	−0.039
Constant	1.652**	0.549	

**$P < 0.01$.

more people in nursing or residential homes; however, it also appears to suggest that (at least at the beginning of the 1990s) utilisation was negatively related to access to beds, but – almost to the same extent – positively related to accessibility to GPs. While one can indeed 'spin a story', for example based on the easier access to day care facilities, clearly there were complex interactions in the use of services at that time – which mitigates against any simple analysis.

In interpreting this model, it is also important to remember that the HES database recorded discharges in 1991–1992, many of which related to very long episodes. At that time, health authorities were seeking to close many long-term beds and so discharged many long-stay patients into the community. The apparent pattern of need this suggests may therefore be misleading, particularly if discharge destinations – the basis for ward of residence in the HES – are clustered into certain wards. However, similar results were obtained from the analysis applied to the 1990–1991 data.

Most of the 'needs' variables that are included are intuitively plausible. The areas with high mortality have higher use (after adjusting for supply), as do areas with: higher proportions of ethnic minorities; elderly people living alone; people in lone parent families; dependants with no carers; permanently sick adults; and people in manual socio-economic groups. However, the negative association between the level of 17-year-olds in full-time education and the proportion of the population living in urban areas with use in the non-acute specialities is less easy to understand.

The needs variables in Table 5.2 were taken as the legitimate drivers of normative utilisation of psychiatric beds. As a preliminary to the multi-level stage of the analysis, least squares regression was carried out on these variables, resulting in the coefficients shown in the right-hand column of Table 5.3. At this stage, the two least intuitively plausible variables became statistically insignificant and so were dropped. This model explains 40% of the variance in utilisation. In the multi-level model itself, there is a substantial district effect, with the proportion of overall variance attributable to the district level being roughly 38%. It was therefore important to re-estimate the OLS equation using multi-level estimation methods. The results are presented in the first two columns of Table 5.3. The results indicate that in general there is a higher response to needs than would have been indicated by the OLS regression, suggesting that the response to need across wards *within* districts is steeper than the average response across all wards. This phenomenon is likely to arise when

TABLE 5.3
Multi-level estimation and OLS regression of use on needs, England, 1990–1992

Variable	Coefficient	Standard error	OLS value
Proportion of households headed by lone parent	0.185	0.015	0.152
Proportion of dependants with no carer	0.143	0.021	0.113
Proportion with head born in New Commonwealth	0.107	0.007	0.049
Proportion of pensionable age living alone	0.361	0.047	0.375
SMR for ages 0–74	0.243	0.038	0.227
Proportion of adult population permanently sick	0.262	0.022	0.267
Constant	1.127	0.241	0.731

districts operate at different absolute levels of provision, and the multi-level procedure is designed to correct for such disparities between districts. This is the reason for recommending these results as the basis for a national formula.

Many alternative specifications were tested under a variety of assumptions. In particular, the acute model was tested by region, by speciality, and by mode of admission (elective *v.* emergency); the full report gives a description of the various sensitivity analyses undertaken.

Scotland

Using average costs across specialities reduces some of the more extreme local variations caused by the uneven distribution of the small number of people in high-cost psychiatric specialities.[7] However, it also removes the variation owing to length of stay. This is an advantage if these variations are owing to differences in local practice, service efficiency and access, but a disadvantage if they reflect genuine differences in need. In developing a similar model for psychiatric utilisation in Scotland using much more recent – and possibly more reliable – data, we were able to reach consistent results using the estimated costs (adjusting for individual length of stay), as shown in Table 5.4.

TABLE 5.4
Scotland: Beta values of typical variables in the two-stage least squares equations (excluding mental handicap, log–log form, using estimated cost as dependant)

	1993–1994	1994–1995	1995–1996
Proportion <64	0.134	0.096	0.214
SMR for ages 0–74	0.206	ni	0.157
Permanent sickness rate	ni	ni	0.194
Dependants with no carer	0.205	0.294	0.144
Unemployment benefit	ni	0.108	ni
Proportion privately renting	0.149	0.139	0.107
Composite deprivation indicator*	0.161	0.199	ni
Adjusted r^2	0.461	0.422	0.512

* Sign reversed.
ni, not included.

---

[7] One could calculate separate average costs for mental health and geriatric psychiatric, but there is not much difference, so there seems little point in that.

Once again, there was a problem about the appearance of density with the 'wrong' sign and, learning from the above experience, it was not included. The major problem appeared to be that – at least in Scotland – density is highly correlated with access variables; in other words, areas with easy access to hospitals tend to be in urban areas.

The runs for the different years lead to a similar level of predictability of mental health care utilisation, with adjusted r^2 varying between 42% and 52%. It is noticeable that the proportion of households with a single carer is never included as a significant variable. Typically, the equations include: the proportion of dependants with no carer; the proportion of the population who are over 64 years; the proportion renting privately; the standardised mortality ratio 0–74; and the composite deprivation indicator.

In proceeding from this model to the second stage, we found that both the composite indicator and the proportion renting privately became insignificant. In fact, we prefer not to use composite indices because they are even less interpretable than the raw variables themselves (Carr-Hill, 1987); and we were suspicious of the private renting variables (because of the small numbers involved).

Because there are only a small number of health boards in Scotland, we adjusted for inter-district variation by using dummy variables rather than the multi-level procedure (Table 5.5).

Reasonably well-specified models can be reached using weighted populations, including health board dummies in both the instrumenting and the 'top' equations. The 'top' equation in the two-stage least-squares procedure has an r^2 of over 0.51, which is more than satisfactory.

TABLE 5.5
Regression of actual costs on chosen needs variables
(coefficients for health board dummies not shown) without density

	1993–1994		1994–1995		1995–1996	
	β	*Standard error*	β	*Standard error*	β	*Standard error*
Constant	3.395	0.372	11.534	1.759	4.419	0.207
SMR for ages 0–74	0.453	0.069				
Proportion aged <64	0.230	0.053	0.141	0.055	0.269	0.060
Dependants with no carer	0.448	0.048	0.540	0.053	0.471	0.048
Composite deprivation indicator			1.371	0.414		
Standardised permanent sickness rate					0.241	0.038

When these 'true' needs variables are entered into the second stage of the process, we retain a high r^2, but some of the variables become insignificant or only just significant. The most consistent set are for runs without density when the proportion of the population over 64 years and the proportion of dependants in no carer households (+) and one other variable enter in all three years.

Conclusions and further developments

There are problems with data, with unmet need and with area level estimation.

Data

There can be coding errors so that admission and discharge may be wrongly coded. Carr-Hill *et al* (1994) adjusted for this with KP70 form, which is the statistical return to the NHS Executive providing annual totals, but this is very crude approximation. Data from more recent years would be more reliable. However, given that the results for Scotland are very similar in terms of the kinds of variables that are included, this increases our confidence in the reliability of the results.

Unmet need

Identifying and planning for unmet need is the holy grail of needs assessment in general and of approaches to resource allocation in particular. Compared with the problem this poses for needs assessment (which might be more familiar to some readers), it needs to be emphasised that the issue here is only the *relative* difference in uncaptured unmet need between areas and not the *absolute* level of uncaptured unmet need. One of the main purposes of starting out with a large set of candidate variables and not just starting out with the old favourites is to explore all the possible inter-correlations between (lack of) utilisation and the socio-demographics of an area. On this basis, we claim that the development of an evidence-based model, rather than simply a statistical regression equation, goes a long way towards solving the problem of relative unmet need.

Area level estimation

While there are good arguments for area level analysis, there also remain arguments for potential problems of inference because of the 'ecological fallacy'. Given the advantages and disadvantages, the best approach is to carry out the estimation at several different levels.

Conclusions

Mental health service utilisation can be predicted reasonably well; but there are complex interactions between need and supply variables that must be taken into account. The procedures adopted in the development of the models currently being used to allocate resources to health authorities have a number of advantages:

- They involve testing for the impact of a wide range of health needs variables on utilisation of psychiatric services.
- Four different aspects of the supply of health care services (both those directly related to psychiatric services and others only indirectly related) have been incorporated into the model.
- Using the multi-level modelling techniques, we have taken into account differences in policies and and practices between health authorities.
- A wide range of social circumstances was included as possible additional determinants of need for health care.
- Statistical methods were technically appropriate.
- The robustness of models has been tested by subjecting them to extensive sensitivity analysis.

We acknowledge that there were a number of limitations:

- We could not address the assumption that the existing national allocation of resources between care groups was appropriate.
- We could not capture variations in health care needs that are not at all reflected in health care utilisation.
- We could not investigate lag structures and an almost limitless number of alternative specifications.

Nevertheless, we would argue that the study reported here produced the best available model of utilisation, given the data available to the team.

Appendix 5.1: Schematic representation of process

The situation described above can be represented algebraically in a simplified way as follows. The level of utilization U_i in locality I is a function of health care needs N_i, the perceived availability of local services P, the actual level of services provided S_i and socio-economic and demographic considerations X:

$$U_i = f_i, \ (N_i, P_i, S_i, X_i) \tag{1}$$

The level of perceived availability is probably itself a function of actual availability and other considerations X:

$$P_i = f_2(S_i, X_i) \qquad (2)$$

and health care needs are a function of socio-economic and demographic conditions:

$$N_i = f_3(X_i) \qquad (3)$$

Finally, supply is a function of utilisation (including both historical patterns of use and current demand) and historical needs, via:

$$S_i = f_4(U_i, U_i^{-1}, N_i^{-1}, X_i) \qquad (4)$$

where the superscript −1 refers to levels of utilisation or needs at some time in the past.

Note that while the needs variables included in equation (1) represent current needs and those in equation (4) represent past needs, this does not affect the argument about simultaneity between supply and utilisation (which is the crux of the problem in estimating unbiased coefficients for the relation between needs and utilisation) because, in practice, the time series data implied by (4) are not available. Therefore, we are forced to assume that current needs are a proxy for past needs, and that current utilisation is a proxy for past utilisation. Then, abandoning the distinction between perceived and actual supply, we obtain the following equations:

$$U_i = g_1(N_i, S_i) \qquad (5)$$

and

$$S_i = g_2(N_i, U_i, X_i) \qquad (6)$$

The simplified model implied by (5) and 6) suggests that utilisation is a function of health care needs and supply. Supply in turn is determined by needs, utilisation and other socio-economic characteristics not directly related to health care needs. The model is illustrated in Fig. 5.2.

Appendix 5.2: Identification of legitimate and illegitimate need

In developing resource allocation formulae, we wish to correct for variations in supply between areas. Effectively, this means assuming that all supply in an area is at some national average level appropriate to the level of needs found in the area. In calculating a measure of relative need, therefore, the variation in utilisation owing to variation in supply variables should be considered only to the extent that supply reflects variations in legitimate need for health care. The requirement is to develop a measure of 'normative utilisation': the utilisation that would be obtained in an area if the response to its needs was at the national average level.

In order to illustrate the problem, consider the model of utilisation developed in Chapter 3, and reproduced as Figure 5.2. Variations in utilisation U arise because of variations in needs N and variations in supply S. Normative utilisation is that part of utilisation which is attributable to needs alone. Now needs can influence utilisation in two ways: first through a direct impact, as indicated by the arrows *a*, and second as mediated through supply (arrows *b* and *c*). The analytic task is to find that part of the supply effect *c* that is attributable to factors X unrelated to needs indicators N, and to remove that part of the supply effect from the model. Thus, we wish to take account of supply. But we only wish to consider supply to the extent that it reflects legitimate health care needs.

The purpose of the two-stage least-squares modelling exercise was to isolate legitimate needs variables N, which have an unambiguous statistical relationship with utilisation. However, the equations derived from this part of the study are not directly helpful from the viewpoint of developing a formula, as the coefficient on supply will reflect both legitimate needs N and extraneous variables X. A technology is therefore needed to isolate the impact of needs alone on utilisation, either directly, or as mediated through supply. The remainder of this section explains the solution to this problem adopted by this study.

Eliminating supply S from equations (1) and (2), the following equation is derived:

$$U_1 = gi(N_i, g_2(N_i, U_i, X_i)).$$

This can be solved to yield the following expression for utilisation:

$$U_i = g_3(N_i, X_i) \qquad (7)$$

Equation (7) is knows as the 'reduced form' expression for U, which explains U in terms of legitimate needs variables N and more general socio-economic variables X. Then, it is noteworthy that the impact of needs N on utilisation U is given by the total derivative: that is, the total effect of needs N on utilisation is found by examining both the direct effect of N on U, and any indirect effect on U associated with X, if X is correlated with N.

The purpose of the two-stage least-squares modelling exercise was to isolate legitimate 'needs' drivers N of utilisation. In order to develop a measure of normative utilisation, it is necessary to estimate the response of utilisation to those needs variables alone, taking account of any covariance the needs variables might have with broader socio-economic circumstances. This is achieved by undertaking an OLS regression of utilisation on the needs variables identified in the modelling work described above. The coefficient on each needs variable will then capture with direct and indirect effect on utilisation.

The legitimate needs variables N (in logarithmic form) are therefore entered in an OLS regression of utilisation as follows:

$$U_1 = \alpha + \sum_{j=1}^{m} \beta_j N_{ij} + \varepsilon$$

The coefficients in the resulting equation reflect the total impact of needs on utilisation, and can therefore be used as the basis for a resource allocation formula. In contrast, in the review of RAWP, the needs coefficients recommended of use were taken from a regression of utilisation on both needs and supply (Department of Health and Social Security, 1988). The strategy used in this study allows for the fact that variations in existing supply might already to some extent reflect variations in legitimate health care needs. By regressing utilisation on needs alone, that part of needs that is correlated with supply has been taken into account.

References

BEVAN, G. (1998) *Using Epidemiological Data as a Basis for Resource Allocation.* Galway: Health Economics Study Group.

BLUNDELL, R. & WINDEMEIJER, F. (1997) Cluster effects and simultaneity in multi-level models. *Health Economic Letters* (electronic version), **1**, 6–13.

CARR-HILL. R. A. (1987) *Health Status, Resource Allocation and Socio-economic Conditions. Interim Report of the Wolverhampton Health Needs Research Study.* Occasional Paper. York: Centre for Health Economics.

——, HARDMAN, G., MARTIN, S., *ET AL* (1994) *A Formula for Distributing NHS Revenues Based on a Small Area Analysis of Hospital In-Patient Utilisation.* Occasional Paper. York: Centre for Health Economics, University of York.

COTGROVE, A. J., BELL, G. & KALONA, G. L. (1992) Psychiatric admissions and social deprivation: is the Jarman under-privileged area score relevant? *Journal of Epidemiology and Community Health*, **46**, 245–247.

CROMWELL, J. & MITCHELL, J. B. (1986) Physician induced demand for surgery. *Journal of Health Economics*, **5**, 293–313.

DEPARTMENT OF HEALTH AND SOCIAL SECURITY (1988) *Review of the Resource Allocation Working Party Formula. Final report by the NHS Management Board.* Internal Departmental Report.

GLOVER, G. R., ROBIN, E., EMANI, J., *ET AL* (1997) A needs index for mental health care. *Social Psychiatry and Psychiatric Epidemiology*, **33**, 89–96.

JARMAN, B. (1984) Underprivileged areas: validation and distribution of scores. *British Medical Journal*, **289**, 1587–1592.

——, HIRSCH, S., WHITE, P., *ET AL* (1992) Predicting psychiatric admission rates. *British Medical Journal*, **304**, 1146–1151.

JOHNSON, J., RAMSAY, R., THORNICROFT, G., *ET AL* (eds) (1997) *London's Mental Health.* The report to the London Commission. London: Kings Fund.

KAMMERLING, R. M. & O'CONNOR, S. (1993) Unemployment rates as predictor of rates of psychiatric admission. *British Medical Journal*, **307**, 1536–1539.

KISELY, S. (1998) More alike than different: comparing the mental health needs of London and other inner city areas. *Journal of Public Health Medicine*, **20**, 318–324.

MELTZER, H., GILL, B. & PETTRIGREW, M. (1994) *The Prevalence of Psychiatric Morbidity among Adults Aged 16–64, Living in Private Households, in Great Britain.* London: Office of Population Censuses and Surveys.

PATERSON, L. & GOLDSTEIN, H. (1991) New statistical models for analysing social structures: an introduction to multi-level models. *British Educational Research Journal*, **17**, 387–393.

ROYAL COLLEGE OF PSYCHIATRISTS (1988) *Psychiatric Beds and Resources: Factors Influencing Bed Use and Service Planning.* Report of a working party of the section for social and community psychiatry (Chair S. Hirsch). London: Gaskell.

SELVIN, H. (1958) Durkheim's Suicide and problems of empirical research. *American Journal of Sociology*, **63**, 61–79.

SHELDON, T. & CARR-HILL, R. (1992) Resource allocation by regression in the NHS: a statistical critique of the RAWP Review. *Journal of the Royal Statistical Society*, Series A, **155**, 403–420.

STRATHDEE, J. & THORNICROFT, G. (1996) *Commissioning Mental Health Services.* London: HMSO.

THORNICROFT, G. (1991) Social deprivation and rates of treated mental disorder. Developing statistics models to predict psychiatry service utilisation, *British Journal of Psychiatry*, **158**, 475–484.

6 Assessing demand for care at district level using a psychiatric case register

MIRELLA RUGGERI, FRANCESCO AMADDEO and MICHELE TANSELLA

The assessment of needs for care is a fundamental step, both in service planning and in routine clinical practice. In the first case, assessment at population level is useful in order to target resource allocation; in the second, needs assessment at the patient level helps understanding if the care provided is adequate and sufficient. While administrators are interested especially in the assessment of need for services of a defined population, clinicians are mainly concerned with the specific needs of the individual patient. Thus, aims and methods to be used do differ in the two perspectives. In this chapter, we shall concentrate mainly on the former type of needs.

Need for services is both a comprehensive and vague concept. It relates to overall estimates of any help or service that can be provided to alleviate the problem detected; no consideration is given to the specific mechanism of the treatment or its content, but the focus is placed on the existence of a disorder of certain severity, which should be possible to treat in some way (Lethinen, 1997).

Needs assessment, at the population level, should be made using *specific instruments*, such as the Camberwell Assessment of Need (CAN; Slade *et al*, 1999) or the MRC Needs for Care Assessment (MRC NCA; Brewin *et al*, 1987), to be completed in representative samples of the general population, as well as *indirect indicators* (Lewis, 1999). However, so far, in most cases needs for services have been detected by using only indirect indicators. The main methods that have been used are population surveys, analyses of social indicators and service utilisation data. Moreover, needs for services have been extrapolated by comparing prevalence rates of psychiatric disorders with treated prevalence. For example, lack of recognition of a mental disorder and lack of treatment for detected mental disorders have been often associated with the presence of unmet needs (for a review, see Ruggeri, 1997). The reduction of relapse or of admission rates owing to specific treatments has been considered as a proxy for the capability of the treatment itself to satisfy patients' needs for services.

Thornicroft & Tansella (1999) suggested a pathway for measuring or estimating local need for care. As a first stage in this pathway, they considered, as best possible information, local epidemiological data on the occurrence of various psychiatric disorders. If these data were not available, as a second stage, they suggested using country/ regional epidemiological data, weighted for local socio-demographic characteristics, or, as a third stage, international data from 'comparator' countries or regions, again weighted as above. When data to be collected using one of the three methods mentioned above would be incomplete or insufficient, it was suggested that a fourth option be used, namely consensus statements produced by a number of experts, taking into account specific local factors. The final stage in Thornicroft & Tansella's pathway is an expert's synthesis of the data arising from all previous stages.

It is evident that all these methods are tentative estimates of needs for services and that their reliability may be limited. Ideally, they should be used only to provide a picture of the overall frame and the context in which to place the more precise and reliable data obtained by the more costly and difficult to complete assessment of individual needs.

This chapter deals with the possible contribution of psychiatric case registers (PCRs) to the assessment of the need for care at the district level. While taking into account the fact that PCRs, being instruments that monitor the care actually provided, cannot supply direct information on the needs for services, we will underline the value of the best proxy information that can be gathered by using the PCR method, that is, the demand for care. We shall first address some issues related to the assessment of needs at the individual and district level; then we shall consider the influence of service organisation on met and unmet needs; and, finally, in order to demonstrate the value of PCR data in the assessment of demand for care, we shall report the results of a three-year follow-up study, based on data from the South Verona PCR.

Assessing the needs for care at the individual and district level

'Need' for care should be kept distinct from 'demand' for care and from 'service utilisation'. Demand for care is an explicit request of an individual to receive some care, while service utilisation refers to the type of care that the individual actually received. As recently shown by surveys completed in the UK and USA (Bebbington *et al*, 1997; Kessler *et al*, 1997; Lin *et al*, 1997), a need does not necessarily imply a demand for care, and the demand for care is not necessarily followed by service utilisation. On the other hand, demand for care and service use do not necessarily imply the presence of a need.

Research done in the past 20 years has shown that the decision to use a health or a social service is influenced by a complex mixture of factors. Some factors are completely unrelated to needs, others can reasonably be considered as linked to their presence (Thornicroft & Tansella, 1999). Overall, these factors belong to four main groups: (a) the environment where the patient lives; (b) the characteristics of health and mental health services in the area; (c) the socio-demographic and (d) the clinical characteristics of the patient.

It has been shown that, among the environmental factors, the degree of *urbanisation* has a direct relationship with the demand for psychiatric services, with higher rates of treated disorders in urban than in rural areas (Lewis *et al*, 1992). Other factors that may affect the use of services (Thornicroft, 1991) are: *non-professional help* by institutions outside mental health; *support* from primary health care and other medical services; characteristics of the *referral* system; and knowledge of and *attitudes* towards psychiatry, including the view that people have about mental disorders, their expectations for care and their satisfaction with previously attended health services.

On the other hand, many factors have been found to have a role in determining the use of services by patients. As a general finding, it has been shown that a small proportion of patients use a large proportion of available resources (Tansella *et al*, 1986; Hansson & Sandlund, 1992). High service utilisation seems to be related to *diagnosis* and *severity of illness*. Often, many factors are combined and form quite complicated sets of predictors. For example, consistent patterns of associations between social and demographic predictors and rates of psychiatric service utilisation have been found for schizophrenic but not for neurotic disorders (Tansella *et al*, 1993; Thornicorft *et al*, 1993). Socio-demographic factors, such as living alone or having no occupation, predict a higher utilisation in some cases, but this finding was not reported in all studies. A diagnosis of psychosis predicts higher utilisation in most existing studies, but these studies have the limitation that they do not consider clinical variables such as illness severity. When both variables are considered, the role of diagnosis is strongly hampered by the effect of illness severity, with highly differentiated patterns of service utilisation in the same diagnostic group (Thornicroft & Tansella, 1999).

The influence of service organisation on met and unmet needs

The way services are organised is likely to have a powerful influence not only on service utilisation but also on the capability of a service to meet the needs of the patients. Availability, accessibility and acceptability of mental health services have been shown to be important factors that affect the demand for care (Balestrieri *et al*, 1989; Sytema *et al*, 1989; Marriott *et al*, 1993). Simon *et al* (1994) have shown that, among primary care patients, mental health service utilisation increases with higher General Health Questionnnaire (GHQ; Goldberg, 1972) scores, but it can, at the same time, be decreased by organisational factors such as the introduction in the health system of out-of-pocket costs.

Thornicroft & Tansella (1999) conceptualised the impact of organisational aspects in modulating the capability of a service to meet satisfactorily the needs of a population. They identified two types of service organisation: the 'segmental' and the 'systemic'. In a service organised according to a segmental approach, each treatment facility or programme is essentially a separate functioning entity, with specific aims, operational policies, funding sources and selection criteria (for example, in terms of patient age, diagnosis or disability). In a service organised according to a systemic approach, each individual facility or programme is part of the wider system of care, and explicitly takes into account the interrelationships between the constituent parts. It is important to understand that these facilities or programmes do have important effects upon each other in any local area, whether or not they are conceptualised as having such effects.

In the segmental approach, the needs of individual institutions or particular types of patients are taken one at a time, without putting these needs in a general framework of the other services available in the same area. In the system approach, planning is often population-based and aims to organise for defined populations a system of care that underlines the connections between different components, and even the relationships with other health as well as social and private services in the same area. In other words, the system approach to planning is the practical consequence of taking a public health approach to assessing the mental health needs of a population.

Thornicroft & Tansella (1999) described nine leading principles that affect mental health service organisation:

(a) *autonomy*, i.e. the capability of the service to preserve and pro-
    mote independence by positive experiences, and to reinforce
    the strengths or healthy aspects of each patient, especially the
    most severely disabled, while controlling symptoms;

(b) *continuity*, i.e. the ability of the relevant services to offer interventions, at the patient or at the local level; refers to the coherence of interventions over a shorter time period, both within and between teams (*cross-sectional continuity*), or which are an uninterrupted series of contacts over a longer time period (*longitudinal continuity*);

(c) *effectiveness*, i.e. the extent to which a specific intervention, when used under ordinary clinical circumstances, does what it is intended to do;

(d) *accessibility*, i.e. a service characteristic experienced by users and their carers that enables them to receive care where and when the care is needed;

(e) *comprehensiveness*, i.e. how far a service extends across the whole range of severity of mental illnesses, and across a wide range of patient characteristics (*horizontal comprehensiveness*), or the availability of the basic components of care (out-patient and community care; day care; acute in-patient and longer-term residential care; and interfaces with other services) and their use by prioritised groups of patients (*vertical comprehensiveness*);

(f) *equity*, i.e. the fair distribution of resources;

(g) *accountability*, i.e. a function that consists of complex, dynamic relationships between mental health services and patients, their families and the wider public, who all have legitimate expectations of how the service should act responsibly;

(h) *coordination*, i.e. a service characteristic that is manifested by coherent treatment plans for individual patients; and

(i) *efficiency*, i.e. a service characteristic that minimises the inputs needed to achieve a given level of outcomes, or which maximises the outcomes for a given level of inputs.

The segmental and systemic models of service planning have many substantial differential characteristics in relation to how far each model considers and satisfies the nine guiding principles. Neither autonomy nor effectiveness is differentially affected by the two approaches, but as far as the other principles are concerned, the systemic approach is much more likely to fulfil these requirements satisfactorily as compared with the segmental approach (Thornicroft & Tansella, 1999). This conceptualisation makes clear that the impact of the organisational aspects in determining the capability of a service to meet patients' needs is potentially enormous; further effort should be dedicated, in future research, in order to provide a solid evidence-based knowledge on this issue.

PCRs can contribute to clarifying these issues. As reported above, they are not adequate tools for measuring needs for care. However, the detailed monitoring of service utilisation that they supply, which concerns not only the intensity but also the typology of care provided, can be useful for building up a comprehensive picture of the strengths and weaknesses that lag behind, in the particular district concerned, the model of service provided. For instance, it is helpful to differentiate service activities mainly influenced by availability or supply of care from activities mainly influenced by demand of care.

Demand for psychiatric care at the district level

As stressed in the previous sections, at the district level, in a community-based system of care, it is important to study the demand for psychiatric care and to try to differentiate service activities mainly influenced by this demand from activities mainly influenced by availability or supply of care (Balestrieri *et al*, 1987; Tansella *et al*, 1989). One way to approach this problem is to analyse separately community contacts that have been made on an urgent basis or without an appointment (unplanned contacts), those which are influenced mainly by demand, and those contacts which were previously booked (planned contacts) and that may be considered as subject to the influence of both supply and demand.

PCRs, where they monitor contacts by differentiating planned and unplanned activities, can therefore be used for assessing longitudinally demand for care at the district level.

A longitudinal case register study on planned and unplanned contacts

In this section, we shall present the results of a longitudinal case register study, completed in South Verona, with the aim of identifying which patients most often use psychiatric services on an unplanned basis and which variables are most often associated with this use, that is, with a use influenced mainly by demand for care.

Methods

The area and the South Verona mental health services

South Verona is an area that includes part of Verona (a city of about 260 000 inhabitants) and two neighbouring small towns. It is a mainly urban area (population density $988/km^2$) with a predominance of service and manufacturing industries.

The South Verona Community-Based Mental Health Service (CMHS) was designed as a systemic service, in which great emphasis is given to communication between all staff members and to integration between the various clinical activities.

Staff members are divided into three multi-disciplinary teams, each serving a subsector of the South Verona catchment area and organised according to a 'single staff module': staff work both inside and outside the hospital and remain responsible for the same patients across different components of the service (to ensure cross-sectional continuity of care) and through the different phases of treatment (to ensure longitudinal continuity of care).

The community mental health centre (CMHC) is the linchpin of the CMHS. Therapeutic programmes include crisis intervention, day care for acute and chronic patients, and social skills groups.

The psychiatric ward is an open ward of 16 beds located in the academic general hospital, which has about 1000 beds. It is a traditional hospital ward, similar to all other medical wards in the hospital and its door is locked when there are patients who have been compulsorily admitted.

The out-patient department provides psychiatric consultations and individual and family therapy. Offices are located in the general hospital and in the CMHC.

The consultation liaison service is dedicated to other medical and surgical departments, but ensures continuing contact with our patients when hospitalised for medical reasons.

There is a psychiatric emergency room service at the general hospital, open 24 hours a day, seven days a week. There is also an emergency night and weekend service, run by two psychiatric nurses.

Home visits can be made to provide crisis intervention, but for chronic patients these are usually planned in advance and offer regular, long-term support and care to patients and their families.

Two residential facilities are available in South Verona, as part of the CMHS. One is a 24-hour staffed supervised hostel with six places for users in need of continuous supervision. The other, a group home, provides six-hour staff supervision on working days, and offers four places (for more details, see Tansella *et al* (1998)).

The psychiatric case register

The South Verona PCR started on 31 December 1978 with a prevalence count and has been operating ever since. At first contact, socio-demographic information, past psychiatric and medical history and clinical data are routinely collected for those aged 14 years and over contacting the psychiatric services. Contacts with psychiatrists, psychologists, social workers and psychiatric nurses are recorded. Each attendance at an out-patient clinic and each domiciliary visit is counted as a contact.

Diagnoses are assigned according to ICD–9 (ICD–10 since 1992) (World Health Organization (WHO), 1978, 1992) and then coded into 12 standard diagnostic groups. The diagnoses of all new cases are routinely reviewed by the director of the case register (M.T.). All psychiatric services of South Verona and the larger province of Verona provide data for the PCR for South Verona residents. Special care and precautions are taken to ensure both accuracy and confidentiality of records.

Subjects

All patients who had at least one contact with the South Verona CMHS and received an ICD diagnosis during the period 1990–1994 (1841 patients) were included in the study. These subjects were followed for three years from the index contact. During the three-year follow-up, 54 956 contacts with the psychiatric services (916 admissions to the psychiatric ward or to the sheltered apartments and 54 040 extramural contacts) were recorded. For the purpose of this study, only extramural contacts are considered.

Results

Patients were classified into five groups, based on the number of contacts made during the three-year follow-up (see Table 6.1). This way of grouping our patients was chosen to obtain homogeneity within them. In each group, the coefficient of variation (a measure of dispersion correcting for the magnitude of the average value of the variable) was under the acceptable limit of 0.8.

In our cohort, out of 54 040 extramural contacts, 4339 were unplanned (8%). The distribution of planned and unplanned contacts over the three years of follow-up within the South Verona Community-Based Psychiatric Service is shown in Table 6.2.

Table 6.3 shows the relationships between the proportion of unplanned contacts and five socio-demographic and clinical patient characteristics. All variables were significantly related to the proportion of extramural contacts made on an unplanned basis, as shown by the confidence intervals.

Male patients had a significantly higher percentage of unplanned contacts compared with females. The patients in the miscellaneous group 'other diagnosis' had the highest percentage (11%) of unplanned contacts; when looking at the de-segregated diagnostic

TABLE 6.1
Distribution of extramural contacts

	No. of patients	Mean no. of contacts	s.d.	95%	CI	CV*
Single consulters	430	1.0				0.00
2–4 contacts	437	2.7	0.8	2.7	2.80	0.30
5–14 contacts	419	8.3	2.8	8.1	8.60	0.34
15–125 contacts	458	41.1	25.2	38.8	43.4	0.61
>125 contacts	97	319.8	217.7	275.9	363.60	0.68
Total	1841	29.9	87.0	25.9	33.80	2.91

* CV is the coeffiecient of variation defined as the standard deviation divided by the mean of the distribution. The acceptable limit of CV is 0.8.

subgroups, the patients most frequently receiving unplanned contacts were those with a diagnosis of drug addiction (20.2%), mental retardation (20.6%) or dementia (26.0%).

The number of unplanned contacts has an inverse trend compared with the intensity of service contacts; in fact, patients with continuous care had less unplanned contacts (5.3%) than single consulters (28.3%) or low users (2–4 contacts) (21.7%) of the service; all these groups are significantly different.

The joint effects of all five patient-related variables (gender, age, occupational status, diagnosis and intensity of contacts) on the likelihood of having unplanned contacts were examined using a generalised linear model (GLM; McCullagh & Nelder, 1989). The

TABLE 6.2
Cohort 1990–1994 (n=1841 patients): extramural contacts with the South Verona CMHS by type of care

	Unplanned (%)	Planned (%)
Out-patient care	7.4	92.6
Day patient care	0.2	99.8
Home visits	8.1	91.9
Emergency service	96.7	3.3
Telephone calls	51.8	48.2
Total	8.0	92.0

TABLE 6.3

1990–1994 cohort: planned and unplanned contacts (n=4339) by socio-demographic variables and clinical variables

	Unplanned (%)	Planned (%)	95% CI
All	8.0	92.0	–
Gender			
Male	8.5	91.5	8.2–8.9
Female	7.7	92.3	7.4–8.0
Occupational status			
Employed	7.5	92.5	7.0–7.9
Unemployed	6.5	93.5	6.1–7.0
Other	8.6	91.4	8.3–9.0
Diagnosis			
Schizophrenia	6.8	93.2	6.4–6.2
Affective disorders	8.1	91.9	7.6–8.5
Neurosis and somatoform disorders	6.5	93.5	5.9–7.0
Personality disorders	9.6	90.4	8.9–10.1
Other diagnoses	11.0	89.0	10.3–11.7
Age, years			
14–24	10.1	89.9	9.2–11.0
25–44	8.2	91.8	7.8–8.5
45–64	6.6	93.4	6.3–7.0
65+	11.8	88.2	10.8–12.8
Type of user			
Single consulters	28.3	71.7	24.1–32.6
2–4 contacts	21.7	78.3	19.3–24.1
5–14 contacts	13.1	86.9	11.9–14.2
15–125 contacts	10.3	89.7	9.9–10.7
High users (>125)	5.3	94.7	5.0–5.5

results are reported in Table 6.4. The GLM allows us to estimate the relationship between patient characteristics introduced into the model and the proportion of unplanned contacts for each patient, using contacts as grouped data. The model shows the negative effect of having a diagnosis of affective disorder or neurosis, being 45 years of age or older, being female and being continuously in contact with the services.

Patients with more frequent contacts with the service had less unplanned contacts. Positive effect was found for patients within the diagnostic group 'other diagnoses'.

The capacity of the model to predict unplanned contacts was also tested (Table 6.5). The 10 most frequently observed subgroups, with

TABLE 6.4
Generalised linear model coefficients

Variable	Coefficient	s.d. error	z	P>|z|
Unemployed	0.000	0.04234	0.003	0.998
Affective disiorder	−0.100	0.04436	−2.261	0.024
Neurosis and somato- form disorders	−0.449	0.05661	−7.931	0.000
Other diagnoses	0.115	0.04171	2.745	0.006
Age ≥45	−0.166	0.03457	−4.789	0.000
2–4 contacts	−0.204	0.13195	−1.548	0.122
5–14 contacts	−0.786	0.12216	−6.431	0.000
15–125 contacts	−1.085	0.11481	−9.453	0.000
>125 contacts	−1.913	0.11608	−16.484	0.000
Female	−0.085	0.03231	−2.682	0.009
Constant	−0.755	0.12101	−6.236	0.000

All variables are entered in the model as dummy variables.

at least 10 patients, obtained using the patient characteristics introduced into the model, are presented. The observed proportion was compared with the expected values obtained, using the co-efficients of the GLM in a linear prediction. Single consulters and patients under 45 years of age were seen more frequently on an unplanned basis and were correctly identified by the model.

Conclusion

In community-based psychiatric services, demand for services and clinical needs generate a continuous flux of planned and unplanned clinical activities. To have information on this flux is one of the key challenges for service providers, as well as for administrators and planners. The categorisation that we used of planned *versus* unplanned appointments needs to be discussed. It is obvious that, to some extent, 'unplanned' care depends on the flexibility of 'planned' services. For instance, if the service is flexible enough to consider, in principle, the possibility of providing prompt response to all requests for intervention, it may be difficult to classify a request for an assessment to be made, for example, in three or four hours' time. Is that to be considered planned or unplanned?

TABLE 6.5

Predicted proportion of unplanned contacts by the GLM model

Observed %	Expected %	n	Gender	Age	Diagnosis	Occupational status	Frequency of contacts
34.5	30.1	28	M	<45	Schizophrenia	Employed	2–4 contacts
33.3	29.8	12	M	<45	Affective disorder	Employed	Single consulters
31.3	28.1	16	F	<45	Affective disorder	Employed	Single consulters
30.4	32.6	46	F	<45	Other diagnosis	Employed	Single consulters
30.0	23.1	20	M	<45	Neurosis	Employed	Single consulters
27.8	21.6	36	F	<45	Neurosis	Employed	Single consulters
26.8	34.5	41	M	<45	Other diagnosis	Employed	Single consulters
24.7	18.3	29	F	≥45	Neurosis	Employed	2–4 contacts
21.0	16.9	21	M	>45	Other diagnosis	Employed	5–14 contacts
20.6	19.7	21	M	<45	Neurosis	Employed	2–4 contacts

Only data concerning groups with more than 10 patients are reported.

When the forms for data collection for the South Verona PCR, used in the present study, were designed, it was decided to adopt a clear-cut definition of planned contacts, that is, all contacts that were scheduled in advance, using our appointment schedule. All other contacts were defined as unplanned. The latter, as defined in the present study, therefore include a full range of contacts, from 'casual' through non-scheduled self-referrals and requests for assessing a patient the same day or before the first available date for booked appointments, to urgent and emergency contacts.

It is clear that related to the issue of 'time' to arrange an appointment are also the issues of 'self-referral' and 'emergency'. From our data-set, it is not possible to identify 'urgent' contacts among those classified as unplanned.

On the other hand, from the point of view of service organisation, casual contacts, self-presentations seeking immediate help (often perceived as urgent by the patient or by the referrer), contacts merely for the patient's convenience and all other non-scheduled contacts that would probably not be defined as urgent from the psychiatrist's point of view impose a higher burden on services than planned appointments (Smith *et al*, 1996). Indeed, at the service level, the 'unplanned' characteristic of a psychiatric contact is highly informative, quite independently from the associated (or not associated) 'urgent' characteristic; all unplanned, non-scheduled interventions, whether or not they are also urgent, are not only mainly influenced by the demand for care made by patients themselves and by their relatives, but, because they interfere with the normal daily activities of mental health services, are also more demanding and more 'expensive' than planned contacts.

The South Verona PCR is one of the few case registers that allows us to analyse separately unplanned and previously booked contacts. Previous research showed that, in our area, 36% of first-ever psychiatric contacts are unplanned (Tansella & Micciolo, 1998), indicating that a large proportion of first-episode patients use available services in a way more directly related to demand for care.

In the present study, 8% of all extramural contacts made in three years were unplanned. This type of contact was more often made by males, patients aged 14–24 years or 65 and over, patients retired, housewives and students, patients with a diagnosis of personality disorder, drug addiction, mental retardation or dementia, and finally by single consulters. Patients with a higher number of contacts over the three-year period tend to have less unplanned contacts, which suggests that for patients receiving a greater amount of care the demand for care is replaced by supply of care made by a responsible service.

Our data show also that when the joint effects of all variables on the amount of unplanned care were examined, female gender, diagnosis of affective disorder or neurosis and somatoform disorder, age of 45 years or more and high use of services were all independently associated with a lower proportion of unplanned care, that is, with a low demand for care.

Some limits of the present study need to be underlined. Being a case register study, no distinction was made between need and demand for services. We should stress again that case registers simply monitor the amount of care provided for a geographically defined population and leave unanswered the question of whether there is a demand for the service (e.g. emergency or unplanned contacts) because it is there or because of need. Other studies, designed to assess demand and need of services independently from service provision, may address this question. However, it is difficult to run such longitudinal studies over a long period of time, and to take into account all services providing care to a defined population. PCRs are therefore useful tools for monitoring, at the district level, the amount and the characteristics of care actually provided, which in turn are, *per se,* important variables for understanding present use of resources and for planning a more rational utilisation of these resources.

References

BALESTRIERI, M., WILLIAMS, P., MICCIOLO, R., *ET AL* (1987) Monthly variation in the pattern of extramural psychiatric care. *Social Psychiatry*, **22**, 160–166.

——, SYTEMA, S., GAVIOLI, I., *ET AL* (1989) Patterns of psychiatric care in South-Verona and Groningen. A case-register follow-up study. *Acta Psychiatrica Scandinavica*, **80**, 437–444.

BEBBINGTON, P. F., MARDSEN, L. & BREWIN C. R. (1997) The need for psychiatric treatment in the general population: the Camberwell Needs for Care survey. *Psychological Medicine*, **27**, 821–834.

BREWIN C. R., WING J. K., MANGEN S. P., *ET AL* (1987) Principles and practice of measuring needs in the long-term mentally ill: the MRC Needs for Care Assessment. *Psychological Medicine*, **17**, 971–981.

GOLDBERG, D. P. (1972) *The Detection of Psychiatric Illness by Questionnaire (GHQ)*. Maudsley Monograph 21. London: Oxford University Press.

HANSSON, L. & SANDLUND, M. (1992) Utilization and patterns of care in comprehensive psychiatric care organizations. A review of studies and some methodological considerations. *Acta Psychiatrica Scandinavica*, **86**, 255–261.

KESSLER, R. C., FRANK, R. G., EDLUND, M., *ET AL* (1997) Differences in the use of psychiatric outpatients services between the United States and Ontario. *New England Journal of Medicine*, **336**, 551–557.

LETHINEN, V. (1997) Population needs for mental health services: introduction to the theme. In: *Making Rational Mental Health Services* (ed. M. Tansella), pp. 3–20. Rome: Il Pensiero Scientifico Editore.

Lewis, G. (1999) Population-based needs assessment. *Current Opinion in Psychiatry*, **12**, 191–194.

—, David, A., Andreasson, S., *et al* (1992) Schizophrenia and city life. *Lancet*, **340**, 137–140.

Lin, E., Goering, P. N., Lesage, A., *et al* (1997) Epidemiological assessment of overmet need in mental health care. *Social Psychiatry and Psychiatric Epidemiology*, **32**, 355–362.

Marriott, S., Malone, S., Onyett, S., *et al* (1993) The consequences of an open referral system to a community mental health service. *Acta Psychiatrica Scandinavica*, **88**, 93–97.

McCullagh, P. & Nelder, J. A. (1989) *Generalised Linear Model*. 2nd edition. London: Chapman & Hall.

Ruggeri, M. (1997) Service utilisation: a pivotal measure in assessing needs and service outcome. In: *Making Rational Mental Health Services* (ed. M. Tansella). Rome: Il Pensiero Scientifico Editore.

Simon, G. E., Von Korff, M. & Durham M. L. (1994) Predictors of outpatient mental health utilization by primary care patients in a health maintenance organization. *American Journal of Psychiatry*, **151**, 908–913.

Slade, M., Thornicroft G., Loftus L., *et al* (1999) *CAN: Camberwell Assessment of Need*. London: Gaskell.

Smith, P., Sheldon, T. A. & Martin, S. (1996) An index of need for psychiatric services based on in-patient utilisation. *British Journal of Psychiatry*, **169**, 308–316.

Sytema, S., Giel, R. & ten Horn G. H. M. M. (1989) Patterns of care in the field of mental health. Conceptual definition and research methods. *Acta Psychiatrica Scandinavica*, **79**, 1–10.

Tansella, M. & Micciolo, R. (1998) Unplanned first contact as a predictor of future intensive use of mental health services. *Social Psychiatry and Psychiatric Epidemiology*, **33**, 174–180.

— , — , Balestrieri, M., *et al* (1986) High and long-term users of the mental health services. A case-register study in Italy. *Social Psychiatry*, **21**, 96–103.

—, — & Zimmermann-Tansella, Ch. (1989) The demand for extramural psychiatric intervention in a community-based service. *European Archives of Psychiatry and Neurological Sciences*, **238**, 220–224.

—, Bisoffi, G. & Thornicroft, G. (1993) Are social deprivation and psychiatric service utilization associated in neurotic disorders? A case-register study in South-Verona. *Social Psychiatry and Psychiatric Epidemiology*, **28**, 225–230.

—, Amaddeo, F., Burti, L., *et al* (1998) Community-based mental health care in Verona, Italy. In: *Mental Health in Our Future Cities* (eds D. Goldberg & G. Thornicroft), pp. 239–262. Hove: Psychological Press.

Thornicroft, G. (1991) Social deprivation and rates of treated mental disorder. Developing statistical models to predict psychiatric service utilisation. *British Journal of Psychiatry*, **158**, 475–484.

— & Tansella, M. (1999) *The Mental Health Matrix. A Manual to Improve Services*. Cambridge: Cambridge University Press.

—, Bisoffi, G., De Salvia, D., *et al* (1993) Urban–rural differences in the associations between social deprivation and psychiatric service utilization in schizophrenia all diagnoses: a case-register study in Northern Italy. *Psychological Medicine*, **23**, 487–496.

World Health Organization (1992) *International Classification of Diseases and Related Health Problems. Tenth revision (ICD–10)*. Geneva: WHO.

7 Assessing the need for psychiatric services at district level: using the results of community surveys

PAUL BEBBINGTON and SIAN REES

In psychiatry, the English word 'need' can be used in various ways to express the relationship between psychiatric disorder, the behaviour of those who suffer from it and the response of those with the task of alleviating it. Need itself is often subdivided into the following types: 'perceived' need or what individuals believe they require; 'expressed' need, which is the demand for services represented by utilisation data; comparative need; and normative need. Comparative need can be defined at the individual or population level: an individual or population may be said to be in need if they share characteristics with others who are receiving a service at a different level of provision, for instance in comparison with national levels.

Normative need is need defined by professionals. It can only be said to exist if there is a known effective intervention that can reasonably be applied to the cause of the need. It has also been described as the capacity to benefit from treatment or care. This is different from comparative need, which assumes that particular levels of provision (the comparison level) are in fact the correct ones. Normative need should be based on evidence of the effectiveness of interventions and is therefore essentially linked to the evidential basis of psychiatry.

Not only is the concept of need itself complex, but it is difficult to arrive at empirical statements about need that would be of use to those responsible for planning psychiatric services. The rationality of decision-making in this area is constrained by the availability of empirical data.

Determining need

There are five main ways of determining need that may be of help in service planning. The first is epidemiological needs assessment. Epidemiology describes the occurrence of disease in a population in terms of person, place and time by determining the incidence and prevalence of disease. These measures do not necessarily equate with need, but are a valuable starting point. Information may be gathered by local surveys (which are expensive) or by extrapolating the results of research to a local population. Extrapolation must take into account, wherever possible, relevant differences between the research and local populations, for example, in terms of age/gender structures, ethnicity and deprivation. An understanding of the risk factors for the development of disorder is therefore essential. This approach does not delineate the actual needs of individuals within the population, but can provide an estimate of the likely numbers in need.

A second way of evaluating need is by using a proxy sociodemographic approach. An understanding of risk factors for disorder allows the assumption to be made that a population that displays high levels of the relevant variables will also have high levels of morbidity. For example, measures of social deprivation, such as homelessness and unemployment, are associated with mental disorder, and inner cities that have high levels of these variables also have high levels of mental ill health. Composite measures that indicate social deprivation, such as those of Jarman (1983) and Townsend *et al* (1985), are also associated with levels of mental ill health.

A third approach is through the analysis of service usage. Data are collected on aspects of service utilisation that may be considered a proxy for need. This approach may produce a skewed picture of need, as not all individuals that could benefit may be in touch with services, and not all those in touch with services may benefit. The information can be compared with data from other services, particularly those that cover similar populations. Analysis that provides evidence of services under strain may be especially valuable, for instance bed occupancy, compulsory admission rates, three-month re-admission rates, numbers of new long-stay patients occupying acute beds and patient diagnostic profiles skewed towards severe mental illness.

It is also possible to arrive at an idea of population need by recruiting key informants. The views of a variety of individuals and groups of people may be of value in attempting to define need, both in terms of how many people (prevalence/incidence) and of how much they may benefit (effectiveness). Informants range from clinicians and service planners to service users. There are a number of mechanisms by which their views can be elicited, for instance, individual or group interviews using structured or semi-structured questionnaires, focus groups and search conferences.

The final, most intensive and most expensive method is to aggregate data from the direct determination of need in individuals. If the population in question can be accurately delineated, data from individual assessments of need can be aggregated to produce an overall picture of need. This approach may utilise clinical assessments for those in touch with services, for example analysis of care planning assessments or formal assessments of need such as the Camberwell Assessment of Need (CAN; Slade *et al*, 1999). Alternatively, a whole population approach may be taken, using a research instrument such as the community version of the MRC Needs for Care Assessment (MRC NCA; Brewin *et al*, 1987).

Needs assessment is inevitably an imperfect science. It is, however, always better to attempt to triangulate data from multiple sources than to rely on guesswork. The determination of need is a starting point for service planning. It should therefore be seen as part of a dynamic set of processes and not as an isolated piece of work. It is important to remember that need is not static; it may change over time, and so projections of future need ought to be considered as part of the exercise.

Related procedures

There are a number of other essential related processes. These include resource mapping, that is, the establishment of precise knowledge of the services (structures, staff and skills) currently available and how much is spent on them. An essential part of this process is that clear definitions of services and interventions are made in order that information collected is comparable across different areas.

Similarly, if need is to be determined by the capacity to benefit from interventions, some knowledge of the effectiveness of any inter-ventions must be known in order to determine need. Thus, an essential part of the establishment of need is reviews of the effectiveness literature, that is, identification of the interventions and services that are beneficial. This information is likely to be partial at best, but should be used wherever possible. It is also essential to determine unmet need and gaps in services, and to link this information to service planning.

Configuration of care systems and the evaluation of need

It is important when assessing and planning services that all aspects of service provision are seen within the context of the whole system. Inevitably, the need for any one component, for example in-patient beds or day care, will be a function of levels of morbidity and the availability of other service components; unacceptably high levels of in-patient bed usage reflect the need for more beds if the patients occupying those beds are all considered to be appropriately placed. However, there is evidence to suggest that as many as 20–30% of acute mental illness beds in London are occupied by new long-term patients (with a length of stay greater than six months). This use of acute beds cannot be considered appropriate, and therefore reflects gaps in service provision for this group, such as staffed and non-staffed community-based residential accommodation. Similarly, the availability of alternatives to acute admission, such as crisis or respite beds, home-treatment services or extended day hospital programmes, may all have an impact on the need for in-patient facilities. It is, however, difficult to predict the precise impact, given the lack of research data for the effectiveness of such services in local inner-city areas as opposed to the model services on which research outcomes have been determined.

Community surveys and the estimation of need

In the rest of this chapter, we shall consider the ways in which community surveys can be used to provide estimates of needs for treatment and, in particular, the extent to which this need goes unmet. The first survey we shall use for this purpose is the British National Survey of Psychiatric Morbidity, in particular its household component, which was based on a sample over 10 000 randomly selected respondents. This has been well described elsewhere (Jenkins *et al*, 1997*a,b*). Its purposes did not include a direct estimate of need, but data were collected that allow indirect assessments of need in the general population.

The prevalence of psychiatric disorders can be taken as a rough indication of the overall need for psychiatric treatment in a general population. Some kind of service contact is required before most treatments can be given, and even then they may not be provided. While most people in the UK general population identified as having a psychiatric disorder will not have sought professional help, those who do will mainly be seen by primary care physicians.

The household component of the National Survey collected information about diagnosis, service use and the receipt of pharmacological and psychological treatments. Combining these does at least allow reasonable estimates of the extent to which needs are *not* being met by services. Two recent papers have focused on the first stage in obtaining treatment, that is, contact with a primary care physician for a mental health problem, and, once this has been made, on the influences that bear on the provision of pharmacological and psychological treatments (Bebbington *et al*, 2000*a,b*).

Within the British National Health Service (NHS), the twin principles of equity and proportionality are held to be particularly important. If only a minority of people diagnosed as cases of psychiatric disorder seek professional help for their symptoms and receive treatment for them, one would at least hope that these principles would exert an appreciable influence. In other words, a greater proportion of severe disorders would receive treatment than mild ones, and disorders of equivalent severity would be equally likely to be treated, whatever the attributes of the person suffering from them. The application of both principles would tend to result in severity being the major determinant of treatment, and treatment access would not vary in relation to socio-demographic variables.

The severity of psychiatric disorders can be conceptualised in more ways than one. Bebbington and his colleagues (2000*a,b*) used as measures of severity the number of psychiatric symptoms and the degree of social impairment. These attributes, while correlated, are sufficiently separate to merit using both as independent variables (Bebbington *et al*, 2000*c*). These authors therefore examined the association of symptom severity, social impairment and socio-demographic variables with seeking help from primary care physicians for a psychiatric problem and with the receipt of various treatments once medical help had been sought. It was expected that the major determinant of contacting a general practitioner (GP) for a psychiatric problem would be the severity of the problem, and thus the proportion of people contacting would be little affected by demographic variables, once severity was accounted for.

In the National Survey, neurotic psychiatric disorder was assessed using the Revised Clinical Interview Schedule (CIS–R; Lewis *et al*, 1992), which is made up of 14 sections, each covering a particular area of neurotic symptoms. Scores on each section can be summed to produce a total score indicative of the severity of neurotic symptoms. CIS–R data can also be subjected to a computer algorithm providing ICD–10 diagnoses (World Health Organization(WHO), 1992*a*). Social impairment was assessed as described by Bebbington and his colleagues (2000*c*). Scores on seven areas of social performance were summed to produce an overall measure of social impairment. Informants were also asked if they had spoken to their GP in the past year, and whether it was for physical or for mental and emotional complaints.

Making contact with health professionals

The authors found that quite large numbers of people with neurotic disorders had not in fact consulted their GP for a mental complaint. Relatively high levels of contacting were seen among subjects with major depressive episode (around 50%), although the highest rate of contacting in females was actually in those with obsessive–compulsive disorder.

There was a very strong relationship between symptom severity and whether subjects attended their GP for reasons of mental health in the previous year. This emerged despite the possibility that people attending earlier in the year might have lost some or all of their psychiatric symptoms by the time they were interviewed. There was also a strong relationship between social impairment and contacting, although not so marked. Thus, the severity of disorder was a major influence on whether people in the general population sought help from their primary care physicians for mental problems.

The authors performed a logistic regression examining the effect of severity of illness on contacting behaviour, but including key socio-demographic variables: age, gender, marital status, employment status, ethnicity, social class, and whether the subject also reported suffering from a physical illness. The major contribution came from psychiatric symptoms, and subjects scoring 18 or over on the CIS–R were nearly eight times as likely to have been in contact with their primary care physician for mental health reasons than people scoring 5 or less. Social impairment also provided a significant independent contribution. Thus, the authors' argument that the severity of disorder is the major determinant of contacting behaviour was supported.

Nevertheless, there were also significant demographic variations (Table 7.1). Women were considerably more likely than men to contact their family doctor with a mental health problem, even after severity of illness was controlled. The presence of a physical illness also had an impact in increasing the likelihood of contact. People who suffered from a physical illness were more than twice as likely to contact their GP with a mental health problem. Other variables that contributed significantly to the model of best fit included age, marital status and employment status. There was a significant, but small, contribution from ethnic group. It is, however, notable that social class was not required in the model. The tendency of women to be allocated to lower social economic groups accounted wholly for the relationship between socio-economic status and contact with a GP for mental health problems.

The peak of contacting occurred in people aged 45–54 years, and the likelihood of contact increased gradually from the youngest age group up to this point. Single people were less likely to contact their GP for mental problems than their married counterparts, although the difference was small. However, contacting was appreciably increased in the divorced, widowed and separated. The South Asian group were particularly unlikely to consult their family doctor for a psychiatric problem, and this applied even after allowing for their comparatively reduced level of symptoms. Finally, those in full-time employment were noticeably different from all other employment groups in their reluctance to consult their GPs for a mental problem, understandable in terms of the practical difficulty of fitting in such a visit.

Other studies have presented similarly worrying results. Shapiro and his colleagues (1984) reported on utilisation data from three centres of the epidemiological catchment area surveys. In the six months before interview, between 6% and 7% of adults in the three centres had made visits to health care providers for reasons of mental health, while 3% had visited mental health specialists. Fifteen to twenty per cent of those with a recent DSM–III disorder (American Psychiatric Association (APA), 1980) had made mental health visits, with around 10% visiting specialists. Of subjects with no history of a DSM–III disorder, 3% had still made visits for mental health reasons, 1% to specialists. This compares with the National Survey finding that 16% of the total sample received a current diagnosis of a neurotic disorder, while 12% of the sample made mental health related visits in the previous year. However, less than half the people with current disorder had made such visits. Only 5% of people with a neurotic disorder saw clinicians working in secondary services. Thus, the comparison between the US and British studies suggests that the central position of primary care in Britain does allow easier medical contact for neurotic disorders.

In another US study, Pollard and colleagues (1989) reported that, of people in the general population suffering from DSM–III agoraphobia, obsessive–compulsive disorder or social phobia, only 40%, 28% and 8% respectively sought the help of a clinician. Finally, a recent British survey conducted by telephone found that only 12.5% of people with depressive disorder had sought help from their GP, although this low rate might be partly owing to over-recognition of the disorder (Ohayon *et al*, 1999).

Despite variations in service structure and provision, these studies consistently indicate that most people with neurotic disorders do not make contact with professional clinicians who might offer

TABLE 7.1

Determinants of contacting primary care physicians for mental health problems and of different sorts of treatment for neurotic disorders (derived from Bebbington et al, 2000a,b)

Symptom	Symptom function-severity	Impaired Physical functioning	Physical illness	Age	Social Gender	Social class	Marital status	Employment Ethnicity	Employment status
Contacting	+	+	+	+	+	0	+	+	+
Antidepresants	+	0	+	+	0	0	+	0	+
Hypnotics/anxiolytics	+	0	+	+	0	0	+	0	0
Counselling/psychotherapy	+	+	0	+	0	0	0	0	+

treatment. The available treatments would be effective for many of the people with neurotic disorders identified in our study. Even on a conservative estimation of actual needs, this represents a considerable amount of unnecessary suffering and disability.

The first concern of Bebbington *et al* (2000*a*) in making these analyses has therefore been confirmed. What of the second, that the data on contacting might reveal inequalities of access? Access certainly appears to vary within the different groupings studied, but this is not always easy to attribute to inequality. If there were significant inequality, one might expect it to be reflected in a social class gradient, but no such gradient was found. The greater access of post-marital groups to primary care physicians for mental health problems may actually indicate need increased by social isolation, and may therefore be appropriate. Likewise, people with dual physical and mental problems may need more help, and their increased contact with primary care might again be appropriate. Young people and those in work do seem relatively to neglect themselves or to be neglected, as do men in general, and this requires consideration by those responsible for delivering services and treatment. There is also an appreciable concern that people of South Asian origin may be suffering unnecessarily. There is confusion about whether people from the Indian subcontinent living in Britain are more or less likely to contact their GPs for psychiatric problems than expected (Gilliam *et al*, 1989; Lloyd, 1992; Jacobs *et al*, 1998). The work of Bebbington and his colleagues (2000*a*) has shown that on a national scale they contact less and that this is independent of symptom level.

Obtaining treatment for psychiatric disorders

The receipt of treatment is the second stage of the process of service utilisation. In Britain, most treatment is provided by primary care physicians. Again, information about this can be gleaned from the National Survey. All subjects classed as having an ICD–10 diagnosis were asked about the medication and other forms of treatment they were receiving. Two broad categories of psychotropic medication were distinguished: antidepressants, and hypnotics and anxiolytics. There were two other forms of treatment: therapy and counselling. Although the interviewers sought to distinguish these treatments more precisely, most responses were not very detailed. For this reason, the two categories therapy and counselling were amalgamated in the published results.

The authors found that relatively few of any of these groups of patients were receiving psychiatric treatment (Bebbington *et al*, 2000*b*). In the case of depressive episode, less than a third were receiving any form of treatment, and around a quarter were receiving medication. These figures were less for the other diagnostic categories (Table 7.2). Thus, of those with the relatively mild conditions, mixed anxiety and depressive disorder and generalised anxiety disorder, only 11% and 10% respectively were getting treatment. For people with depressive episodes, antidepressants were prescribed more often than anxiolytics. This is not so for the other diagnoses, in which there was little evidence of specificity of treatment: the ratio between the prescription of antidepressants and anxiolytics varied little by diagnostic class.

The question may be asked to what extent the likelihood of treatment is increased if people actually report seeking help from a clinician. The National Survey results suggest that the effect was to double the rates for the various treatments compared with the groups of people with neurotic disorders as a whole. Nearly half the people suffering from depressive episode were in receipt of some kind of treatment, a value approached by those with phobias. A third of the people who had been to see their GP with a depressive episode were being treated with an antidepressant – which of course still means that two-thirds were not. Thus, contacting a primary care physician does increase the likelihood of an effective treatment, but only to levels that remain worrying.

Once more, Bebbington and his colleagues (2000*b*) analysed the effect of severity, in terms of symptoms and of social impairment. Both had an impact on the likelihood of receiving treatment. Even so, only 30% of people scoring a high 25+ on the CIS–R were in receipt of any form of psychiatric treatment. Thus, over two-thirds of people in this severe category received no treatment at all. The number of psychiatric symptoms strongly influenced receipt of all three treatments. Thus, the most severe category was nearly five times as likely as the least severe to receive antidepressants. Once symptom severity was accounted for, impaired social functioning was only associated with an increased receipt of psychological therapies.

These results make two points strongly. First, even among extremely symptomatic people in the general population, psychiatric treatment is given only to a small minority. Second, severity, however measured, is a major determinant of the likelihood that treatment is given.

There were other clinical and demographic variables that affected the receipt of treatment. The existence of physical illness made an independent contribution to whether people with neurotic disorder received psychotropic drug treatment, but had no effect on referral for counselling. Marital status also had an effect on pharmacological treatments. In parallel with primary care contact, the least likely to be treated with drugs were again the single, the most likely the divorced,

TABLE 7.2

Treatment given to subjects identified as having psychiatric disorders in the British National Surveys of Psychiatric Morbidity (from Meltzer et al (1995))

	Mixed anxiety and depressive disorder (%)	Generalised anxiety disorder (%)	Depressive episode (%)	Phobia (%)	Obsessive– compulsive disorder (%)	Panic (%)
Any medication	6	12	21	21	16	13
Antidepressants	3	8	16	15	12	11
Anxiolytics and hypnotics	2	7	10	11	9	3
Any counselling or therapy	4	7	11	14	9	6
Any treatment	9	16	25	28	19	15

widowed and separated. Marital status had no effect on who received counselling. Age had a consistent effect. However, the salient age for receiving antidepressants and counselling was 45–54 years, while the pattern for anxiolytics and hypnotics was for a continuing increase with age. The latter was largely owing to the more general use of hypnotics in older populations. Nevertheless, there appeared to be a general trend for younger people to have relatively little access to treatment, and this paralleled their reduced likelihood of making clinical contact for a mental health problem in the first place (Bebbington *et al*, 2000*a*).

Employment made antidepressant and psychological treatment less likely. The economically inactive were over twice as likely to be receiving these drugs. It was notable that neither gender nor social class had any effect on the receipt of any of these treatments (see Table 7.1).

The authors of these papers combined information about diagnosis, severity of disorder and contact with services to draw conclusions about needs for treatment and the extent to which they are unmet. Despite the pitfalls in this process, they found that only a small proportion of people diagnosed as having a neurotic disorder in Britain actually consulted their family doctor for treatment. The direct assessment of treatment in the National Survey was reasonably detailed, and the data suggest very strongly that only a small fraction of people diagnosed as having a neurotic disorder in Britain receive anything that could be described as treatment. The available treatments would be effective for many of the people with neurotic disorders identified in this study. Consultation with a primary care physician roughly doubled the chance of receiving all types of psychiatric treatment, but still left over two-thirds of people with depressive episode without the benefit of an antidepressant. Similar results have recently been reported by Ohayon *et al* (1998) in a British telephone survey.

It is possible that in some cases more detailed psychiatric evaluation of some individuals in the National Survey sample might lead to a conclusion that no treatment was required. This might lie behind the very large proportion of people with mixed anxiety and depressive states who were not in receipt of treatment. However, the findings were so dramatic that one must conclude that they represent a large reservoir of untreated psychiatric disorders.

The purpose of the study of Bebbington *et al* (2000*b*) was also to identify influences on the receipt of treatment. In no case did gender, social class or ethnicity have an effect on who received treatment, once other clinical and demographic variables had been taken into account. These results are surprising in themselves. It is clear that the major determinant of who received treatment was symptomatic severity, although this had somewhat less effect on the receipt of counselling. Social impairment, which is another measure of clinical severity, had no effect additional to symptom severity, except in the case of counselling; people with some social impairment were more likely to be referred for counselling. Marital status affected antidepressant and anxiolytic prescribing, with single people having much less access to these treatments. This probably does represent some inequality of provision, as there is no reason why the single should have less need after controlling for severity of disorder. The reduced access to treatment with antidepressants and to counselling by those who are in employment may actually reflect reduced need, even after controlling for disorder severity, but it may also indicate that the demands of work prevent attention to health needs. Overall, the powerful impact of severity, with relatively little contribution from key measures of social disadvantage (gender, ethnicity and social class) does suggest that, even in the context of low treatment uptake, the principles of equity and proportionality apply reasonably well.

Assessment of needs for treatment from other community surveys

Very few other studies have attempted to evaluate needs for psychiatric care, and indeed only three are worth describing in the context of this chapter.

Epidemiologic Catchment Area Survey

Shapiro and his colleagues (1985) made an attempt to use the data from the Baltimore site of the Epidemiologic Catchment Area Survey to assess actual needs for treatment. They defined need as mental health service use in the last six months or two of three indicators of poor mental health. These indicators were a diagnosis of a DSM–III disorder in the last six months, a score of 4 or more on a 20-item version of the General Health Questionnaire (GHQ; Goldberg, 1972), and the respondent's report that they had been unable to carry out normal activities for at least one whole day in the last three months. Around 14% of the population were defined as having a need for treatment on this basis. Of these, nearly half had made no recent visits for mental health problems and were thus regarded as having an unmet need. These results are of interest, but the study clearly confuses the definition of need with the definition of unmet need; put another way, it carries the assumption that visits to health professionals for mental health reasons indicate a need for treatment, and a failure to make such a visit implies an unmet need. At least their index of need does include some attempt to measure social functioning.

Mini Finland Health Survey

Lehtinen and his colleagues (1990) evaluated the need for treatment in the Mini Finland Health Survey. Need for specialist treatment was judged to be present if the case was *definite* according to the PSE9–ID–CATEGO system (i.e. ID level 6 and above; Wing *et al*, 1978), *or* if the interviewer thought that treatment was needed. Interviewers also made judgements about the need for treatment by primary care physicians in cases of less severity. The subject's own judgements about whether they needed treatment were also recorded.

The results of this study are again interesting. The need for treatment assessed by the interviewers was less than the prevalence of disorders, and that assessed by the subjects themselves was lower still. The interviewers estimated that around 9% of subjects were in need of specialist treatment, whereas only 1% thought so themselves; a further 6%, however, felt that they were 'probably' in need of treatment. Taking all forms of treatment, around 4% of subjects were receiving adequate treatment, and 14% showed an unmet need. This study is a useful attempt at a more direct measure of need. Its drawback is that it still confuses need with mere prevalence: it assumes that an ID level of 6 or over is an absolute indication of a need for treatment. Moreover, the structuring of the assessment of need is not described. Finally, no attempt is made to say exactly what treatment is needed, or by whom it might be provided.

Camberwell Needs for Care Survey

Only one direct investigation of needs for specific psychiatric treatment and the extent to which they have been met has been published (Bebbington *et al*, 1997, 1999). This was carried out in an area of inner-south London with high levels of deprivation. A wide range of clinical information was used to rate the community version of the Needs for Care Assessment (MRC NFCAS–C).

The sample was randomly selected from the electoral roll. There was a two-stage design. At stage two, people were assessed using Schedules for Clinical Assessment in Neuropsychiatry (SCAN; WHO, 1992*B*), the MRC Social Role Performance Schedule (Hurry & Sturt, 1981), the Life Events and Difficulties Schedule (Brown & Harris, 1978), and a treatment inventory specially developed for the study.

Over 700 people were assessed at stage one, and over 400 interviewed at stage two.

The information obtained from the various assessment instruments was then used as a basis for rating needs for care with the NFCAS–C. This instrument has seven clinical domains: psychosis, depression, anxiety, alcohol misuse, drug misuse, eating disorders and adjustment disorders. The actual items of treatment provided are compared with an explicit model of care based on current clinical consensus and the literature on treatment effectiveness. Each item of care is rated according to whether it is provided and whether it is appropriate and effective in the context of a given level of disability. The ratings allow the establishment of a primary need status falling in the potential categories: met need, unmet need, no need and no meetable need. There is also a facility for rating over-provision. There is an elaborate rating for each individual actual or potential item of care for a given clinical domain. It should be noted that the convention of the assessment is to record 'no need' where there is no effective treatment available, even if there is a clear disability. In other words, needs are only recorded when there is a practical treatment. The ratings were made by a psychologist and psychiatrist following presentations of case vignettes describing disabilities, symptoms and treatments.

While the prevalence of meetable need for treatment in this survey was very similar to the prevalence of all ICD–10 disorders, the people with needs for treatment did not wholly overlap with diagnosed cases. Unmet needs outnumbered met needs, and unmeetable needs comprised an appreciable minority of all needs.

There is obviously considerable clinical interest in looking in more detail at the items of care that were assessed (Bebbington *et al*, 1999). Thus, for example, 30 subjects in total were assessed in the depression section. In 21 of these, the provision of antidepressant medication was evaluated, in relation to 26 care periods. In only six instances (23%) was effective medication provided, while in a further case it was provided but not regarded as being fully effective. Many subjects did not like to medicalise their low mood, and this is reflected in 12 instances (46%) where the whole idea of medical treatment was rejected. There were, however, six cases (23%) where medication would have been acceptable but had not been prescribed. Of these, two had seen their GP for 'nerves'. Most subjects would have welcomed some professional support, but this had rarely been provided. Interestingly, in two cases where psychotherapy was thought appropriate, it was rejected by the subject. In three others, there was felt to be an unmet need for psychotherapy, cases in which the depressive condition emerged from a long-standing depressive personality and a history of early adversity of various sorts.

In the view of the assessment team, 12 subjects (40% of the total individuals assessed for depression) would have benefited from cognitive therapy because of persistent problems with self-esteem and recurrent depressed mood. In most cases, this was rated as an unmet need. No subject was actually receiving this form of treatment for depression, and the need was rated as unmet in over 80%. Two subjects rejected the whole idea of treatment and would not consider cognitive therapy.

Again, many care episodes of anxiety (54% of 24) were characterised by an unmet need for treatment. The authors were reluctant to consider medication for such conditions, unless they were likely to be short-lasting and pharmacotherapy would serve a useful function in the short term. An unmet need for medication was identified in two subjects, and in four others medication that had been prescribed was seen as appropriate and fully or partly effective. There was an interesting contrast to subjects with depression: those with anxiety were unlikely to reject the idea of treatment (only two of the 17 did so). Unmet needs for cognitive therapy were identified in eight individuals, and three subjects (25% of the 12 in which it was regarded as appropriate) were actually receiving treatment of this type.

The two surveys used in this chapter to illustrate needs for psychiatric treatment complement each other. In the smaller, more intensive study, needs were assessed directly using a specially developed standardised technique. This revealed that many needs for treatment were not being met in the community, and that this applied to the two commonest groups of disorder, depression and anxiety. In the large British National Survey, needs were not measured directly. However, it is reasonable to assume that an appreciable proportion, particularly of the more severe disorders like depressive episode, would have been adjudged in need of treatment. This can then be set against the utilisation of services and the provision of treatment, and the findings relating to this are so striking that one is left with the inevitable inference that only a minority are getting the treatment they need.

Thus, in the Needs for Care Survey, the proportion of meetable needs for the treatment of depression that were actually met was less than a quarter, and for anxiety it was not much more than 10%. This tallies quite well with the National Survey, in which 75% of cases of depressive episode were completely untreated, and even more for other neurotic diagnoses.

It is of particular interest that antidepressant medication was given infrequently, and that this often came about because the subjects themselves were very wary of it. They were less wary of psychological treatments, but these were rarely available. There is evidence from elsewhere that people with anxiety disorders are often not treated, and when they are, they do not get the right treatment (Hunt, 1997), despite the cost-effectiveness of cognitive–behavioural therapy. The problem of anti-treatment attitudes has also been identified by others. Lin & Parich (1997) showed that much under-treated depression comes about because of the anti-treatment attitudes of those who suffer from it. A national survey in Australia confirms that members of the general public have a low opinion of the effectiveness and appropriateness of antidepressants as a treatment for depression (Jorm *et al*, 1997), and similar findings were obtained in Germany (Wittchen, 1997).

Finally, the effect of severity, as reflected in comorbidity, in increasing the likelihood that treatment is provided has also been noted in the Munich Prospective Community Survey. The number of comorbid anxiety disorders predicted utilisation.

The issue of severity illuminates the moral dilemma posed by these results. More severe cases are more likely to receive treatment, and in a cash-limited service one might be inclined to approve this trend, feeling that the service has at least some claims to be a just one. However, some severe disorders are nevertheless untreated, and the general under-treatment of milder conditions is neither humane nor just.

How could we rectify the state of affairs described in this chapter, and if we could, how might we pay for it? In fact, the costs of increased recognition and treatment might not be too great, as the primary care services for mental ill health represent a small proportion of the overall costs of mental health care in the UK (NHS Executive, 1996). Thus, an increase in provision might not greatly extend primary care budgets. Moreover, there are potential savings to be made. First, it may be cost-effective to treat disorders of all severities, partly because treatment might pre-empt deterioration, and partly because even these disorders impose a burden of disability and cost. Second, those with psychiatric symptoms make considerable demands on primary care physicians for reasons ostensibly other than their mental problems. In the British National Household Survey described here, people identified as having a neurotic disorder were 40% more likely to have contacted their GP for a physical complaint than respondents with no such disorder (Meltzer *et al*, 1995). Thus, more effective targeting of GPs' time might reduce the frequency of ineffective contacts.

The inappropriately low levels of primary care consultation identified in this chapter almost certainly indicate an education gap, and this is likely to be shared by primary care physicians and the general public. The best way to augment the education of GPs about mental health has been the subject of study for years, and yet deficiencies almost certainly remain. There is thus a major problem of designing services that are capable of delivering treatments known from specific studies to be effective, and this problem includes the financing of the service in a way that is free from perverse incentives. A major benefit of focusing on needs for treatment is that it initiates debate on how these problems might be overcome. Considerable effort has also been invested in the mental health education of the public, for example, in the UK, the Royal College of Psychiatrists' 'Defeat Depression' campaign. These efforts clearly need to be unrelenting. Without these educational improvements, the question of meeting the costs of increased levels of care may be irrelevant.

References

AMERICAN PSYCHIATRIC ASSOCIATION (1980) *Diagnostic and Statistical Manual of Mental Disorders. Third revision (DSM–III)*. Washington, DC: APA.

BEBBINGTON, P. E., MARSDEN, L. & BREWIN, C. R. (1997) The need for psychiatric treatment in the general population: the Camberwell Needs for Care Survey. *Psychological Medicine*, **27**, 821–834.

—, — & — (1999) The treatment of psychiatric disorder in the community: Report from the Camberwell Needs for Care Survey. *Journal of Mental Health*, **8**, 7–17.

—, BRUGHA, T., JENKINS, R., *ET AL* (2000*a*) Unequal access and unmet need: Neurotic disorders and the use of primary care services. *Psychological Medicine*, **30**, 1359–1367.

—, —, —, *ET AL* (2000*b*) Neurotic disorders and the receipt of psychiatric treatment. *Psychological Medicine*, **30**, 1369–1376.

—, —, —, *ET AL* (2000*c*) Psychiatric disorder and dysfunction in the National Survey of Psychiatric Morbidity. *Social Psychiatry and Psychiatric Epidemiology*, **35**, 191–197.

BREWIN, C., WING, J. K., MANGEN, S. P., *ET AL* (1987) Principles and practice of measuring need in the long-term mentally ill: The MRC Needs for Care Assessment. *Psychological Medicine*, **17**, 971–982.

BROWN, G. W. & HARRIS, T. (1978) *Social Origins of Depression: A Study of Psychiatric Disorders in Women*. London: Tavistock.

GILLIAM, S. J., JARMAN, B., WHITE, P., *ET AL* (1989) Ethnic differences in consultation rates in urban general practice. *British Medical Journal*, **299**, 953–957.

GOLDBERG, D. P. (1972) *The Detection of Psychiatric Illness by Questionnaire (GHQ)*. Maudsley Monograph 21. London. Oxford University Press.

HUNT, C. (1997) *The Unmet Need for Treatment in the Anxiety Disorders*. Paper presented at WPA Section of Epidemiology and Community Psychiatry Symposium: The Unmet Need for Treatment. Sydney 19–22 October.

HURRY, J. & STURT, E. (1981) Social performance in a population sample: relation to psychiatric symptoms.. In: *What is a Case? The Problem of Definition in Psychiatric Community Surveys* (eds J. K. Wing, P. E. Bebbington & L. N. Robins), pp. 202–213. London: Grant MacIntyre.

JACOBS, K. S., BHUGRA, D., LLOYD, K. R., *ET AL* (1998) Common mental disorders, explanatory models and consultation behaviour among Indian women living in the UK. *Journal of the Royal Society of Medicine*, **91**, 66–71.

JARMAN, B. (1983) Identification of underprivileged areas. *British Medical Journal*, **256**, 1587–1592.

JENKINS, R., BEBBINGTON, P. E., BRUGHA, T., *ET AL* (1997*a*) The National Psychiatric Morbidity Surveys of Great Britain – strategy and methods. *Psychological Medicine*, **27**, 765–774.

——, LEWIS, G., BEBBINGTON, P. E., *ET AL* (1997*b*) The National Psychiatric Morbidity Surveys of Great Britain – initial findings from the Household Survey. *Psychological Medicine*, **27**, 775–790.

JORM, A. F., KORTEN, A. E., JACOMB, P. A., *ET AL* (1997) *The Australian National Survey of Mental Health Literacy*. Paper presented at WPA Section of Epidemiology and Community Psychiatry Symposium: The Unmet Need for Treatment. Sydney 19–22 October.

LEHTINEN, V., JOUKAMAA, M., JYRKINEN, E., *ET AL* (1990) Need for mental health services of the adult population in Finland: results from the Mini Finland Health Survey. *Acta Psychiatrica Scandinavica*, **81**, 426–431.

LEWIS, G., PELOSI, A. J., ARAYA, R. C., *ET AL* (1992) Measuring psychiatric disorder in the community: a standardized assessment for use by lay-interviewers. *Psychological Medicine*, **22**, 465–486.

LIN, E. & PARICH, S. (1997) *Sociodemographic, Clinical and Attitudinal Characteristics of the Untreated Depressed in Ontario*. Paper presented at WPA Section of Epidemiology and Community Psychiatry Symposium: The Unmet Need for Treatment. Sydney 19–22 October.

LLOYD, K. (1992) Ethnicity, primary care and non-psychotic disorders. *International Review of Psychiatry*, **4**, 257–265.

MELTZER, H., GILL, B., PETTICREW, M., *ET AL* (1995) *The Prevalence of Psychiatric Morbidity Among Adults Living in Private Households*. OPCS Survey of Psychiatric Morbidity in Great Britain. *Report 1*. London: HMSO.

NHS EXECUTIVE (1996) *Burdens of Disease*. Leeds: NHSE.

OHAYON, M., CAULET, M., PRIEST, R. G., *ET AL* (1998) Psychotropic medication consumption patterns in the UK general population. *Journal of Clinical Epidemiology*, **51**, 273–283.

——, PRIEST, R., GUILLEMINAULT, C., *ET AL* (1999) The prevalance of depressive disorders in the United Kingdom. *Biological Psychiatry*, **45**, 300–307.

POLLARD, C., HENDERSON JR, J., FRANK, M., *ET AL* (1989) Help-seeking patterns of anxiety-disordered individuals in the general population. *Journal of Anxiety Disorders*, **3**, 131–138.

SHAPIRO, S., SKINNER, E. A., KESSLER, L. G., *ET AL* (1984) Utilization of health and mental health services: Three epidemiologic catchment area sites. *Archives of General Psychiatry*, **41**, 971–978.

——, ——, KRAMER, M., *ET AL* (1985) Measuring need for mental health services in a general population. *Medical Care*, **23**, 1033–1043.

SLADE, M., THORNICROFT, G., PHELAN, M., ET AL (1999) *Camberwell Assessment of Need (CAN)*. London: Gaskell.

TOWNSEND, P., SIMPSON, D. & TIBBS, N. (1985) Inequalities in health in the city of Bristol: a preliminary review of statistical evidence. *International Journal of Health Services*, **15**, 637–663.

WING, J. K., MANN, S. A., LEFF, J. P., *ET AL* (1978) The concept of a case in psychiatric population surveys. *Psychological Medicine*, **8**, 203–219.

WITTCHEN, H. U. (1997) *The Unmet Need for Treatment in Anxiety Disorders: From Early Stage Interventions to the Chronic Patient*. Paper presented at WPA Section of Epidemiology and Community Psychiatry Symposium: The Unmet Need for Treatment. Sydney 19–22 October.

WORLD HEALTH ORGANIZATION (1992*a*) *International Classification of Diseases and Related Health Problems. Tenth revision (ICD–10)*. Geneva: WHO.

—— (1992*b*) *SCAN Schedules for Clinical Assessment in Neuropsychiatry*, Geneva: WHO.

8 Setting priorities during the development of local psychiatric services

ELAINE MURPHY

What is service planning and how is it done?

The content of health policy will always reflect the values of those who create it. The process of setting priorities in health care planning brings sharply into focus the conflicts between organisational and professional groups, whose aspirations are founded on differing philosophical values. Over the past 30 years, mental health care services have been especially vulnerable to planning 'blight' as a result of a failure to reconcile differences between the professions, statutory agencies, voluntary organisations, the general public and those who use the services. The planning process is hindered further by the fact that there is no easy way of discerning, still less proving, that there is a clear causal link between levels of health care expenditure and states of mental health. Professionals working in mental health have been poor advocates for the development of their services, because they have been unable to articulate a coherent vision of the specific outcomes they were aiming to achieve for individuals, beyond the traditional goals of improvements in symptoms and behaviour and social independence. Priorities arise out of specific service objectives that have their roots in a clear vision of the service's aims. This chapter describes the process by which the agency or agencies responsible for planning local services can decide on their own local priorities.

In 1990, the district health authority (DHA) became the lead agency responsible for planning and commissioning specialist hospital and community health services for local people with severe mental illness. The elected local authority was responsible for planning social

144

rehabilitation and care services for the same group. Joint planning and commissioning of mental health services was encouraged through the duty of the health and local authorities to publish annually an agreed Community Care Plan. In some areas, largely through the commitment of determined individuals in both agencies, a truly joint plan for mental health services was achieved. In many areas, however, the Community Care Plan had the appearance of two separately written documents loosely woven together for the annual publication deadline. As more authorities perceived the wisdom of having a real joint plan, frustration with the existing ad hoc and voluntary joint planning mechanisms grew. The new Labour government of 1997 introduced a number of Green and White Papers (Department of Health, 1998*a,b,c*, 1999*a,b*), enshrining the Duty of Partnership between the statutory agencies responsible for health care planning, and introduced mechanisms to ensure that financial and management systems could support effective joint planning. This should make a significant difference to the overall shape of service plans.

Doctors, and others educated in a rational, scientific tradition, sometimes have difficulty with the concept of health policy planning as a process of decision-making that accommodates multiple conflicting interests. Planning has two parts to it: first, a rational, scientific judgement is made about what service is required, based on hard information gleaned from local demographic data, epidemiological studies, case registers and current usage of services; but the second, more difficult, part of planning is concerned with making a political judgement about what is realistically achievable locally, given the existing dominant influences, the funds available and the time to achieve the objectives. Setting priorities is a fundamental part of the planning process in which explicit choices are made; it involves a political and social process for reconciling goals and objectives.

Health services have generally adopted an 'incrementalist' approach to planning. The first assumption underlying this approach is that what now exists must remain and that as extra growth money becomes available there will be marginal improvements by the addition of an extra consultant here, a couple of community nurses there, a new day centre perhaps, and so on. These marginal improvements are usually determined by local influential people within the service system, such as a group of consultant psychiatrists. Each year, a set of disjointed decisions muddles up through the planning hierarchy to senior managers, who choose from the assorted menu of excessive bids presented to them. In lean times, when public expenditure drops or the service falls out of favour locally, an equally ad hoc converse process of expenditure cuts are proposed that will have the least impact on the most influential people in the service. Under these circumstances, reduced funding nibbles around the edge of the service, creating internal staff resentment, but rarely influencing the overall pattern of care. This was the commonest style of planning before the National Health Service (NHS) reforms of 1990 separated the responsibility for planning from the responsibility of providing a service.

A contrasting style of planning is the 'rationalist' approach. Those who are impatient with the incrementalist shuffling of existing services may aim instead at comprehensive, rational problem-solving, and try to tackle the important issues in one fell swoop, in a short series of strategic planning meetings, assuming capacities of analysis and powers of implementation that do not exist within public health and social care organisations. Some ambitious health authorities, keen to flex their new purchasing muscles, tried to impose such 'rational' planning processes in the early years of the purchaser/provider split, meeting predictable antagonism and resistance from the service providers.

In the health service, 'incrementalism' has consistently won out over 'rationalism' because of low expectations of real change, the influence of senior professionals in the health service, who have very good reasons for resisting major change, and the continual disappointments afforded to 'rationalists' by the ever-changing economic and organisational climate in which planning is carried out. There are, however, feasible ways of achieving significant changes within public sector services, if priorities can be agreed on and a cultural change effected across the service to support the chosen priorities.

One of the most effective ways to achieve the necessary cultural and attitudinal changes is to use the planning process itself as a vehicle for change (Nichol, 1986). Plans are merely statements of preferred options at a given point in time and must change in response to the changing environment. It is possible to keep options fairly flexible in order to accommodate change and to adopt a pragmatic approach to changing specific plans as new circumstances arise, as long as the overall service priorities remain steady and are universally acknowledged and 'owned' by those who will implement them.

The final practical task of planning is to appraise a range of no more than three or four carefully costed options for local action against a set of criteria that are believed to best describe the priority objectives. The manner in which the technical task is achieved, through widespread participation, consultation and education of the local community, is at least as important as interpreting correctly local information.

In this chapter, the task of priority setting has been divided into the following key areas:

- understanding the current focus of the service;
- establishing principles and goals, developing a vision;
- interpretation of local information;
- participation and consultation, joint planning, locality planning';
- the impact of the NHS and Community Care Act 1990 and subsequent legislation; and
- maintaining flexibility and responsiveness.

Understanding the current focus of the service

An important barrier to change is the tendency of service providers to believe their own rhetoric about the characteristics of their own service. Almost all districts now claim to provide a 'community-oriented psychiatric service', but the pattern of allocation of financial resources tells a different story. The first step in accepting that change must occur is accepting the reality of the present focus of the service.

All services have an existing philosophy of care, usually unstated but implicit in the way services are delivered. Over the past 30 years, since the policy of community care was officially adopted, two linked themes were emphasised in government policy documents. The dominant theme was a plan for short-term treatment of mental illness in district general hospital units, out-patient clinics, day hospitals and community mental health centres. The second theme, played *sotto voce* and much less forcefully presented, was the plan for local government to provide a network of hostel and home accommodation, social work support, day care, and sheltered work for chronically disabled people, to provide a real alternative to the back wards of the mental hospital. The first theme grew into a major symphonic work, the second theme was scarcely audible until the 1980s.

District health authorities have shifted very large amounts of money originally invested in care for people with long-term severe disabilities living in large old mental hospitals into the development of acute psychiatric services for the local community, which focused mainly on those patients with short-term, treatable conditions. To assess the balance in a target district, the focus of the health service component of mental health services can be measured along two dimensions. The first dimension is the distribution of services between acute short-term patients and those in need of long-term care.

The second dimension is the proportion of services devoted to providing specific health care services for diagnosis, treatment and rehabilitation and the proportion of the service devoted to 'social care', that is, meeting patients' basic human needs for adequate financial resources, a home, work, friendships and ensuring that all the daily activities of normal life are satisfactorily achieved. This latter distinction is extremely important, since a large part of community service development in the past 30 years has been concerned solely with promoting health care through the appointment of community psychiatric nurses (CPNs), psychologists, occupational therapists and other therapists, and there has been much less investment in comprehensive social care. The majority of patients with serious mental illness will require help with one or more of the following aspects of daily life: income entitlement, accommodation and daily occupation. Neither health nor social services have invested much in welfare rights workers, home-finders, work development schemes, staff to develop befriending and leisure schemes, and personal and domestic care staff.

The analysis of the division of services between acute, short-term patients and long-term chronic patients is not quite so straightforward as the paragraph above might suggest. There are many patients with long-term problems who suffer intermittent episodes of acute psychiatric illness that may recur as frequently as every few weeks, or may return after a gap of several months or years. The phrase 'revolving door' refers to those patients who at one time would have remained continuously in hospital for many years, but who are now readmitted frequently to acute psychiatric units and are rapidly discharged again, once the acute phase of the illness is settled. Planning must therefore take account of the acute health care needs of long-term patients in addition to their social care needs.

Resources in mental health

In 1996/1997, approximately £2800 million was spent by the NHS directly on mental health services, some 12.4% of total health service expenditure (Patel & Knapp, 1998; Mental Health Foundation, 1999). In addition to this, social services departments spent £421 million on residential, day care and personal social services, to which a further £73 million (1998) was added in the form of a Mental Illness Specific Grant (Chartered Institute of Public Finance Accounts (CIPFA, 1997; Mental Health Foundation, 1999). A further £760 million is spent by the Department of Social Security on income support and, finally, a considerable but difficult to estimate amount of money is expended by the courts, prisons and the police (Office for National Statistics (ONS), 1995). A further £500–600 million was spent supporting elderly people with dementia in private residential care homes and nursing homes. Approximately £5000 million in total from the public purse is spent on disabling mental disorder.

Most of the spending on adult mental health services is through the health service (NHS Executive, 1998), although significantly less than prior to the mid-1970s, when a new government initiative made high levels of welfare benefit from Social Security funds available for board and lodgings payments, enabling the transfer of patients from state institutions into private residential care and substantially altering the balance of provision of long-term care. In the 1960s and 70s, it was assumed that as long-stay hospital beds closed, money would transfer from the health service to local authorities in order to provide alternative facilities. But all bureaucracies have a tendency to hang on to their own funds, and the NHS successfully retained mental health funds to cover the rapidly growing costs of in-patient beds and new acute services.

Health managers and professionals have potent reasons for wishing to retain funds within services directly under their own control. The larger the unit budget, the greater the pay and status of its managers, but also the more flexibility that can be created within the budget: an expanding budget in general acute psychiatry attracts personnel to extend professional departments; large professional departments attract trainees and postgraduate students; professional esteem is enhanced; and the influence of the professional group grows within the local health service. It is not surprising then to find that during a period when thousands of long-stay beds closed, mental health's share of the NHS cake has remained steady and the proportion of funds for mental health spent on in-patient beds and professional services has remained much the same, with very little movement of resources into local authority and other community services.

However, over this period, the cost of an in-patient bed for a mentally ill person doubled. There are two main reasons for the rise in proportion of costs attributable to the 'acute' arm of mental health services. In part, it was owing to increased staffing levels on acute psychiatric wards and improvements in community psychiatric nursing and other professional services. Another reason was the direct shift of resources out of long-stay care beds into new acute units in district general hsopitals, the growth of community health centres and community assessment teams. The realisation that this shift in resources had occurred led to a reappraisal of strategic plans in some districts, but in many others the shift was neither recognised nor tackled. As long-stay patients died or left hospital, there were only marginal savings on the overall costs of running a hospital and as a consequence the unit costs of each long-stay patient rose. The overall cost of in-patient beds increased, both because of the rising cost of long-stay beds and the cost of new in-patient services.

The result of this gradual shift in use of health service resources is that most health districts in Britain in the 1990s spent approximately half of their total mental health service budget on those parts of the service that can broadly be designated as 'health care' rather than 'social care'. Half the budget now funds doctors, psychologists, occupational therapists, other therapists, nurses on acute psychiatric wards and catchment area CPNs, whereas in pre-hospital-closure days, prior to the 1960s, approximately 20% of funds were spent on direct health care, the rest on social care. The vital social care elements of the service have not therefore been able to grow at the required pace, through lack of investment.

Stein & Test (1980) argued that 85% of resources for mental health services should be allocated to community-based services rather than hospital in-patient services, and perhaps this is broadly correct. Most services still allocate over half the total NHS expenditure on mental health to in-patient beds (nationally £1.7 billion out of the total £2.8 billion) (Health Select Committee Minutes & RO3 Return, 1998). The proportionate allocation required for future plans will depend on the relative values afforded to health care beds and community health services on the one hand and to social care services on the other. What is needed is an explicit consideration of the balance of care, how the balance has come about and what degree of shift, if any, is desirable. A further crucial decision is the proportion of the allocation of community-based resources to health and social care respectively.

The failure of a significant proportion of health districts and social services authorities to make any meaningful improvement in the provision of social care, particularly in the housing needs of people requiring 24-hour supported care, eventually persuaded successive governments from the early 1990s that central money must be 'ring-fenced', that is, allocated specifically for certain projects only in response to collaborative bids from the statutory authorities. The first targeted initiative, which began in 1995, the Mental Illness Specific Grant, was health service finance allocated for social care projects only, available only for projects designed for people with serious mental disorder. Schemes had to be jointly agreed and tailored to suit local circumstances. The responsibility to plan services remains a local task.

Establishing principles and goals, developing a vision

Developments will tend to be unplanned and haphazard if there is no target to aim for, so this section is placed before the section on participation and consultation, but the two processes must be closely linked. There is no point in a local mental health service developing its own vision in isolation from other key 'stakeholders' in the service. Following the NHS and Community Care Act (House of Commons, 1990), the responsibility for developing a vision of the future service lies jointly with the two purchasing agencies, the DHA and the corresponding local authority, and the authorities therefore carry a joint responsibility for ensuring that real participation of community groups occurs. From 1999, a 'duty of partnership' has been enshrined in legislation, but it remains to be seen whether the incentives will be sufficient to weld together authorities reluctant to work together.

A vision must be rooted in values and moral principles. Clinicians tend to view 'mission statements' with distaste, probably rightly if they have not been involved in developing them; too often, mission statements are full of grandiose notions of good intent to 'care', but have no recognisable hard content. But it is important to be explicit about principles, if only because they are so rarely shared at the outset by all the interested parties inside and outside the service. A service that has as its main aim:

> "the alleviation of mental distress by accurate diagnosis, assessment and treatment; the provision of shelter, asylum, safety from harm; a service that is readily accessible twenty four hours a day"

may end up looking very different from one that:

> "aspires to provide individuals with as fulfilling and rewarding a life as possible and provides for the ordinary needs of life – a home, daily occupation, emotional support through friendships and social contacts and recognises individuals' rights as citizens".

And yet, both mission statements contain legitimate principles in which services can be rooted. Many districts will wish to target as their first priority those patients who experience the greatest personal burden of mental illness for long periods of their lives, and second, those who impose the greatest emotional burden and distress on relatives, neighbours and the community at large. Inevitably, those individuals who pose the greatest economic burden on their families and statutory agencies will also be a priority for consideration, because setting priorities is an explicit rationing and control procedure aimed at containment of costs and getting better value for money. In the late 1990s, the government added a new and overriding principle – the safety of the general public – which, while not a new concern as an issue for consideration in the design of services, assumed far greater emphasis than previously, and inevitably led to a change in the overall philosophy of mental health services in the UK and to a shift of priorities from the most distressed to the most dangerous. These priorities are not of course mutually exclusive, but do impact on the overall design of a service.

The choice of setting local priorities between several needy groups is undoubtedly difficult but essential. Increasingly, the central Department of Health allocates finances in such a way to determine what those priorities should be. *Modernising Mental Health Services* (Department of Health, 1999*b*) was the first comprehensive statement from government about the future direction of mental health policy since the 1970s and is likely to remain the key guidance for the next decade. It was highly prescriptive, designed to address public concern about the perceived failures of community care and put public safety as the highest priority. The specific guidance is designed to strengthen the safety, comprehensiveness and supportiveness of services for people with severe mental illness. This is to be achieved through ensuring that there are: sufficient acute admission beds; an increased number of secure beds; sufficient high-support 24-hour 'nursed care' places in long-term homes and hostels; new 'assertive outreach' teams to work with that minority of patients with highly complex needs, who are exceptionally hard to engage in services; and a rapidly available crisis intervention service available round the clock, seven days a week.

The guidance is weaker on the specific content of social care provision. It stresses mechanisms for developing inter-agency planning partnerships, improving the use of information technology and recruiting and training staff. The core basics of how patients can be helped to spend their day in a fulfilling way and how daily needs are to be met are not prescribed, leaving plenty of flexibility for local service planners to innovate.

The issue of treatability, so dear to the hearts of doctors, is irrelevant for planning the total comprehensive health and social care service, but becomes important in assessing the emphasis that service planners should give to funding specific treatment activities for each of their priority groups. The health service traditionally has funded those parts of the service that its existing staff of doctors, nurses and therapists felt most able to treat or cure. Future plans need to take a broader view of the needs of mentally disordered people across the total local population. Specific medical and nursing interventions may form a relatively small part of the requirement for many priority groups.

Priorities need to be described in detail for the district as a whole, and also for different localities within the district. The following descriptive dimensions are useful:

- *target groups*: age range; gender; income group; ethnic or cultural group; and geographical area within district

- *client groups*: diagnostic group; type of illness or disability; short-term/long-term; and severity level
- *type of function needed*: preventive and educational work; treatment; social support; financial benefit assistance; accommodation; work opportunities; education; leisure; and family support.

Interpretation of local information

There is a wealth of data available on the epidemiology of mental disorders in the community and in institutions and a good deal of information about existing patterns of service use. Unfortunately, the former is generally unhelpful in predicting demand or highlighting current need for specialist services, and the latter only reflects historical and current patterns of service provision. Goldberg & Huxley (1980) demonstrated that referral 'filters' modify the decision of individuals with psychiatric morbidity to attend general practitioners (GPs), and further selection factors determine which GP patients will be directed to psychiatric services. Many potential patients will not seek help from their GPs, for example members of certain ethnic groups, for fear of acknowledging mental disorder within the family. Factors such as the patient's age, gender, social class and type of disorder heavily influence patterns of referral by GPs. Furthermore, community surveys are often flawed methodologically from the point of view of assessing the prevalence of relatively rare conditions. Community surveys, in which as many as several thousand of the population have been surveyed or interviewed, will reveal only a handful of individuals in need of the specialist mental health services. Even for common conditions such as senile dementia, where perhaps 3% or 4% of the population over 65 years may be expected to suffer from the condition, local surveys are rarely sufficiently large to produce statistically significant results with anything but very broad confidence limits, which when applied to the whole resident population of a district may be too broad to be useful. Furthermore, demand for specific psychiatric treatments from professionals is notoriously hard to predict from surveys. Individuals with short-lived episodes of disorder may be severely disabled and require expensive treatments for a short time only, but a point prevalence survey is unlikely to detect such cases.

Current patterns of service use will be influenced by the accessibility of the service to local users. Access is affected by the willingness of the service to accept referrals of certain categories of patients, the availability of in-patient beds and treatment facilities, the existence of specialist services, such as services for drug misuse or old age psychiatry, and the popularity of the service with local GPs and social workers.

The one area where data on current usage of services are useful is that of need for treatment and care of individuals with the most severely disabling acute disorders, since these individuals have a high likelihood of being admitted to hospital, and therefore usage may reflect need. But, even for this group, local prisons may be providing containment for seriously disturbed people if local hospital services are insufficient to meet the need, so information on current usage would have to be supplemented by information from the local criminal justice system and prison medical service. Current data on bed usage also highlight where in-patient resources are being used, perhaps inappropriately, for example to provide long-term accommodation for those in need of further rehabilitation and support.

For detailed planning, a district mental health information system is required, which performs three separate tasks. First, managers need information to assess and monitor service performance against objectives. Second, clinicians need relevant information for delivering the clinical service to individuals, and third, social services authorities need relevant information on social care needs of the population. Information systems, however, are expensive to develop and maintain. While districts should invest in the right technology and systems in order to assist them to deliver an efficient service, the practical process of planning and priority setting can rarely wait for the systems to be established. Furthermore, the 'perfect' information system will still mainly reflect the existing pattern of service use and will not provide guidance on future planning of priorities. Planning nearly always has to be done using imperfect information. Other chapters in this book focus on methods of assessment of mental health needs and the interpretation of information; all that needs to be repeated here is the vital importance for every district of developing a strategy for gathering information for planning purposes and for monitoring the implementation of plans.

Participation and consultation, joint planning and locality planning

Health service planning has conventionally been a centralising process that concentrates control over priority setting in the hands of a few senior personnel. It is natural that those who hold the purse strings should wish to retain sovereignty over the way money is spent. A central planning approach in mental health service development is almost bound to lead to widespread conflicts at the official consultation stage, when other agencies and the local population are confronted with documents that reflect only the attitudes and values of existing senior health service staff. Loosening the reins of control over priority setting by a participative planning process both improves the quality of decision-making and also fosters the local commitment needed to implement plans. A 'democratic' participation approach can also be seen as promoting ideals of social justice, redressing in part the balance of power between the community of people on the receiving end of the service and those who control its delivery. Whether or not senior managers espouse an underlying philosophy that underpins commitment to participative planning, a pragmatic realisation of the practical benefits should encourage districts and local authorities to adopt a partnership approach that includes service users, carers and the wider community. National Priorities Guidance (Department of Health, 1998*a*) specified that mental health services should be a 'shared lead priority' for both health and local social services authorities.

Who should participate and how? Joint planning teams are usually too big to be effective. The balance between inclusiveness and effectiveness is a difficult one. In general, it is better to have a multi-layered structure of consultative groups, each with the right to be heard. Focus groups, citizen's juries, public debates and 'Question Time' open days can all play a useful part in widening the opportunities for community and staff involvement.

Avoiding the pitfalls is not easy, but the process can be made easier. First, we need to recognise that the practical administrative work of planning can only be done by one or two people with the help perhaps of an inner circle of five or six key players. Second, we need to ensure that there are mechanisms for involving on a continuing basis the appropriate groups, in addition to health and social services staff. Local community planning using sectors is described in Chapter 9.

The impact of the NHS and Community Care Act 1990 and subsequent legislation

From 1 April 1990, the DHA's role has been to establish local priorities, decide on the shape of local services and then to purchase a spectrum of services from whatever 'providers' can best match their requirements for the lowest cost and the highest quality. In theory, the local DHA and local authority should jointly agree a set of strategic planning priorities for mental health services for their resident population and then decide from which statutory agencies, hospitals, community services and independent sector organisations they will purchase services. In reality, much of the local expertise and the enthusiasm, drive and commitment required to change mental health services lies with existing service providers.

The creation of primary care groups, eventually primary care trusts, in the White Paper *The New NHS: Modern, Dependable* (Department of Health, 1997) transferred much of the day-to-day planning of health services from the DHA to the new groups. Health authorities, however, retain a key role in strategic planning and, with the local authority, are responsible for monitoring the effectiveness of GP group purchasing and for commissioning specialist mental health services. It is likely that there will be further legislation facilitating the direct linkage of health and social care services (Department of Health, 1998*b*). Health Action Zone areas, created to channel development monies into areas with serious social deprivation, already have the ability to ask for certain financial rules on the transfer of funds between authorities to be waived, and it is likely that more initiatives of this kind will be introduced to facilitate statutory and independent sector collaboration.

The Community Care part of the 1990 Act was implemented in 1993. Local authorities became responsible for the allocation to individuals of social security welfare benefits for board and lodging. The role of the local authority is to assess the needs of its resident population for community care support, set local priorities and service objectives and arrange the required care by designing, organising and purchasing care. In order to allow it to do this effectively, former social security benefit and community care grant monies were channelled via social services. These funds have increasingly been used to support people at home as well as in institutions, one of the positive benefits of the 1990 changes.

When professionals who work in mental health services talk of an 'integrated, comprehensive, seamless service', they mean a service where acute hospital beds, hostels, residential homes, community teams and services for people in their own homes are all managed as one service, with an identified team of people having responsibility for delivering care. This has been achieved by a handful of health and local authorities, but very rarely have the private and voluntary sectors been included as part of the team – an unfortunate omission when the independent sector plays such a vital role in total service provision in many parts of the country. Nevertheless, most professionals aspire to a flexible, easily accessible service where 'users' can move rapidly between home, day care and hospital when the need arises. One of the major disadvantages of the NHS changes of 1990, which introduced the 'purchaser/provider split', was the fragmentation of services between competitive providers and in some areas a distancing of planning from providing, which was counter-productive. The swing of the pendulum in the late 1990s towards closer collaboration and cooperation between health service agencies was welcomed, but it carries the danger of creating once more a monolithic centralised bureaucracy that stifles innovation and originality. It remains to be seen what overall impact the centralist shift will have on shape of services.

Some statutory authorities have created a new joint organisation for purchasing mental health services; some have pooled budgets for providing services. These new organisations are pointing the way all services are likely to go before long. Apart from the clear advantages of having a joint strategic plan for mental health services, a joint commissioning agency has much enhanced buying power and can make considerable economies in developing information systems and pooling skills in service development and the maintenance of standards of care.

Maintaining flexibility and responsiveness

Health care planning is often carried out assuming that the planning systems will remain stable and that the characteristics of the population to be served will remain steady. But, in the real world, we cannot assure political or economic stability; health service personnel often complain that 'the goalposts keep moving'. Public sector services operate in a permanent climate of upheaval and change, imposed both from above as a result of political change and from pressure upwards from the changing nature of populations and disorders. For example, in East London, the inner-city area has witnessed in the past 10 years the influx of a large and shifting refugee population, a dramatic rise in the population of over 85-year-olds and a sharply increased incidence of acquired immunodeficiency syndrome and tuberculosis. Within one decade, very significant changes can derail a 10-year strategic plan. Because of the changing needs of mental health patients, it is important to have plans that are sufficiently flexible that facilities and services are appropriate for future generations of users. This is especially important when planning for the resettlement outside of hospital of the old 'long-stay' population.

Flexibility is improved, first, by developing services that do not depend on specific purpose-designed capital building developments, but which whenever possible use ordinary housing and small-scale developments that can be turned to alternative purposes in the future. Second, it is important to maintain a workforce that possesses core skills common to serving a wide range of types of disability, not so highly specialised that it cannot turn its skills to people with related disorders.

There is a tendency to develop specific and quite separate 'community teams' for rehabilitation of adults with long-term mental disorders, people with mental handicap, elderly people with mental disorder and so on, all of which develop operational policies exclusively focused on one care group. Since the members of these teams may be performing very similar work, a service can retain future flexibility by enhancing the cross-training and exchange of staff. Champions of specific services can create a separatist ethos of service development that tends to set the existing services in concrete until the 'champion' retires, unless this specific problem of maintaining flexibility is addressed at the outset.

Priorities will change as the years pass and no plan should remain static. Setting priorities is part of a cyclical process of current service analysis, joint planning, analysis of options, implementation, review of progress, re-analysis of service and new priority setting. What must not change is the vision and aspirations of the individuals who lead the priority-setting process.

References

CIPFA (Chartered Institute of Public Finance Accountants) (1997) *Personal Social Services Actuals* 1996/7.

Department of Health (1997) *The New NHS: Modern, Dependable.* Cm 3807. London: The Stationery Office.

—— (1998a) *Modernising Health and Social Services: National Priorities Guidance 1999/00–2001/02.* LAC (98)22. London: The Stationery Office.

—— (1998b) *Partnership in Action: New Opportunities for Joint Working between Health and Social Services.* London: The Stationery Office.

—— (1998c) *Modernising Social Services: Promoting Independence, Improving Protection, Raising Standards.* Cm 4169. London: The Stationery Office.

—— (1999a) *National Service Framework for Mental Health Services* HSC (99) Cm 624. LASSLL (99)x. London: The Stationery Office.

—— (1999b) *Modernising Mental Health Services.* 14356 HSD. London: The Stationery Office.

Goldberg, D. & Huxley, P. (1980) *Mental Illness in the Community.* London: Tavistock.

Health Select Committee Minutes and RO3 Return (1998) quoted in *The Fundamental Facts,* p. 37 (Mental Health Foundation, 1999).

House of Commons (1990) *NHS and Community Care Act.* London: HMSO.

Mental Health Foundation (1999) *The Fundamental Facts,* pp. 33–38. London: Mental Health Foundation Publications.

NHS Executive (1998) Burdens of Disease, quoted in *Our Healthier Nation: A Contract for Health.* Cm 3852 (Department of Health, 1998).

Nichol, D. K. (1986) Action research and development in strategic planning. In: *Managers as Strategists* (ed. G. Parston). London: King's Fund.

Office for National Statistics (1995) *Surveys of Psychiatric Morbidity in Great Britain. Report No 3: Economic Activity and Social Functioning of Adults with Psychiatric Disorders.* London: The Stationery Office.

Patel, A. & Knapp, M. (1998) *The Cost of Mental Health in England. Mental Health Research Review No 5.* London: Centre for the Economics of Mental Health.

Stein, L. I. & Test, M. A. (1980) Alternatives to hospital treatment. 1. Conceptual model, treatment program and clinical evaluation. *Archives of General Psychiatry,* **37**, 392–397.

9 The Care Programme Approach: prioritising according to need in policy and practice

JONATHAN BINDMAN and GYLES GLOVER

The Care Programme Approach (CPA) is the policy framework within which all specialist mental health services in England are provided (Department of Health, 1990, 1995). It sets out the way in which the approximately 180 trusts that provide mental health services should work together with their local authority social service departments (LASSDs), and the processes by which patients should be assessed and treated. It aims to prioritise individuals according to need and to ensure that resources are targeted to those in greatest need, with a focus on severe, enduring mental illness (SMI; Slade *et al*, 1997). This chapter describes the CPA policy, its implementation in practice and its implications for needs assessment.

Origins of the Care Programme Approach

The CPA was introduced by the Department of Health in 1990, and arose out of a number of related developments. First, in England, as elsewhere, the development of Community Care, with care being provided increasingly by multiple agencies in multiple locations, led to increasing recognition of the importance of continuity of care (Johnson *et al*, 1997). Second, inquiries into incidents of failures of care, such as the Spokes Inquiry into the care and treatment of Sharon Campbell, emphasised the importance of maintaining follow-up after discharge from hospital, and of clarifying the responsibility for maintaining it (Department of Health and Social Security (DHSS), 1988). Third, the introduction of the National Health Service (NHS) and Community Care Act (1990) established new requirements for health and social services to work together in the care of those with enduring mental illness, resulting in a need for a framework for cooperation. Finally, research into models of community care in the USA and elsewhere led to recognition of the possible role of individual case managers (providing direct care) or care managers (coordinating or 'brokering' care provided by others) (Holloway *et al*, 1991).

CPA principles and practice

Principles

The policy incorporates a number of principles, which are described in Table 9.1.

CPA elements

The CPA consists of five elements (Table 9.2). The intention of the policy is that every patient under the care of a trust (providing specialist psychiatric services to an average population of 280 000) should be recorded on a register. All patients should then receive each of the remaining elements: a needs assessment, a care plan, a keyworker and a care plan review.

TABLE 9.1
Principles of the Care Programme Approach (CPA)

Communication: inter-agency and interdisciplinary	Communication between all those involved in the care of the patient, both within the multi-disciplinary mental health team and between different agencies providing care in the community
Severe mental illness (SMI)	Specialist services should be focused on the needs of those with SMI
Continuity	Follow-up should be provided for all those who need continuing care, and an appropriate degree of assertiveness should be used to ensure it happens
Comprehensiveness	The policy should be applied to all patients of the specialist psychiatric services
Non-prescriptive	The policy is an approach, and is not intended to be prescriptive about how its aims should be achieved at a local level
Involvement of users and carers	The care plan should be developed in discussion with, and with the agreement of, users and carers

TABLE 9.2
Elements of the Care Programme Approach (CPA)

CPA register	In each trust; register of all patients and details of the other CPA elements
Needs assessment	Jointly carried out with social services where appropriate. Needs for which no service can be offered should also be identified to assist in service planning. Risk should also be considered
Care plan	Written record of appropriate response to identified needs
Keyworker	Individual reponsible for ensuring delivery of care plan; usually direct care provider also, e.g. community psychiatric nurse
Review	Regular review of the effectiveness and appropriateness of the care plan, which should be revised if necessary

The 'tiered' CPA and the supervision register

Soon after its introduction, it was recognised that, in addition to identifying those individuals who should receive a specialist psychiatric service, the CPA could also incorporate levels of further prioritisation within it (Department of Health, 1993). This led to the development of the 'tiered' CPA (Department of Health, 1995), in which the majority of patients could be provided with a 'minimal' level of CPA. This might involve only a single member of the treatment team carrying out all the necessary tasks: assessing needs; recording the plan of treatment offered; taking the keyworker responsibility for the patient's care; and offering the review appointment. A 'more complex' level of CPA could then be reserved for a smaller number of patients, perhaps those for whom more than one member of the treatment team would be involved, increasing the requirements for communication. Finally, a 'full multi-disciplinary' tier could be used for those individuals with the greatest number of staff involved, the greatest level of needs, or the greatest need for coordination of care between multiple agencies or professional carers. The policy is not prescriptive about the criteria to be used to distinguish between the tiers; the number of staff or agencies involved, the complexity or level of the patients needs, and the assessed level of risk are all possible criteria.

Supervision register

In 1994, following concern over high-profile incidents of failures of care (Ritchie *et al*, 1994), the government introduced a requirement of all mental health provider trusts that they should introduce a 'supervision register' of individuals "in greatest need and at greatest risk" of self-harm, of harming others, or of serious self-neglect (Holloway, 1994; NHS Executive, 1994). This register (which could either be a separate record or a 'flagging' system within the CPA register) was intended to ensure that the identified individuals received the elements of the CPA. The supervision register could be regarded as a further, or fourth, tier of the CPA, but was more usually regarded as a subset of those on the topmost tier.

Needs assessment and the CPA

Two distinct forms of needs assessment are described within the CPA policy: individual needs assessments, and also the assessment of the needs of the population for specialist psychiatric care.

Individual needs assessment

Individual needs assessment is a central element of the CPA. However, in keeping with the principle of the policy that it should offer an approach rather than be prescriptive, the way in which needs assessment is carried out is left to the discretion of local services (Department of Health, 1995). The importance of agreeing a process of needs assessment between social and health services, so that their separate responsibilities can be met without duplication of effort, is stressed, as is the importance of assessing risk as part of the needs assessment.

The Camberwell Assessment of Needs (CAN; Phelan *et al*, 1995; also Slade *et al*, 1999*a*) has been designed as a standardised instrument for assessing needs in a manner compatible with the requirements of the CPA. However, the majority of individual needs assessments carried out are not standardised, but carried out according to local clinical practice.

Population needs assessment

The CPA policy makes explicit the need to identify those patients with the most severe mental illnesses, and to target resources towards them. The health authority, the agency with the responsibility to purchase a comprehensive range of mental health services for all the population (averaging 500 000) in its area, should agree with the

LASSDs, provider trusts and voluntary sector organisations in its area what the needs for services are at the population level.

Evaluation of the CPA

A number of evaluations of the CPA have been carried out. The Audit Commission (1994) investigated the extent of its implementation by trusts soon after its introduction. Although examples of good practice were identified, it was also clear that many services had not yet implemented it. Marshall *et al* (1995) suggested that the inclusion of keyworking in the CPA was misguided, as experimental studies of case management had failed to support its effectiveness. Tyrer and colleagues (1995) examined this issue directly in a randomised controlled trial comparing the effect of allocating a CPA keyworker to patients on a case register to the previously existing standard care. A significantly higher proportion of patients allocated to standard care (64/197; 32.5%) were lost to follow-up than those who received a keyworker (40/196; 20.4%, $P<0.01$). Patients with keyworkers had significantly more hospital admissions (30% *v.* 18%, $P<0.01$) and spent 68% more days in hospital than the standard group. This suggests that although the CPA may be effective in achieving one of its aims, that of ensuring continuing care, it does not have the effect, described in some experimental studies, of assertive community treatment, of reducing use of hospital beds (Kluiter, 1997). The author suggest that CPA keyworking may be different from the intensive case management applied in experimental studies, in which case managers work with higher levels of support from multi-disciplinary teams. Burns (1997) emphasised the difficulty of drawing conclusions about the effectiveness of the CPA policy as a whole from experimental studies of well-defined interventions, such as case management, as the actual treatment interventions offered under the CPA could vary widely and need not be directly equivalent to specific experimental models. As part of the PRiSM Evaluation of Supervision Registers, a study of the impact of the supervision register policy carried out in 1997 (Bindman *et al*, 1999, 2000), we examined the extent and variability of implementation of the CPA and supervision register, as described below.

Numbers prioritised for care under the CPA

Method

We surveyed the 180 trusts in England who were providing mental health services in 1996/1997. A postal questionnaire was sent to key informants, and a shortened form of the questionnaire was administered by telephone to those who had not responded after six months. We asked informants to report the number of people in their local area who had been assessed, according to the CPA policy, as requiring a specialist mental health service, and how many of these had been placed on a higher tier, or on the supervision register. The total population of the area served by the trust was also obtained.

Results

Of the 180 trusts surveyed (all of which responded), 59% were allocating patients to three CPA tiers, 36% to two tiers, and 5% were using a single tier (Bindman *et al*, 1999). All but five trusts (3%) were operating a supervision register. Fig. 9.1 shows the numbers allocated to the various tiers; where there were two upper tiers, these are shown as combined. On average, about 1.2% of the total population were receiving specialist psychiatric care. About 0.25% were assessed as requiring higher levels of care, and less than 0.01% were regarded as 'in greatest need and at greatest risk'. These figures represent an administrative point prevalence, and

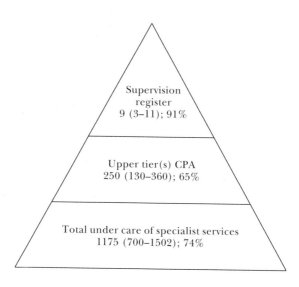

Fig. 9.1 CPA 'pyramid'; patients per 100 000 total population (25th–75th centiles); percentage of trusts responding

are not strictly comparable with measures of period prevalence of psychiatric disorder. However, as Table 9.3 shows, the number of patients being offered care under the CPA is broadly consistent with other measures of mental illness with relatively high levels of severity, suggesting that, with the possible exception of those trusts with the largest numbers on the CPA, care is focused on SMI as intended.

The numbers varied considerably between trusts. As Fig. 9.1 shows, the range between the 25th and 75th percentiles was about twofold for the total under care of the services, but was proportionately greater at the higher level, with a threefold interquartile range for the upper tiers of the CPA and a fourfold range for the supervision register. This suggests that the assessment of population need for psychiatric services at the population level is inconsistent between trusts. This inconsistency is more pronounced when higher levels of need are identified, and the addition of a risk criterion in the very explicit way attempted by the supervision register policy

TABLE 9.3

Use of the Care Programme Approach (CPA) and prevalence estimates for mental disorder

Definition of group	Prevalence (population/period of prevalence)
Total morbidity	2.4% (population at risk per year)[1]
CPA (need for specialist psychiatric care)	1.2% (total population, administrative)
Psychiatric out-patient attenders	0.8–1.4% (population aged 15–64 years per year)[2]
All functional psychoses	0.4% (range 0.2–0.9%) (total population per year)[3]
Clinical diagnosis of schizophrenia, rural Scotland	0.28% (total population, annual period)[4]
Clinical diagnosis of schizophrenia, urban area	0.35% (total population, annual period)[4]
Upper tier CPA (need for priority care from specialist services), England, 1997	0.25% (total population, administrative)

1. Goldberg & Huxley, 1991.
2. Wing, 1994.
3. OPCS, 1995.
4. McCreadie *et al*, 1997.

(although risk assessment may also form a part of needs assessments at lower levels of the CPA) results in even greater inconsistency.

Numbers on the CPA and population need

The variation, shown above, in the numbers of individuals prioritised to receive care under the CPA does not take account of the variation that would be expected as a consequence of variations in the population need for psychiatric services, arising from differences in morbidity and socio-economic deprivation. It was impossible to examine the relationship between the numbers shown in Fig. 9.1 and population need directly, because there is no national source of data concerning levels of population need in each trust. However, it was possible to address the question indirectly, using data collected centrally concerning the numbers subject to the CPA, and those included on supervision registers, in each health authority purchasing area.

The level of need for specialist psychiatric services in each health authority area was measured using the Mental Health Needs Index (MINI; Glover *et al*, 1998) score. The index was derived by analysis of the association between admission prevalence and a range of socio-demographic variables in the former North East Thames health region. The score for each health authority varies between 160.6 and 454.6, and is closely correlated with the resources made available by central government to purchase mental health services.

We analysed the extent to which variation in the numbers on the CPA and supervision register is explained by variation in need, as estimated by the MINI predicted prevalence score, in the 84 (of a total of 100) health authorities for which full data were available, using the MINI score as a predictor variable in negative binomial regressions, with the CPA and supervision register rates as the dependent variables. Table 9.4 gives estimated rate ratios for a 100-point increase in MINI predicted prevalence score, as well as the estimates of α, the coefficient of scatter additional to the Poisson distribution. The MINI predicted prevalence score is only weakly associated with the CPA rate, and the association is not significant at the 5% level. The supervision register rate is significantly predicted by the MINI score, but there is considerable unexplained variation. The apparently strong relationship between the rate on the supervision register and need is largely attributable to a few health authorities with socially deprived populations and high supervision register rates. Excluding the three purchasers with over 200 patients on the supervision register per 100 000 reduces the supervision register rate ratio for a 100-point increase in the MINI

TABLE 9.4

Association between population need and numbers of patients per 100 000 population on the CPA and supervision register in purchasing areas (n=84)

No. of people	Estimated ratio per 10-point increase in MINI (95% CI)	P	Estimate of α (P)
On supervision register	1.71 (1.39–2.1)	<0.001	0.48 (<0.001)
On the CPA	1.14 (0.99–1.31)	0.06	0.19 (<0.001)

score from 71% to 33% (95% CI 3–73), only just significant at the 5% level.

Individual needs assessment, the CPA and supervision register

The results described above suggest that the variation in the numbers subject to the CPA in different trusts is due to inconsistencies in the methods of needs assessment adopted, rather than to differences in population need. This can also be demonstrated at the level of individual needs assessments. As part of the PRiSM Evaluation of Supervision Registers, we compared 133 patients on the supervision register in a random sample of 14 trusts with 126 patients on the (locally defined) top tier of the CPA, matched for responsible medical officer (Bindman *et al*, 1998; Slade *et al*, 1999*a*). All patients on the supervision register from the eight trusts with less than 15 supervision register cases in total were included, and a random sample of 15 from the remainder. Keyworkers were asked to rate their patients' needs, and whether these were met or unmet, using the short form of the CAN, the CANSAS (Phelan *et al*, 1995; Slade *et al*, 1999*b*). The response rate was 92% for the supervision register cases and 91% for the CPA comparison patients. In the sample as a whole, the total number of needs of the supervision register cases was only slightly higher than that of the CPA comparison group (8.1 *v.* 7.1, *P*=0.01), providing weak evidence that the supervision register cases were being prioritised appropriately on the basis of greater need. However, the number of needs was highly variable between sites, for both the supervision register cases and the CPA comparison group. For supervision register cases, the total number of needs at each case varied between an average of 6.4 and 10.4 (excluding three sites with less than five patients on the supervision register). For the CPA patients, the range was 4.4–9.5

(excluding the same three sites). Similarly, both met needs (ranging from 3.4–7.8 in supervision register cases, 1.9–7.3 in CPA comparisons) and unmet needs (supervision register 1.8–4.1; CPA 1.4–3.9) varied considerably more between different trusts than they did between the two levels of CPA prioritisation. Although the number of patients sampled at each site was small (an average of 10 cases and comparison patients in each site included in the figures above), the figures suggest wide differences in the threshold of needs that results in prioritisation to the upper tier of the CPA or supervision register at the various trusts.

Conclusions: equity, needs assessment and the CPA

The CPA continues to grow and develop rapidly, as it has done considerably in the 10 years since its implementation. The most recent changes (Department of Health, 1999) include a recommendation to use only two tiers and simplify the application of the lower tier, and permission for trusts to discontinue supervision registers, provided thst adequate alternative risk assessment procedures are in place. Practice also varies widely between services. For both these reasons, it is hard to draw firm conclusions about the effectiveness of the CPA policy as a whole in ensuring prioritisation of patients with SMI on the basis of need, and effective targeting of resources to them. However, some conclusions can be drawn from the above:

(a) The CPA policy has been implemented nationally, and all specialist services are aware of the importance of identifying and registering all patients under their care and providing long-term follow-up to those who need it, in a way which they were clearly not before the policy was introduced.
(b) The average number of patients identified by services, 1.2% of the total population at any one time, is consistent with the targeting of specialist care to a group with relative SMI.
(c) There is considerable variation between services in the number of patients they care for, and the number they prioritise to receive more intensive levels of care. This variation does not seem to be explained by variations in the need of the local population they serve. This suggests that the levels of individual need that result in a patient crossing the threshold into specialist care, or receiving higher levels of input, vary between services.
(d) The threshold level of need that results in prioritisation of an individual to the upper tier of the CPA or supervision register can also be shown to vary between trusts, when a standardised measure of need is applied to patients on the same tier of the CPA in different trusts.

The variable level of need that results in the receipt of specialist care has important implications for equity, recently re-emphasised as a priority for UK health services (Acheson, 1998). Equity demands that individuals with the same levels of need should receive the same level of care in any part of the country. The resources allocated to health authorities to purchase psychiatric services are distributed according to population need on this assumption (Glover, 1999). If services apply different thresholds of need for entry to their services, or for prioritisation within them, equity cannot be achieved.

A possible approach to achieving more consistency between services in the way they assess need would be to introduce a standardised measure of need such as the CANSAS (Slade *et al*, 1999*b*) into routine practice. Even if it is not feasible to do this for all patients, if it were applied to representative samples of patients on the various CPA tiers in different trusts, and the results compared, consistency in needs assessment could be progressively improved.

References

ACHESON, D. (1998) *Report of the Independent Inquiry into Inequalities in Health.* London: The Stationery Office.

AUDIT COMMISSION (1994) *Finding a Place. A Review of Mental Health Services for Adults.* London: HMSO.

BINDMAN, J., BECK, A. & THORNICROFT, G. (1998) *PRiSM Evaluation of Supervision Registers.* Report to the NHS Executive Research and Development Directorate. London: Institute of Psychiatry.

—, —, GLOVER, G., ET AL (1999) Evaluating mental health policy in England. Care Programme Approach and supervision registers. *British Journal of Psychiatry*, **175**, 327–330.

—, —, THORNICROFT, G., ET AL (2000) Psychiatric patients at greatest risk and in greatest need. Impact of the Supervision Register Policy. *British Journal of Psychiatry*, **177**, 33–37.

BURNS, T. (1997) Case management, care management and care programming (editorial). *British Journal of Psychiatry*, **170**, 393–395.

DEPARTMENT OF HEALTH (1990) *The Care Programme Approach for People with a Mental Illness Referred to the Specialist Psychiatric Services.* HC(90)23/HASSL(90)11. London: Department of Health.

— (1993) *Health of the Nation: Key Area Handbook Mental Illness* (1st edition), p. 129. London: HMSO.

— (1995) *Building Bridges. A Guide to Arrangements for Inter-Agency Working for the Care and Protection of Severely Mentally Ill People.* London: Department of Health.

— (1999) *Effective Care Co-ordination in Mental Health Services. Modernising Mental Health Services.* London: Department of Health.

DEPARTMENT OF HEALTH AND SOCIAL SECURITY (1988) *Report of the Committee of Inquiry into the Care and Aftercare of Miss Sharon Campbell.* Presented to parliament by the secretary of state for social services by command of Her Majesty, July 1988 (Chairman J. Spokes). Cm 440. London: DHSS.

GLOVER, G. R. (1999) How much English authorities are allocated for mental health care. *British Journal of Psychiatry*, **175**, 402–406.

——, Robin, E., Emami, J., *et al* (1998) A needs index for mental health care. *Social Psychiatry and Psychiatric Epidemiology*, **33**, 89–96.

Goldberg, D. & Huxley, P. (1991) *Common Mental Disorders*. London: Routledge.

Holloway, F. (1994) Supervision registers. Recent government policy and legislation. *Psychiatric Bulletin*, **18**, 593–596.

——, McLean, E. K. & Robertson, J. A. (1991) Case management. *British Journal of Psychiatry*, **159**, 142–148.

Johnson, S., Prosser, D., Bindman, J., *et al* (1997) Continuity of care for the severely mentally ill: concepts and measures. *Social Psychiatry and Psychiatric Epidemiology*, **32**, 137–142.

Kluiter, H. (1997) In-patient treatment and care arrangements to replace or avoid it – searching for an evidence-based balance. *Current Opinion in Psychiatry*, **10**, 160–167.

McCreadie, R. G., Leese, M., Tilak-Singh, D., *et al* (1997) Nithsdale, Nunhead and Norwood: similarities and differences in prevalence of schizophrenia and utilisation of services in rural and urban areas. *British Journal of Psychiatry*, **170**, 31–36.

Marshall, M., Lockwood, A. & Gath, D. (1995) Social services case-management for long-term mental disorders: a randomised controlled trial. *Lancet*, **345**, 409–412.

NHS Executive (1994) *Introduction of Supervision Registers for Mentally Ill People from 1 April 1994*. (HSG(94)5.) Leeds: NHSE.

Office of Population Censuses and Surveys (1995) *Report 1: The Prevalence of Psychiatric Morbidity among Adults Living in Private Households*. London: HMSO.

Phelan, M., Slade, M., Thornicroft, G., *et al* (1995) The Camberwell Assessment of Need: the validity and reliability of an instrument to assess the needs of people with severe mental illness. *British Journal of Psychiatry*, **167**, 589–595.

Ritchie, J., Dick, D. & Lingham, R. (1994) *The Report of the Inquiry into the Care and Treatment of Christopher Clunis*. London: HMSO.

Slade, M., Powell, R. & Strathdee, G. (1997) Current approaches to identifying the severely mentally ill. *Social Psychiatry and Psychiatric Epidemiology*, **32**, 177–184.

——, Thornicroft, G., Loftus, L., *et al* (1999a) *CAN: The Camberwell Assessment of Need. A Comprehensive Needs Assessment Tool for People with Severe Mental Illness*. London: Gaskell.

——, Beck, A., Bindman, J., *et al* (1999b) Routine outcome measures for patients with severe mental illness: CANSAS and HoNOS. *British Journal of Psychiatry*, **174**, 404–408.

Tyrer, P., Morgan, J., Van Horn, E., *et al* (1995) A randomised controlled study of close monitoring of vulnerable psychiatric patients. *Lancet*, **345**, 756–759.

Wing, J. K. (1994) Mental illness. In: *Health Care Needs Assessment* (eds A. Stevens & J. Raftery), pp. 202–304. Oxford: Radcliffe.

10 Local catchment areas for needs-led mental health services

GERALDINE STRATHDEE
and GRAHAM THORNICROFT

This chapter is written from the perspective of clinicians involved in the development of community-based mental health services. We shall consider here how needs assessment relates to the planning, implementation and evaluation of routine clinical services. We shall focus on the stages required to establish services that are locality-oriented rather than hospital-oriented. We wish to see in place services that reflect those principles for the development of community mental health services that have a widespread measure of agreement, as shown in Box 10.1 (Department of Health, 1999).

We have framed our discussion in terms of the geographical sector, as we consider this catchment area to be the most useful local level of organisation for service needs assessment, and the most manageable

---

Box 10.1
Fundamental principles for planning services for people with mental health problems in the National Service Framework for Mental Health in England (Department of Health, 1999)

People with mental health problems can expect that services providing their care and treatment will:

- show openness and honesty
- demonstrate respect and offer courtesy
- be allocated fairly and provided equitably
- be proportional to their needs
- be open to learning and change.

---

level of analysis for mental health service evaluation. Two basic themes have underpinned government policies for the practice of community care for the past three decades. These are that policies should be needs-led, rather than service-led, and that this objective can best be met by replacing the large psychiatric institutions with a more balanced and flexible range of local alternative services (Strathdee, 1990). There has been little expert guidance from academics on the application of standardised assessment techniques suitable for use by hard-pressed clinicians in the rigours of busy clinical practice. Indeed, the tendency for otherwise excellent texts (Talbot, 1983; National Institute of Mental Health, 1987; Torrey *et al*, 1990) to focus on qualitative rather than quantitative descriptions of the needs in community psychiatric services has drawn criticism from Andrews (1990) in his own vigorous attempt to redress their deficiencies. With a similar lack of focus, clinicians, while accustomed to making ad hoc assessments of an individual's need before prescribing treatment, have been slow to incorporate this approach into planning terms (Stevens & Gabbay, 1991; and Chapter 4 of this book).

Although there has been a qualified consensus that closure of the large psychiatric hospitals is a preferred option (Jones, 1972; Thornicroft & Bebbington, 1988), little agreement has been reached on how best to structure the services that replace them. The traditional path of service developments in medicine owes as much to serendipity and opportunism as to rational strategic planning (Todd, 1984). In current practice, community developments are frequently determined by financial expediency, lacking any theoretical basis, and focus more on buildings than on the flexible recruitment and deployment of personnel (Holloway, 1988).

Mental health service developments in Great Britain have tended to be based on replications (often uncritical) of models in America or Europe, rather than being a product of a well-considered local strategy (for a fuller discussion of these issues see: Muijen *et al*, 1992*a,b*; Lehman *et al*, 1995; Kluiter, 1997; Lewis, 1997; Marshall *et al*, 1997*a,b*; Becker *et al*, 1998; Holloway & Carson, 1998; Lehman *et al*, 1998; Mueser *et al*, 1998; Stein & Santos, 1998; Teague *et al*, 1998; Thornicroft *et al*, 1998*a,b*, 1999; Burns & Priebe, 1999; UK700 Group, 1999). As Kingdon (1989) found, only three-fifths of health districts had an up-to-date mental health strategic plan. Nevertheless, there are indications that at the level of grass-roots clinicians, locally relevant developments do occur, either in response to crisis management or based on accumulated knowledge of local needs and resources (Strathdee & Williams, 1984).

Establishing sector boundaries

The early proponents of community care concentrated less on specifying the components of care than on developing the organisational framework within which such services could be effectively delivered. Philippe Paumelle, working in Paris, formulated three essential principles: that services should provide continuity of care, coordination of care and integration of care (Walsh, 1987). In order to fulfil these requirements, it was his view that the planning and operation of services should take place at a defined local level. Thus, the concept of a 'sector' as the denominator in local planning evolved and has subsequently gained wide support. The term 'sector' now generally refers to a delineated geographical area, with a defined catchment population.

Internationally, the concept of the sector permeates community service development. Following the emergence of the first sectors in France in 1947, by 1961 over 300 had been established. In the USA, the Community Mental Health Centers Act (Levine, 1981) introduced the principle of a catchment area for each community mental health centre, and by 1975 40% of the population had sectorised services. In Europe, throughout the 1970s, sector development grew but sizes varied between countries (Lindholm, 1983; Hansson *et al*, 1995; Saarento *et al*, 1998). Germany has sector sizes in the range of 250 000, The Netherlands around 300 000, while the areas for the Scandinavian countries are smaller, with Denmark averaging 60 000–120 000, Finland 100 000, Norway 40 000 and Sweden 25 000–50 000. Of all the countries, however, Italy has most comprehensively adopted the concept by virtue of Law 178, passed in 1978, which established sectors in the range of 50 000–200 000 population. Tansella (1989), in recognition of the vital role of such an infrastructure, reiterates that "what is important in community care is not only the number and characteristics of various services but the way in which they are arranged and integrated".

In Great Britain, as in many other European countries, sectorisation is regarded by many as an essential prerequisite for the development of effective community psychiatric services (Strathdee & Thornicroft, 1992). A study in England and Wales (Johnson & Thornicroft, 1993, 1995) indicated that 81% of districts nationally have divided their catchment areas into sectors. Many of the claimed advantages for the sector as the basic unit of planning, organisation and service delivery are shown below, although there has been little rigorous evaluation for most of these claims.

Planning advantages

    (a) high identification rates of patients
    (b) a feasible scale for clinical and social assessments
    (c) assists appropriate and planned development of services
    (d) development of a wide range of local service components
    (e) improved knowledge and use of community resources
    (f) greater budgetary clarity.

Service delivery advantages

    (a) less patients lost to follow-up
    (b) individually tailored inter-agency patient programmes
    (c) facilitates home treatment
    (d) improved identity of staff with locality
    (e) clarity of functions of district teams
    (f) facilitates inter-agency liaison, training and working
    (g) allows comparative research and evaluation.

Quality of service advantages

    (a) less use of crisis and in-patient facilities
    (b) improved patient education and intervention
    (c) greater support of relatives and carers
    (d) defined responsibility for each patient
    (e) improved communication for staff, patients and carers
    (f) improved primary–secondary service communication.

Research has concentrated almost exclusively on establishing whether sectorisation facilitates the development of community alternatives to in-patient hospital treatment. In Nottingham, for example, Tyrer *et al* (1989) found the following reductions after sectorisation: number of admissions (5%), duration of admissions (4%) and use of in-patient beds (38%). One Swedish study (Hansson, 1989) found a decrease in the number of admissions (20%), bed days used (40%), and compulsory admissions (25%). Another study (Lindholm, 1983) found similar, but non-significant trends.

Factors influencing sector size

The division of a district into sectors is influenced by many considerations. In practice, the need to be coterminous with either social service boundaries or general practice locations is often the primary rationale for defining the area within the sector. However, equally important issues are the rural or urban nature of the area, and the presence of rivers, main roads and other significant natural local geographical structures that impair access. Factors that influence sector size and location are outlined below.

Factors in the population

    (a) socio-demographic composition
    (b) social deprivation indices
    (c) ethnic composition
    (d) age and gender structure
    (e) knowledge of identified psychiatric morbidity
    (f) knowledge of existing service utilisation patterns
    (g) assessment of model of service needed.

Factors in the organisation of services

    (a) social services boundaries
    (b) primary care organisation
    (c) extent of sheltered housing
    (d) number of old/new long-stay
    (e) presence of a large institution
    (f) presence of a district general hospital (DGH)
    (g) manpower and other resource parameters.

Factors in the locality

    (a) significant geographical structures
    (b) inherent community cultures
    (c) presence of sites for development.

There is strong evidence that such social and demographic factors are closely associated with the measured rates of psychiatric disorder (Thornicroft, 1991; Jarman *et al,* 1992; Glover, 1996). The age structure of the population also serves as a pointer for service needs. Overrepresentation in the age range 20–29 years will predict a higher rate of population at risk of developing psychotic disorders. The association between psychiatric disorders and social class (particularly for schizophrenia and depression) is one of the most consistent findings in psychiatric epidemiology (Eaton, 1985; Jablensky, 1986). The Jarman combined index of social deprivation has been shown to be highly correlated with psychiatric admission rates for health districts in the South East Thames region, and may be used to estimate the degree of excess morbidity (Jarman, 1983, 1984; Hirsch, 1988; Thornicroft, 1992).

It seems reasonable therefore to use a deprivation-weighted population score to estimate morbidity within psychiatric sectors. Ethnicity also has a powerful influence on service utilisation, with non-White ethnic groups having a higher risk than their White neighbours of being admitted to psychiatric hospital, an increased risk of compulsory admission and a substantially increased risk of being diagnosed as suffering from schizophrenia (Ineichen *et al*, 1984; Harrison *et al*, 1988, 1989).

A further modifier of service use is the presence within a district of a large psychiatric institution and the nature of local psychiatric resettlement facilities (Paykel, 1990). The acceptability and appropriateness of the service model to be implemented is an important consideration. For example, in some areas, general practices are seen as the non-stigmatising facility that the local population traditionally uses as the pathway into mental health services. In other localities, the pathways into care are less defined, with less use of statutory services and more presentation to voluntary organisations and ethnic group facilities. This appears to be particularly likely in areas where the ethnic composition is not homogeneous. In such cases, rational division into patches should take into account the need for development of innovative services, which reflect the likely help-seeking behaviour acceptable to the local population. One approach to the question of how many beds and residential places are required in different of areas of England has been provided by Johnson *et al* (1997), as shown in Table 1.3 in Chapter 1.

Clarifying service priorities

The range of services needs to be considered when planning for the sector begins. The scheme outlined is not intended as a comprehensive, sequential pathway to a 'sector development blueprint', but seeks to delineate the routine elements of clinical, training, organisational and evaluation work likely to be encountered, with some suggested mechanisms for action.

An issue that needs to be addressed early in planning needs-led services is which patient groups are to be prioritised, and, by implication, which will not be targeted (Patmore & Weaver, 1990). Although the broad grouping of 'the seriously mentally ill' is often set as the highest priority, this is rarely specifically defined, with notable exceptions. Operational definitions of severe mental illness used by health service providers are outlined in Box 10.2. These are all health service only definitions, but it could be argued that in order to implement the current legislation on community care, which has an

Box 10.2
Definitions of severe mental illness

Goldman et al (1981)
(i) Diagnosis (DSM–III–R; American Psychiatric Association (APA), 1980) of:
  - schizophrenia and schizoaffective disorder   295.*x*
  - bipolar disorders and major depression   296.*x*
  - delusional (paranoid) disorder   297.*x*
(ii) Duration: at least one year since onset of disorder
(iii) Disability: sufficiently severe disability to seriously impair functioning or performance in at least one of the following areas:
  - occupation
  - family responsibilities
  - accommodation.

McLean & Liebowitz (1989)
At least one of the following must be present:
  (i)   two or more years contact with services
  (ii) depot prescribed
  (iii) ICD–10 295.*x* or 297.*x* (World Health Organization (WHO), 1992)
  (iv) three or more in-patient admissions in last two years
  (v)   three or more day patient episodes in last two years
  (vi) DSM–III highest level of adaptive functioning in the past year rates 5 or more

Tyrer (1985)
  - Patients with chronic psychosis
  - Two or more in-patient admissions in the past year
  - Contact with two or more psychiatric agencies in past year
  - Frequent consultations
  - Risk of being homeless/imprisoned

Ruggeri et al (2000)
  - two or more years duration of mental disorder
  - Global Assessment of Function Score ≤50

inherent assumption that agencies will form closer working links, there is a need to identify a common language to define service priorities. If the target group of severely mentally ill is defined, then the service can be assessed to establish whether it is targeting this group well or poorly (Figs 10.1 and 10.2; Thornicroft & Tansella, 1999).

The information infrastructure

To set up and monitor locally based mental health services, it is necessary to estimate the numbers of patients who fall within the priority group. One approach to this issue is to conduct a case

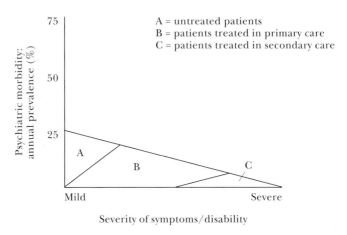

Fig. 10.1 Relationship between degree of disability and treatment setting (primary or secondary care) for a well-targeted service

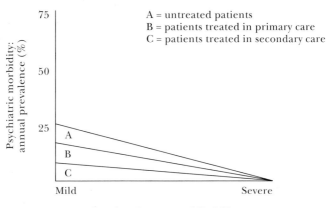

Fig. 10.2 Relationship between degree of disability and treatment setting (primary or secondary care) for poorly targeted services

identification exercise, drawing upon contacts by people with severely disabling mental illness with a wide range of services. A clear, systematic and consistent method of collecting clinical and social need and service usage data is required to inform the planning of the most appropriate service model for the local situation. As Shapiro *et al* (1985) conclude, there are limitations in each of the three methods most commonly used for this assessment. First, there are the broad estimates and projections derived from utilisation rates of services by defined patients (Goldberg *et al*, 1980; Goldman *et al*, 1981). Second, there are calculations based on the relationships of mental health disorders to age, gender, race, marital status, economic status and other social variables (Rosen & Goldsmith, 1981). Finally, needs are often defined by a focus on the seriously impaired chronically mentally ill (US Department of Health, 1980).

The most comprehensive method of eliciting, coding and storing the data listed above is the case register (Wing, 1989). Although such systems were formerly labour-intensive and tended to be used primarily as research and epidemiological tools, the recent availability of on-site microcomputers and minicomputers has made their widespread use for clinical service delivery a practical option in many areas. A rapidly growing number of general practices now have such systems, and there is increasing evidence that the establishment of health promotion or disease registers such as those for asthma and diabetes improve the quality of patient care. Kendrick *et al* (1991) present convincing evidence that this method is equally applicable to the care of individuals with mental health disorders.

Inter-agency planning and organisation

Between sectors and districts, there are wide variations in the functions served by different agencies. In general, health authorities have provided the bulk of in-patient and acute care, with day care being administered by a combination of statutory agencies. In the case of sheltered housing and work facilities, the situation is more variable, and in some areas it is social services or the voluntary sector that provide the majority of facilities. Likewise, individuals suffering from psychological and social distress can present initially to housing, policy, and social services, as well as to mental health facilities. In Britain, general practitioners (GPs) also play a major role in the care of those with both acute and chronic psychological disorders (Murray Parkes *et al*, 1962; Shepherd *et al*, 1966; Goldberg & Blackwell, 1970; Johnstone *et al*, 1984; Brown *et al*, 1988; Strathdee, 1992*a*; Department of Health, 1999). In many districts, the GP surgery constitutes the front-line for patients in crisis, whether or not they are concurrently in contact with the mental health teams.

In the absence of any core agency responsible for assuring the delivery and coordination of all services, informal joint working patterns are vital to meet the full range of needs, to achieve jointly owned policies and to avoid unnecessary duplication of services through parallel developments. At a strategic level, many local areas now have health improvement programmes and joint investment plans, which negotiate joint financing and management initiatives. Work with social services at the ground level has been improved by the development of community mental health centres, which allow joint crisis and assessment initiatives to flourish (Sayce *et al*, 1991). In addition, the development of case management (Thornicroft, 1991), and care coordination fora (Strathdee, 1992a) appear likely to facilitate the development of joint assessment instruments and the organisation of joint training.

Effective delivery of community care

Some fundamental questions remain. What constitutes the most effective form of organisation between patients, relatives, and statutory and non-statutory agencies, in the assessment of need? What is the best way to form an active partnership to provide a comprehensive range of services? As mentioned earlier, Philippe Paumelle, one of the first proponents of community care, provides some guidance for the theoretical resolution of this dilemma (Bennett, 1978). He considered that effective services were those that offered continuity of care, coordination of care, and integration of care. *Continuity of care,* he believed, could best be achieved by ensuring that persons and families were dealt with at all stages and at all levels of illness by the same team who had their own associated structures such as beds and clinics. Given the range of needs of individuals with mental health problems, *coordination of care* requires the introduction of multi-disciplinary and interagency teams to ensure that the range of treatments necessary to overcome the impairment and disability of the mentally ill be delivered.

The need for *integration of care* is underpinned by the premise that in any community, first contact for individuals in distress is often not with the psychiatric specialist team, but rather with persons in key positions of responsibility in the community, such as teachers, police, public health nurses, community nurses, social workers, and GPs (WHO, 1983). Any specialist team must therefore integrate its efforts with those of the non-specialists, as well as taking the lead in educating and counselling non-specialists.

Dichotomies in relation to the development of sector services

Within each agency, a similar issue requires attention. What is the most appropriate configuration of services provided by any single agency? Four dichotomies arise.

The sectorisation–district-wide dichotomy

How do we achieve the most appropriate balance between services that should be provided within the local sector and those that should have a district-wide remit? This applies particularly to rehabilitation services and crisis intervention services.

The specialist–generalist dichotomy

What is the optimal method of integrating specialist and generic staff both within sectors, for an entirely sectorised service, and between district and sector services for other configurations. For example, specialist rehabilitation outreach or drug and alcohol teams might primarily be a district service, but have identified members who provide continuity for patients by dual membership with specific sector teams. Similar issues apply to forensic facilities and psycho-therapy services.

The acute–continuing care dichotomy

What is the best distribution of workload and skills mix within the sector teams? A one-team sector model could, for example, care for the whole range of psychiatric morbidity within a small defined area; or, alternatively, two teams might divide responsibilities, with one providing primary care and acute assessment and treatment services, including acute in-patient work, and a second team accepting responsibility for the longer-term patients, including respite, rehabilitation, outreach, support and crisis intervention.

The primary care–mental health specialist dichotomy

How should integration and clear definition of responsibilities between primary and secondary care teams be developed? First contact for patients presenting in crisis or in the early signs of relapse is often with the primary care agencies (Strathdee, 1992*b*), including GPs and primary health teams, social workers and housing officers. Therefore, to what extent should mental health team personnel be attached to, or integrated within, the primary care framework? How can they ensure their commitments to the priority patient group against competing demands? Traditionally, this dilemma has confronted community psychiatric nurse (CPN) services.

The resolution of the final dichotomy is likely to be facilitated in future by the presence of large health centres and group practices that provide the critical number of incumbent GPs, referring an adequate number of patients and providing adequate space for these 'attached' specialist clinicians. These forms of integration are taking place insidiously with the move of psychologists (Broadhurst, 1972; Earl & Kincey, 1979), nurse therapists (Paykel *et al*, 1982; Marks, 1985), CPNs (Robertson & Scott, 1985; Oyebode *et al*, 1990), social workers (Corney & Bowen, 1980) and counsellors (Marsh & Barr, 1975; Martin & Mitchell, 1983) into primary care teams. Furthermore, there has been a relocation of psychiatric out-patient clinics to health centres (Strathdee & Williams, 1984; Tyrer, 1985; Pullen & Yellowlees, 1988).

An important element for the future is the indication in the National Service Framework that primary care groups (PCGs) and primary care trusts (PCTs) that fulfil the criteria shown in Box 10.3 may provide the range of adult mental health services that in the past have been provided by secondary mental health care.

Commissioning clinical teams and their bases

Fundamental to the success of a sectorised service is the nature and functioning of its multi-disciplinary team(s). Although the various

---

Box 10.3
Criteria necessary for PCGs and PCTs to provide adult mental health services

- Service user and carer involvement
- Advocacy arrangements
- Integration of care management and the Care Programme Approach (CPA)
- Effective partnerships with primary health care, social services, housing and other agencies including, where appropriate, the independent sector
- Board membership includes competent management of specialist mental health services
- Proportioned representation of mental health professionals on the executive of the PCT

disciplines were established to perform specific tasks, discussion about multi-disciplinary teams has taken place in the absence of close analysis. Ambelas (1991) proposes two approaches for determining the skills and discipline mix within any team: to focus on the needs for treatment, or to focus on the coordination of treatment and management. Ovretveit *et al* (1986*a*) have suggested that these and other relevant issues, such as responsibility, degree of autonomy, accountability, leadership and management, are best determined by the creation of an operational policy that includes such practical issues as aims, criteria for referral and discharge, nature and format of meetings and agendas, case allocation and management, reporting of workload, and development, support and training. The net effect of these considerations is that planners are faced with a range of options for the provision of community mental health teams, now in the context of the NHS Plan (Department of Health, 2000) (Thornicroft & Tansella, 1999; Thornicroft *et al*, 1999), as shown in Box 10.4.

The siting of the team-base is a fundamental decision that often reflects the philosophy of the model of service being developed, but is influenced by many variables. First, there is the need for efficient resource allocation. Central, highly resourced facilities, for example, hospital-based units, may appear more efficient and effective in terms of easy movement of staff between wards, training, information gathering and reduction in staff isolation, but be inflexible in addressing patients' needs. Second, the degree to which local statutory and non-statutory agencies inter-relate is vital; and third, the availability of suitable sites for the chosen model may be a decisive and pragmatic local factor.

Box 10.4
Seven types of community mental health team configuration in clinical practice

(1) Generic, multi-disciplinary community-based mental health teams (CMHTs)
(2) Generic CMHTs, supplemented by a crisis/home treatment team
(3) Generic CMHTs, supplemented by an assertive community treatment (ACT) team
(4) Generic CMHTs with assertive community treatment team and crisis/home treatment team
(5) Generic CMHT including augmented crisis or ACT functions
(6) Separate specialist teams providing specialist forms of treatment to subgroups of patients
(7) Specialist staff in particular evidence-based treatments placed in generic teams

Needs for training

In a review, Sturt & Waters (1985) advocated that for work in community-based settings, clinicians are required to develop skills beyond the purely clinical. In particular, they advocated the development of the ability to "recognise alternative resources to those found in hospital settings, obtain the skills of networking and the ability to administrate and manage". Ignorance of each other's training background may lead to difficulties in resolving issues of authority and responsibility within multi-disciplinary teams. They advocate that a regular activity within each team should be explanatory sessions when members of each discipline explain the rationale behind their thinking and formulate their concept of discipline-specific skills. The Royal College of Psychiatrists has suggested a valuable range of training experiences in psychiatry. However, there is a clear hiatus in the provision of practical training in service planning, development, implementation and evaluation.

Conclusions

We have argued that a geographical 'sector', with a defined population of about 50 000, forms a workable unit for the planning, provision and evaluation of community-oriented mental health services. So far, there is a dearth of information on the quantitative effects of such an approach to organising services. In our view, these questions are central to the proper implementation of community care for people with severe mental health problems, and to support the implementation of the National Service Framework for Mental Health. It is clear that many different service models can deliver the essential functions required of an at least adequate mental health service, as indicated in Table 10.1.

In future, we expect that a greater degree of flexibility will be required of mental health purchasers and providers in moving staffing resources across sites according to the needs of patients, and we shall see staff decreasingly fixed to beds. Second, we have given a range of places for each category, as we now find strong evidence for variations in local service requirements primarily according to local social and demographic characteristics. Finally, a truly comprehensive service could be expected to have provisions in most or all of the categories, although this is currently far from the case, and indeed many districts have places in only two or three of the categories. There is a clear interdependence between these types of provision, and where whole groups of services are absent, this will produce a greater demand upon, and use of, those services that do exist. In our view, a necessary

TABLE 10.1
The relationship between service functions and service models

Service functions	Service models
Crisis intervention	Domiciliary visits Casualty department Crisis-intervention teams Drop-in services at community mental health centres (CMHCs) Community crisis beds CPN crisis-response service GPs Approved social worker day/night service 24-hour telephone help-line
Acute care/asylum	Local/district intensive care Local/regional medium-secure facilities
Assessment	Hospital out-patient clinics Primary care/health centre liaison clinics CMHC clinics Sessional input to social services, housing, voluntary sector

mechanism to realise such plans is to set clear, realistic and ambitious service development targets (Department of Health, 1999). We expect that among the prime challenges to mental health services for the next decade will be: extending the variety of services offered; diversifying working relationships with voluntary, user, informal carer and statutory services; and carefully measuring the outcomes of these interventions.

References

AMBELAS, A. (1991) The task of treatment and the multidisciplinary team. *Psychiatric Bulletin*, **15**, 77–79.

AMERICAN PSYCHIATRIC ASSOCIATION (1980) *Diagnostic and Statistical Manual of Mental Disorders. Third revision (DSM–III–R)*. Washington, DC: APA.

ANDREWS, G. (1990) *The Tolkien Report. A Description of a Model Mental Health Service*. Sydney: University of New South Wales.

BECKER, T., HOLLOWAY, F., MCCRONE, P., ET AL (1998) Evolving service interventions in Nunhead and Norwood. PRiSM Psychosis Study 2. *British Journal of Psychiatry*, **173**, 371–375.

BENNETT, D. (1978) Community psychiatry. *British Journal of Psychiatry*, **132**, 209–220.

BROADHURST, A. (1972) Clinical psychology and the general practitioner. *British Medical Journal, i*, 793–795.

BROWN, R. M., STRATHDEE, G., CHRISTIE-BROWN, J. R., *ET AL* (1988) A comparison of referrals to primary care and hospital out-patient clinics. *British Journal of Psychiatry,* **153**, 168–173.

BURNS, T. & PRIEBE, S. (1999) Mental health care failure in England. Myth and reality. *British Journal of Psychiatry,* **174**, 191–192.

—— , BEADSMOORE, A., BHAT, A. V., *ET AL* (1993) A controlled trial of home-based acute psychiatric services. I: Clinical and social outcome. *British Journal of Psychiatry,* **163**, 49–54.

CORNEY, R. H. & BOWEN, B. A. (1980) Referrals to social workers: a comparative study of a local authority intake team with a general practice attachment team. *Journal of the Royal College of General Practitioners,* **309**, 139–147.

DEPARTMENT OF HEALTH (1999) *The National Service Framework for Mental Health. Modern Standards and Service Models.* London: Department of Health.

—— (2000) *The NHS Plan.* London: Department of Health.

EARL, L. & KINCEY, J. (1979) Clinical psychology in general practice: a controlled trial evaluation. *Journal of the Royal College of General Practitioners,* **32**, 32–37.

EATON, W. W. (1985) Epidemiology of schizophrenia. *Epidemiologic Reviews,* **7**, 105–126.

FALLOON, I. (1988) The prevention of morbidity in schizophrenia. In: *Handbook of Behavioural Family Therapy* (ed. I. Falloon). London: Hutchinson.

GLOVER, G. (1989) Private sector psychiatric services (letter). *Psychiatric Bulletin,* **13**, 198–199.

—— (1996) The Mental Illness Needs Index (MINI). In: *Commissioning Mental Health Services* (eds G. Thornicroft & G. Strathdee). London: HMSO.

GOLDBERG, D. P. & BLACKWELL, B. (1970) Psychiatric illness in general practice: a detailed study using a new method of case identification. *British Medical Journal, ii,* 439–443.

——, REGIER, D. & BURNS, T. (1980) *Use of Health and Mental Health Outpatient Services in Four Organised Health Care Settings.* Mental Health Services Systems Reports, Series DN No. 1. Washington, DC:US Government Printing Office.

GOLDMAN, H., GATTOZZI, A. & TAUBE, C. (1981) Defining and counting the chronically mentally ill. *Community Psychiatry,* **31**, 21.

HANSSON, L. (1989) Utilisation of psychiatric in-patient care. *Acta Psychiatrica Scandinavica,* **79**, 571–578.

——, ÖIESVOLD, T., GÖSTAS, G., *ET AL* (1995) The Nordic Comparative Study on Sectorized Psychiatry. Part I: Treated point-prevalence and characteristics of the psychiatric services. *Acta Psychiatrica Scandinavica,* **91**, 41–47.

HARRISON, G., OWENS, D., HOLTON, A., *ET AL* (1988) A prospective study of severe mental disorder in Afro-Caribbean patients. *Psychological Medicine,* **18**, 643–657.

——, HOLTON, A., NEILSON, D., *ET AL* (1989) Severe mental disorder in Afro-Caribbean patients: some social demographic and service factors. *Psychological Medicine,* **19**, 683–696.

HIRSCH, S. (1988) *Psychiatric Beds and Resources: Factors Influencing Bed Use and Service Planning.* London: Gaskell.

HOLLOWAY, F. (1988) Day care and community support. In: *Community Care in Practice* (eds A. Lavender & F. Holloway). Chichester: Wiley.

—— & CARSON, J. (1998) Intensive case management for the severely mentally ill. A controlled trial. *British Journal of Psychiatry,* **172**, 19–22.

INEICHEN, B., HARRISON, G. & MORGAN, H. G. (1984) Psychiatric hospital admissions in Bristol. I. Geographic and ethnic factors. *British Journal of Psychiatry,* **145**, 600–604.

JABLENSKY, A. (1986) Epidemiology of schizophrenia: A European perspective. *Schizophrenia Bulletin,* **12**, 52–73.

JARMAN, B. (1983) Identification of underprivileged areas. *British Medical Journal,* **286**, 1705–1709.

—— (1984) Underprivileged areas: validation and distribution of scores. *British Medical Journal,* **289**, 1587–1592.

——, HIRSCH, S. & WHITE, P. (1992) Predicting psychiatric admission rates. *British Medical Journal*, **304**, 1146–1150.

JOHNSON, S. & THORNICROFT, G. (1993) The sectorisation of psychiatric services in England and Wales. *Social Psychiatry and Psychiatric Epidemiology*, **28**, 45–47.

—— & —— (1995) Emergency psychiatric services in England and Wales. *British Medical Journal*, **311**, 287–288.

——, BROOKS E., RAMSAY R., *ET AL* (1997) The structure and functioning of London's mental health services. In: *London's Mental Health* (eds S. Johnson, R. Ramsay, G. Thornicroft, *et al*), pp. 22–249). London: King's Fund.

JOHNSTONE, E. C., OWENS, D. G. C., GOLD, A., *ET AL* (1984) Schizophrenic patients discharged from hospital – a follow-up study. *British Journal of Psychiatry*, **145**, 586–590.

JONES, K. (1972) *A History of the Mental Health Services*. London: Routledge and Kegan Paul.

KENDRICK, A., SIBBALD, B., BURNS, T., *ET AL* (1991) Role of general practitioners in care of long term mentally ill patients. *British Medical Journal*, **302**, 508–511.

KINGDON, D. (1989) Mental health services: results of a survey of English district plans. *Psychiatric Bulletin*, **13**, 77–78.

KLUITER, H. (1997) Inpatient treatment and care arrangements to replace or avoid it – searching for an evidence-based balance. *Current Opinion in Psychiatry*, **10**, 160–167.

LEHMAN A. F., STEINWACH D. M. AND THE CO-INVESTIGATORS OF THE PORT PROJECT (1998) Translating research into practice: the schizophrenia Patient Outcomes Research Team (PORT) treatment recommendations. *Schizophrenia Bulletin*, **24**, 1–10.

LEHMAN, A. G., THOMPSON, J. W., DIXON, L. B., *ET AL* (1995) Schizophrenia: treatment outcomes research – editor's introduction. *Schizophrenia Bulletin*, **21**, 561–566.

LEWIS G. (1997) Closing the gap between research and practice: new evidence is required. *British Journal of Psychiatry*, **171**, 227.

LEVINE, M. (1981) *The History and Politics of Community Mental Health*. Oxford: Oxford University Press.

LINDHOLM, H. (1983) Sectorized psychiatry. A methodological study of the effects of reorganization on patients treated at a mental hospital. *Acta Psychiatrica Scandinavica*, **67**, Supplement 304.

MARKS, I. (1985) Controlled trial of psychiatric nurse therapists in primary care. *British Medical Journal*, **240**, 1181–1184.

MARKS, J. N., GOLDBERG, D. P. & HILLIER, V. F. (1979) Determinants of the ability of general practitioners to detect psychiatric illness. *Psychological Medicine*, **9**, 337–353.

MARSH, G. N. & BARR, J. (1975) Marriage guidance counselling in a group practice. *Journal of the Royal College of General Practitioners*, **25**, 73–75.

MARSHALL, M., GRAY, A., LOCKWOOD, A., *ET AL* (1997*a*) Case management for severe mental disorders. In: *Schizophrenia Module of the Cochrane Database Systematic Reviews* (eds C. E. Adams, L. Duggan, J. de Jesus Mari, *et al*). Oxford: Update Software.

——, ——, ——, *ET AL* (1997*b*) Assertive community treatment. In: *Schizophrenia Module of the Cochrane Database Systematic Reviews* (eds C. E. Adams, L. Duggan, J. de Jesus Mari, *et al*). Oxford: Update Software.

MARTIN, E. & MITCHELL, H. (1983) A counsellor in general practice: a one year survey. *Journal of the Royal College of General Practitioners*, **33**, 366–367.

McLEAN, E. K. & LIEBOWITZ, J. A. (1989) Towards a working definition of the long-term mentally ill (letter). *Psychiatric Bulletin*, **13**, 251–252.

MUESER, K. T., BOND, G. R., DRAKE, R. E., *ET AL* (1998) Models of community care for severe mental illness: a review of research on case management. *Schizophrenia Bulletin*, **24**, 37–74.

MUIJEN, M., MARKS, I., CONNOLLY, J., *ET AL* (1992*a*) Home based care versus standard hospital care for patients with severe mental illness: a randomised controlled trial. *British Medical Journal*, **304**, 749–754.

——, ——, ——, *ET AL* (1992*b*) The daily living programme. A preliminary comparison of community versus hospital-based treatment for the seriously mentally ill facing emergency admission. *British Journal of Psychiatry*, **160**, 379–384.

MURRAY PARKES, C., BROWN, G. W. & MONCK, E. M. (1962) The general practitioner and the schizophrenic patient. *British Medial Journal*, i, 972–976.

NATIONAL INSTITUTE OF MENTAL HEALTH (1987) *Towards a Model for a Comprehensive Community-Based Mental Health System*. Washington DC: NIMH.

OVRETVEIT, J. (1986) *Case Responsibility in Multi-Disciplinary Teams*. London: Good Practices in Mental Health.

OYEBODE, F., CUMELLA, S., GARDEN, G., *ET AL* (1990) Diagnosis-related groups: implications for psychiatry. *Psychiatric Bulletin*, **14**, 1–3.

PATMORE, C. & WEAVER, J. (1990) *A Survey of Community Mental Health Centres*. London: Good Practices in Mental Health.

PAYKEL, E. (1990) Innovations in mental health in the primary care system. In: *Mental Health Service Evaluation* (eds I. Marks & R. Scott). Cambridge: Cambridge University Press.

——, MANGEN, S. P., GRIFFITH, J. H., *ET AL* (1982) Community psychiatric nursing for neurotic patients: a controlled trial. *British Journal of Psychiatry*, **140**, 573–581.

PULLEN, I. & YELLOWLEES, A. (1988) Scottish psychiatrists in primary health-care settings. A silent majority. *British Journal of Psychiatry*, **153**, 663–666.

ROBERTSON, H. & SCOTT, D. J. (1985) Community psychiatric nursing: a survey of patients and problems. *Journal of the Royal College of General Practitioners*, **35**, 130–132.

ROSEN, B. & GOLDSMITH, H. (1981) *Evaluation and Program Planning Vol. 4. The Health Demographic Profile System*. Elmsford, NY: Pergamon Press.

RUGGERI, M., LEESE, M., THORNICROFT, G., *ET AL* (2000) Definition and prevalence of severe and persistent mental illness. *British Journal of Psychiatry*, **177**, 149–155.

SAARENTO, O., OIESVOLD, T., SYTEMA, S., *ET AL* (1998) The Nordic comparative study on sectorised psychiatry: continuity of care related to characteristics of the psychiatric services and the patients. *Social Psychiatry and Psychiatric Epidemiology*, **33**, 521–527.

SAYCE, L., CRAIG, T. K. J. & BOARDMAN, A. P. (1991) The development of community mental health centres in the United Kingdom. *Social Psychiatry and Psychiatric Epidemiology*, **26**, 14–20.

SHAPIRO, S., SKINNER, E., KRAMER, M., *ET AL* (1985) Measuring need for mental health services in a general population medical care. *Medical Care*, **23**, 1033–1043.

SHEPHERD, M., COOPER, B., BROWN, A., *ET AL* (1966) *Psychiatric Illness in General Practice*. London: Oxford University Press.

STEIN, L. & SANTOS, A. (1998) *Assertive Community Treatment of Persons with Severe Mental Illness*. New York: Norton.

STEVENS, A. & GABBAY, J. (1991) Needs assessment, needs assessment. *Health Trends*, **23**, 20–23.

STRATHDEE, G. (1990) The delivery of psychiatric care. *Journal of the Royal Society of Medicine*, **83**, 222–225.

—— (1992*a*) The interface between psychiatry and primary care in the management of schizophrenic patients in the community. In: *The Primary Care of Schizophrenia* (eds R. Jenkins, V. Field & R. Young). London: HMSO.

—— (1992*b*) Liaison between general practice and secondary care teams towards the prevention and treatment of neural disorders. In: *The Prevention of Depression and Anxiety in Primary Care* (eds R. Jenkins & J. Newton), pp. 113–124. London: HMSO.

—— & THORNICROFT, G. (1992) Community sectors for needs-led mental health services. In: *Measuring Mental Health Needs* (eds G. Thornicroft, C. R. Brewin & J. Wing), pp. 140–162. London: Gaskell.

—— & WILLIAMS, P. (1984) A survey of psychiatrists in primary care: the silent growth of a new service. *Journal of the Royal College of General Practioners*, **34**, 615–618.

STURT, J. & WATERS, H. (1985) Role of the psychiatrist in community-based mental health care. *Lancet, i,* 507–508.

TALBOT, J. (1983) *Unified Mental Health Systems. Utopia Unrealised.* Washington, DC: Jossey Bass.

TANSELLA, M. (1989) Evaluating community psychiatric services. In: *Epidemiological and Social Psychiatry. Essays in Honour of Michael Shepherd* (eds P. Williams, G. Wilkinson & K. Rawnsley), pp. 386–403. London: Routledge.

TEAGUE, G. B., BOND, G. R. & DRAKE, R. E. (1998) Program fidelity in assertive community treatment: Development and use of a measure. *American Journal of Orthopsychiatry,* **68**, 216–232.

THORNICROFT, G. (1991) Social deprivation and rates of treated mental disorder. Developing statistical models to predict psychiatric service utilisation. *British Journal of Psychiatry,* **158**, 475–484.

—— (1992) The TAPS project. (6): New long-stay psychiatric patients and social deprivation. *British Journal of Psychiatry,* **161**, 621–624.

—— & BEBBINGTON, P. (1988) Deinstitutionalisation: from hospital closure to service development. *British Journal of Psychiatry,* **155**, 739–753.

—— & TANSELLA, M. (1999) *The Mental Health Matrix. A Manual to Improve Service.* Cambridge: Cambridge University Press.

——, STRATHDEE, G., PHELAN, M., *ET AL* (1998*a*) Rationale and design. PRiSM Psychosis Study I. *British Journal of Psychiatry,* **173**, 363–370.

——, WYKES, T., HOLLOWAY F., *ET AL* (1998*b*) From efficacy to effectiveness in community mental health services. PRiSM Psychosis Study 10. *British Journal of Psychiatry,* **173**, 423–427.

——, BECKER, T., HOLLOWAY, F., *ET AL* (1999) Community mental health teams: evidence or belief? *British Journal of Psychiatry,* **175**, 508–513.

TODD, J. W. (1984) Wasted resources. Referral to hospital. *Lancet, ii,* 1089.

TORREY, E., ERDMAN, K. & WOLFE, S. (1990) *Care of the Seriously Mentally Ill. A Rating of Scale Programs* (3rd edition). Washington, DC: Public Citizen Health Research Group and National Alliance for the Mentally Ill.

TYRER, P. (1985) The 'hive' system. A model for a psychiatric service. *British Journal of Psychiatry,* **146**, 571–575.

——, TURNER, R. & JOHNSON, A. (1989) Integrated hospital and community psychiatric services and use of in-patient beds. *British Medical Journal,* **299**, 298–300.

——, MORGAN, J., VAN HORN, E., *ET AL* (1995) A randomised controlled trial of close monitoring of vulnerable psychiatric patients. *Lancet,* **345**, 756–759

UK700 GROUP (1999) Comparison of intensive and standard case management for patients with psychosis. Rationale of the trial. *British Journal of Psychiatry,* **174**, 74–78.

US DEPARTMENT OF HEALTH AND HUMAN SERVICES STEERING COMMITTEE ON THE CHRONICALLY MENTALLY ILL (1980) *Towards a National Plan for the Chronically Mentally Ill.* Washington, DC: US Government Printing Office.

WALSH, D. (1987) Mental health service models in Europe. In: *Mental Health Services in Pilot Study Areas: Report on a European Study.* Copenhagen: WHO.

WING, J. (1989) *Health Services Planning and Research. Contributions from Psychiatric Case Registers.* London: Gaskell.

WORLD HEALTH ORGANIZATION (1983) *First Contact Mental Health Care.* Copenhagen: WHO Regional Office for Europe.

—— (1992) *International Classification of Diseases and Related Health Problems. Tenth revision (ICD–10).* Geneva: WHO.

11 Needs from a user perspective

MARION BEEFORTH and HELEN WOOD

This chapter will describe the service system that is seen as needed, from the viewpoint of the people who use the services. The information has been obtained from two primary sources. First are the issues raised at the Mental Health Task Force User conferences. Ten conferences were held across Britain, with 100 users at each, totalling the views of over 1000 service users/survivors. The second source is a report on an extensive review of user literature (51 articles) commissioned by the Audit Commission for their review of mental health services (Wood, 1994). The need for purchasers and providers to take account of service users views is well noted and acknowledged (Department of Health, 1989; Beeforth *et al*, 1990; Audit Commission, 1994; Mental Health Foundation, 1994). We agree with the view that "user participation is important making the service system effective in meeting individual need" (Audit Commission, 1994, p. 38). From these sources, we have identified 10 priority areas of needs from a user perspective:

- access to information
- presence of a charter
- availability 24 hours a day, seven days a week
- practical help
- flexibility and responsiveness to individual need
- user-run services
- advocacy
- access to specialist help
- something meaningful to do during the day
- an integrated system with continuity of care.

Access to information

A wide range of information needs to be available, in a variety of formats (written, verbal, tape and video) using clear, simple language. It should be available in a range of languages and locations, easily accessible and preferably written by or with service users. Information may need to be given more than once, as at times of distress it can be very difficult to remember things or take it all in. The most commonly described types of information requested include:

- rights: personal and legal rights, rights for redress, how to make complaints and how those complaints will be addressed;
- medication: including risks and benefits, side-effects, the expected duration of prescription, monitoring and review procedures;
- treatment: a range of treatment options available and alternatives to medical treatment and talking therapies;
- care plan: a written copy of people's care plan should be given to them;
- hospital admission: admission procedures, ward procedures and policies, length of stay, facilities, rules, status and visiting;
- services and facilities: what is available locally, both in hospital and in the community across all agencies, including self-help groups, how to access them and when they are open;
- staff: what are the different roles, what they can offer, how to contact them, when they are available and what cover is available for when they are away;
- welfare and benefits: what users' entitlements are, how they apply, how hospital admission might affect their benefits and whether they can work; and
- advocacy: what independent services are available, what type of advocacy, what user forums are around and how to contact them.

Presence of a charter

Many people who come into contact with services would find it extremely helpful to have access to a charter, this being a clear statement of intent, outlining standards of what can be expected. It should include the following.

Statement of intent

Confidentiality of information is important: people need to feel that private and distressing information they pass on to professionals will be kept safe and not passed on to others without their express permission.

Safety

People need to feel that when they come into hospital (or a community facility) personal safety is held as a high priority, from the point of view of both violence and sexual harassment/assault. This is particularly the case for women, many of whom seek women-only units. The importance of safety should also be extended to personal belongings. Provider units should make it explicit how they intend to keep people suffering distress safe. Safety also includes safe use of medication (not overprescribed).

Complaints procedure

People need to know that there are accessible means by which they can express their concerns about the treatment they are receiving, particularly to an independent source. The procedure should clearly state how to make a complaint and to whom, how it is dealt with and how long it might take. A written and verbal response to complaints should be given.

Needs-led service

Service users want to know that the service they receive will reflect their specific needs and situation, and be responsive to age, gender and cultural background. Flexibility and choice in treatment provision is essential, alongside their active involvement in determining the service they receive.

Involvement in decision-making

People want to know that they will have opportunities to be actively involved in making decisions that affect their own lives.

Support

People want to feel confident that they will receive the right level of support necessary to achieve a desirable standard of quality of life. They do not want to feel overpowered or ignored by services.

Availability 24 hours a day, seven days a week

Service users have for many years expressed the viewpoint that they cannot contain their crisis or distress to Monday–Friday, 9.00am–

5.00pm. Help needs to be available and accessible at the time when it is needed. In many instances, this can prevent an escalation of the problem and reduce the demand for hospitalisation and crisis services. In addition to specialist health assistance, there needs to be provision of social supports in the form of evening and weekend activities. Social isolation is a frequent life experience of people in contact with mental health services. Service users need to know that there is somewhere they can go to meet people if they need support and/or social opportunities. Improvements to services would include:

- accessible help in times of crisis: including alternatives to hospital admission, e.g. crisis house, telephone helplines and response 24 hours a day, seven days a week;
- focus on prevention and early intervention work: helping people develop coping strategies, regular contact and monitoring of well-being;
- prompt response: short waiting times;
- access to evening and weekend activities and support;
- extended availability of staff: e.g. 8.00am–8.00pm seven-day cover as a baseline for service provision.

Practical help

One of the most strongly expressed needs is that of access to practical help. In many instances, neglect to attend to basic needs creates crisis situations and enhances feelings of not being able to cope. Services must attend to people's most basic needs first, if they are to make any impact on general emotional well-being. This help should be imaginatively and flexibly offered, in many instances through multi-agency collaborative working practices:

- maximising income: access to welfare and benefits advice to ensure that people have a sustainable income to live on is essential;
- financial assistance: assistance with keeping up to date with bills, rent and negotiating the housing and welfare system; help with money management is also needed;
- help finding appropriate housing;
- activities of daily living: practical help with basic tasks at home, e.g. cooking, home maintenance, shopping, personal care, etc.
- help to build up self-confidence;
- social contacts: support and introduction to social networks that individuals can develop; and
- peer support: creating opportunities for support through social clubs, user groups/forums, peer advocacy and self-help groups.

Flexibility and responsiveness to individual needs

It can be very difficult to objectively monitor a service's ability to be flexible and responsive to needs. It is not a building, nor a number of professionals, the indicators frequently presented as the availability of a service. Purchasers and providers need to identify creative mechanisms for auditing service outcomes in relation to their ability to create appropriate and responsive service provision. Of course, the most candid measure is to ask service users. Flexible and responsive service features might include:

- respect for individuality: every individual's needs will differ according to age, culture, gender, personal background and social supports;
- choice: there should be opportunities for people to have choices over the type and style of treatment/service that might benefit them. This includes having alternatives and choice in location of service, alternatives to being admitted to hospital, choice of workers and treatment interventions including non-medical treatments;
- a multi-disciplinary assessment;
- involvement in decision-making: having their views taken into account;
- an integrated system of health and social care; and
- recording unmet need: for use in future planning.

User-run services

Frequently, people who have been in contact with mental health services have noted that they would prefer services that are run by others who have had similar experiences. Service users as a group seek to have a more equal partnership with providers of services, being actively involved in determining, planning, providing and monitoring services. This may involve having control over their own resources or working in partnership with agencies, either as purchasers or as providers. The literature review for the Audit Commission report (1994) noted a preference for user-run facilities and drop-ins as alternatives to the more traditional medical model of many statutory services. The Mental Health Task Force has produced national guidelines for a framework for local charters for user involvement. Real involvement requires more than just broad-based consultation exercises: it also encompasses people's active participation in decision-making forums:

- broader user involvement: at individual, unit, organisational and purchasing levels;
- services run for and by other service users;
- support for involvement: provision of resources, information, practical assistance, training, forums and structures, views listened to and financial reward for involvement;
- support for workers;
- opportunities: to be involved and for people to get together without professionals/service managers; and
- training: for staff to allow users to be involved fully and for service users to acquire the skills and confidence to do the job.

Advocacy

Access to advocacy is having someone, independent from the service, who will assist individuals in obtaining the services they need, or in making a complaint. It could involve someone speaking on their behalf, or with them, to ensure that their views are heard and individual rights are respected. It cannot be effectively done by a keyworker, other than in pursuing a negotiated care plan. The right to seek an independent advocate (of their own choice), if desired, is seen as extremely important and necessary. This is particularly the case for people under the Mental Health Act. There should be accessible information on how to access an advocate, and this person should be freely able to make contact with the individual concerned. Service users are very clear that a keyworker can not fulfil this role as an independent voice:

- peer/citizen/legal advocacy: these are all different types of advocacy and it should be made clear which is on offer;
- essential for people detained under the Mental Health Act: training available, local charter for standards and support for independent projects.

Access to specialist help

Within the service system, there should be opportunities for people to gain access to specialist help, advice and treatment if and when desired. Involvement with specialist services should be negotiated. People in contact with the mental health service should also have equitable access to good physical care:

- benefits and welfare advice;
- social services staff;

- health professionals: physical and mental health professionals;
- education and employment specialists.

Meaningful activities

People are looking for opportunities to participate in activities that help build skills, confidence and interests that are relevant to their lifestyles. Support needs to be available to help people to use ordinary local resources, to enhance their feeling part of the local community and to re-engage them with community life away from specialist services. Help with employment is extremely important, as well as availability of drop-ins and centres offering support in times of need and activities that:

- are valued, interesting and stimulating;
- assist the development of useful skills: work, social, leisure, educational and spiritual opportunities;
- reflect individuals' lives in terms of race, culture, gender, age and religion;
- promote integration with the community;
- are available in a range of settings: these include naturally occurring community facilities, specialist facilities and people's homes;
- promote choice: people may not want to do exactly the same thing every day; and
- are available evenings and weekends.

Integrated services

Purchasers need to establish an integrated network of services, promoting continuity and collaborative working. People often find it difficult to navigate their way around the range of different service agencies (including health and social services, primary care, housing and welfare). Very often, people feel that they fall between the cracks or end up in a position where two, or often three, agencies are working in opposition, with no one knowing what anyone else is doing – a very confusing and distressing position for the individual concerned to be in. A number of factors contribute to integration of services:

- joint commissioning of health and social care: integrated system of care management and the Care Programme Approach (CPA) with joint needs assessment;

- better collaboration with community agencies: especially local Black and other ethnic minority community groups and voluntary organisations;
- integration with primary care: including better communication between primary and secondary care agencies;
- good communication systems;
- for people with longer-term support needs, there should be one named individual (with holiday cover) responsible for coordination and liaison across agencies and between hospital and community services; and
- evaluation: mechanisms for evaluating effectiveness of service systems should be established and incorporate users as part of this process.

Monitoring user participation

The following is a sample of questions that can be asked in monitoring how both purchaser and provider units facilitate and support users in influencing service provision. They are not in any particular order of merit, but can be used as a baseline for setting standards to ensure user participation.

- Do you provide training to enable users to do this?
- Are all people applying for jobs with your organisation sent information about your policy on user involvement?
- Are there arrangements for involving users in professional training?
- Is there a particular service you are proud of? If so, can you describe it?
- Does your trust involve users in planning groups?
- Does your trust have an independent advocacy service?
- Who runs this service?
- Do you support user groups/patients councils?
- Do all units have user groups or patient councils?
- Do you fund user groups?
- Where do they meet?
- Do you let them use your photocopiers?
- Who pays their telephone bills?
- Who funds them?
- Do you have a user's charter negotiated with local users?
- Do you know the local charter?
- Are your services evaluated by users, so that the services are accountable to users?

- Do you have direct links with user groups?
- Is there a named person responsible for user involvement?
- Are users involved in interviewing new staff members?
- Are they democratically elected?
- Are people able to discuss their preferences about treatment?
- Do people have a choice of worker, or can they change their psychiatrist, for example, to have a woman worker?
- Have there been changes resulting from consultation with users? What evidence can you show for this?

Within the purchasing process, commissioners should ensure that users views are clearly taken account of, and that both the ideology and the practical implementation of user involvement is made explicit in this process.

Acknowledgement

This chapter is adapted from Chapter 18 of *Commissioning Mental Health Services* (eds G. Thornicroft & G. Strathdee, 1996). Crown copyright material is reproduced with the permission of the Controller of Her Majesty's Stationery Office.

References

AUDIT COMMISSION (1994) *Finding a Place. A Review of Mental Health Services for Adults.* London: HMSO.

BEEFORTH, M., CONLON, E. V., HOSER, B., *ET AL* (EDS) (1990) *Whose Service is it Anyway? Users Views on Co-ordinating Community Care.* London: National Unit for Psychiatric Research and Development.

——, CONLON, E. & GRALEY, R. (1994) *Have We Got News for You. User Evaluation of Case Management.* London: Sainsbury Centre for Mental Health.

BERESFORD, E. & HARDING, T. (EDS) (1993) *A Challenge to Change. Practical Experiences of Building User Led Services.* London: National Institute of Social Work.

BRANDON, A. & BRANDON, D. (1992) *Consumers as Colleagues.* London: MIND.

CROFT, S. & BERESFORD, E. (1993) *Getting Involved. A Practical Manual.* London: Open Services Project and Joseph Rowntree Foundation.

DEPARTMENT OF HEALTH (1989) *Caring for People. Community Care in the Next Decade and Beyond.* London: HMSO.

HUTCHISON, M., LINTON, G. & LUCAS, J. (1992) *User Involvement Information Pack. From Policy to Practice.* London: MIND Southeast.

MENTAL HEALTH FOUNDATION (1994) *Creating Community Care. Report of the Mental Health Foundation into Community Care for People with Severe Mental Illness.* London: Mental Health Foundation.

NATIONAL SCHIZOPHRENIA FELLOWSHIP (1992) *How to Involve Users and Carers. Guidelines on Involvement in Planning, Running and Monitoring Care Services.* London: NSF.

ROGERS, A., PILGRIM, D. & LACEY, R. (1993) *Experiencing Psychiatry. Users Views of Services.* London: MIND.

SMITH, H. (1988) *Collaboration for Change. Partnership between Service Users, Planners and Managers for Mental Health Services.* London: King's Fund Centre.

THORNICROFT, G. & STRATHDEE, G. (EDS) (1996) *Commissioning Mental Health Services.* London: HMSO.

USER CENTRED SERVICES GROUP (1993) *Building Bridges between People Who Use Services and People Who Provide Services.* London: National Institute of Social Work.

WOOD, H. (1994) *What do Service Users Want from Mental Health Services. Report to the Audit Commission for Finding a Place. A Review of Mental Health Services for Adults.* London: Audit Commission.

12 Costing psychiatric interventions

JENNIFER BEECHAM and MARTIN KNAPP

When we mean to build,
We first survey the plot, then draw the model;
And when we see the figure of the house,
Then must we rate the cost of the erection;
Which, if we find outweighs ability,
What do we then but draw anew the model
In fewer offices, or at least desist
To build at all? (Shakespeare, *King Henry IV, Part II*)

The demands and needs for cost information in psychiatric contexts have multiplied considerably in recent years, but have often been frustrated by inadequate data. The typical costs data available to the policy-maker, manager, clinical professional or researcher have been dominated until recently by age-old accounting practices and line management arrangements, and constrained by fragmentation of responsibility. Most limiting of all, costs data have rarely been used in making decisions about individual cases. In considering the demands and needs for costs in psychiatry, this chapter describes a research instrument – the Client Service Receipt Inventory (CSRI; Beecham & Knapp, 1992) – which has been developed and extensively applied in order to meet some of these needs. The chapter includes illustrations of applications of data recorded using the CSRI.

Scarcity and costs

It is difficult to think of a health care system, in the present day or in the past, that has not faced resource constraints. Demands and needs for health care almost always exceed available supplies. Indeed, often the pressures of scarcity have forced the complete re-drawing or abandonment of promising plans and laudable aspirations. A current example is the push to develop better community-based mental health services, where the needs-led aspirations of the 1990 National Health Service (NHS) and Community Care Act have been compromised in some localities by severe shortages of appropriate services, giving way to supply-led service arrangements (Johnson *et al*, 1997).

We should not be surprised – or even perhaps particularly depressed – by this and other examples of policy or preferred practice fettered by the scarcity of resources. Any lack of surprise should not be for the cynical reason that there always seems to be a gulf between political rhetoric and actual delivery, but because scarcity is the fundamental reality. Aspiration will and should always run ahead of attainability.

Recognition that there are insufficient resources to meet expressed demands or underlying needs is the prompt to examine carefully how those resources are deployed. Almost every debate in and about Britain's mental health care services boils down to a discussion – sometimes a heated disagreement – about resource use. In particular, can they be employed more productively (that is, with greater efficiency) or more fairly (with greater equity) in one use rather than another? Almost any attempt to answer these efficiency and equity questions will involve collecting and analysing quality evidence on needs, outcomes and of course costs. This chapter focuses on the last of these elements.

Demand

Demands for cost information stem from a variety of policy, practice and research needs. Notwithstanding the well-known difficulties of defining and measuring need, it has been remarked that there have not only been increases in levels of need for mental health services, but also growing gaps between latent or assessed needs and supplies of services to meet them. Certainly, the ageing of the population is increasing the numbers of people with dementia, posing major new challenges for public sector health and social care services (Knapp *et al*, 1998*a*). There is evidence of growing needs for child and adolescent mental health services (Costello *et al*, 1993), and the Psychiatric Morbidity Surveys of 1993/1994 uncovered large residuals of unmet needs (Meltzer *et al*, 1995*a,b*).

Resource limitations, or economic pressures generally, can create their own vicious circles. Needs that are inadequately addressed one year because of supply constraints can return, perhaps with a crisis-like vengeance, to dog providers in subsequent years. Child and adolescent mental health problems are closely associated with psychiatric and other problems in adulthood, unless the continuities can be broken with effective early treatment (Maughan & Rutter, 1998). These growing needs and their attendant problems represent latent demands for economic information. They are the underpinning causes of scarcity, and the underlying reasons for needing to adopt soundly based allocation criteria, such as efficiency and equity.

Increasingly, these latent demands get turned into expressed demands for costs information, although the transition is by no means straightforward (Knapp, 1997). There are many such demands (see Box 12.1). For instance, the substantial changes to the mental health care system announced by UK ministers soon after the Labour government came to power in June 1997, many of them developed in the National Service Framework launched in 1999, clearly need wide-ranging accurate resource utilisation data to inform local and national decisions. Governments always need resource information of this kind, but no more so than during a period of rapid change, as the next few years promise to be. Similarly, the licensing of new drugs and the development of new psychosocial interventions generate demands for information, not just on efficacy but on resource consequences (cost-effectiveness and cost offsets).

The mental health care system in the UK is characterised by pluralism of both provision and funding. On the funding side, the NHS is the major funder of treatment and care services, but in fact comprises quite a large number of fairly autonomous agents, particularly primary care groups and trusts, and health authorities. There are also local authority social services departments, housing departments and the criminal justice system, all financing services. On the provider side, alongside the substantial historical presence of

---

Box 12.1
Expressed demands for cost information

- To check value for money (and best value) for users and purchasers.
- To underpin and guide purchasing and providing decisions within quasi-markets, and for other 'managed care' initiatives.
- To inform, monitor and evaluate current or proposed mental health policies.
- To inform service delivery and practice, and to guide care managers operating within devolved budgets.
- To evaluate the resource implications of new treatment modalities.
- To assist the marketing of new treatments such as pharmacotherapies.
- To inform decisions by formularies, licensing authorities and reimbursement groups.
- To audit service provision and purchasing, and for accountability and probity checks.

the public sector, there are private and voluntary providers, as well as advocacy groups and campaigning organisations. The rapid development of this 'mixed economy' of funding and provision was, of course, a major policy priority for the Conservative governments of the 1980s and 1990s, but the mixed economy is clearly not going to disappear with a Labour government. Consequently, there is an even more pressing need for transparency of information about the costs of different interventions, and the resource consequences of successful and unsuccessful treatment. These are not required simply for cost comparisons between competing providers, but represent cost needs that run throughout Britain's complex care system.

Supply

When the first edition of this book was published in 1992, there was little British evidence on the economics of mental health treatments and services. The position has changed, quite markedly in some fields, even though costs information generally remains relatively scarce. The internal market introduced by the 1990 Act obviously generated a need for costs and price data to be collated and disseminated, because priced contracts drove the quasi-market system, and the response has been quite impressive in some areas. Auditors within and outwith care-providing agencies have increasingly turned their attentions to value-for-money and, more recently, 'best value' criteria, and public health and social care agencies have been able to provide more such evidence. Care managers and keyworkers in many localities have been instructed to work within preset budgets and have been given costs and other data to assist their decision-making. Research-funding bodies have also responded with the explicit recommendation that health services research projects should look not only at outcomes for users but also at the costs for providers and the wider society, with the result that many more study teams include a health economist.

How then is cost information to be gathered? This chapter focuses on a research tool (the CSRI) that has been developed and successfully employed in the collection of information on costs, service utilisation, income and related matters. We describe this schedule, illustrating its flexibility for use in many mental health service and evaluation contexts. Collecting such data is the first of three linked tasks, so the next section continues by broadly outlining our methodology for estimating service costs and for calculating the costs of the full care packages recorded on the CSRI.

We will then illustrate the use of the CSRI from some of our own research. Like the plans for the new health and social care systems set in place in the early 1990s, and reinforced by the Labour government in more recent policy pronouncements, the aim of this research tool and its accompanying methodology has been to generate costs data that are client-focused rather than agency-centred, comprehensive rather than partial, consolidated rather than fragmented, and constructively employed in the improvement of efficiency and equity rather than merely employed to monitor probity. In this section, we use data generated by the CSRI to outline the service and cost implications of psychiatric hospital reprovision, look at cost–need associations and explore issues of the relative cost-effectiveness of community-based arrangements.

A costing methodology for research in psychiatry

The basic cost rules

We first recommended four general costing 'rules' for psychiatric research 10 years ago (Knapp & Beecham, 1990). The first rule recommends that costs should be comprehensively measured. They should therefore range over as many service components of care programmes or 'packages' as is relevant in any particular circumstance.

> Unless costs are defined and measured comprehensively, one treatment mode may appear to be less costly than another, when in reality that mode merely shifts costs into forms that have not been measured (Weisbrod *et al*, 1980, p. 403).

The calculation of comprehensive costs is most usefully effected at the individual level, partly because this is the level at which clinical data are collected, and partly because this preserves inter-client variability in the research domain – an essential feature of any needs-based service system. The second costing rule then urges that neither these variations between clients nor the likely variations between facilities or areas of the country should be overlooked. Analysed properly, these cost variations can produce useful policy and practice insights, for costs will usually be linked to differences in individual characteristics and needs and outcomes.

An examination of cost differences encourages conclusions to be drawn about comparative performance. The third rule should then come into play: such comparisons must be made on a like-with-like basis. It is of little value, for example, to report that community care costs less than hospital care if clients in the community have fewer behavioural or health problems than those in hospital. Finally, cost information is far more useful if it does not stand in isolation from other relevant evidence, particularly outcome data. Reliance on cost information alone could be dangerous, just as it is inadvisable to *neglect* costs in policy and practice discussions and decisions. In a radical review of community care that had a major influence on the 1990 health and community care legislation, Griffiths wrote:

> "To talk of policy in matters of care except in the context of available resources and timescales for action owes more to theology than to the purposeful delivery of a caring service." (Griffiths, 1988, p. iv)

For example, underpinning most evaluations is the hoary old question: for whom and under what circumstances is one intervention preferable to another? But to define the criterion 'preferable' solely in clinical outcome terms, without regard to cost, is to invite unnecessary (that is, avoidable) difficulties of implementation.

These cost rules embody two sets of principles: they are consistent with the demands of economic theory as applied to health and social care (Knapp, 1984; Knapp, 1995; Drummond *et al*, 1997), and they are also essentially the costing counterparts to the usual principles of any evaluation. This congruence and the economic theoretical grounding help considerably in the design and interpretation of empirical research. With these four rules tucked under one arm, we will describe the instrumentation developed for collecting service utilisation data and calculating comprehensive support costs. Although the potential undoubtedly exists within care management or care programme frameworks, it is not yet possible to ask any one person about the full cost implications of a client's care package. The process of calculating the full costs of supporting individuals, therefore, is broken down into the three connected tasks described below:

- the collection of service receipt or utilisation data for individual clients or patients over a consistently defined period;
- the costing or pricing of each service used; and
- the combination of these two sets of information in order to calculate the cost of the full care packages.

Each of these tasks is described in general terms below, illustrating the approach in a variety of applications, although focusing primarily on an economic evaluation of psychiatric reprovision with which we have been associated.

Collecting service utilisation data – the CSRI schedule

In order to calculate the costs of community care for people moving from long-stay hospital residence, we developed and employed a new instrument in 1986, the CSRI. The CSRI built on previous research at the Personal Social Services Research Unit (PSSRU), University of Kent at Canterbury, particularly on child care and young offender services (see Knapp & Robertson, 1989, for a partial review), and incorporated relevant parts of previously developed instruments in the mental health field, particularly the Economic Questionnaire of Weisbrod *et al* (1980). Although the instrument needed to be tailor-made to fit the research context, an early requirement, and one that has proved invaluable in subsequent research, was easy adaptability. At the time, the CSRI was to be employed in the PSSRU's evaluation of the Department of Health's Care in the Community demonstration programme of 1984–1989, which concerned all the main adult client groups, and also in the evaluation of the psychiatric reprovision services being established under the closure programmes for Friern and Claybury hospitals in North London.

In both evaluations, we could be certain that most clients would have a key carer or case manager, or would be living in a group home where a diary would be kept of residents' activities (especially contacts with health, social care and related services, and with peripatetic professionals). The questionnaire was therefore originally designed for administration by an interviewer from the research team to the principal carer of the person with mental health problems. For about 10% of the clients, the key carer could not be identified, for example when someone was living independently in domestic accommodation. In these situations, the schedule was successfully completed in an interview with the client. It was also completed during telephone interviews and by staff with no interviewer present, even though not specifically designed for that mode of use. In some research projects, the key questions of the CSRI have been incorporated into other schedules. However, experience has confirmed our initial expectations that a trained interviewer can best tease out accurate and comprehensive information.

The CSRI was piloted in the summer of 1987 in the Maidstone Care in the Community project for people with learning difficulties, where a wide range of services had been developed, affording the chance to test the instrument under different conditions. A second round of instrument refinement was based on use of the CSRI in another three Care in the Community projects. Since its introduction, the CSRI has been used in many evaluation studies, and some of the service contexts are listed in Box 12.2.

The questionnaire is usually printed on six A4 pages and takes approximately 20 minutes to complete. Both factors, however, will vary depending on the client's situation, the research focus, the scope of costs and the extent to which required data are recorded on other

---

Box 12.2
A selection of evaluation contexts in which the CSRI has been used

- A long-term evaluation of an assertive outreach service, the Daily Living Programme (Knapp *et al*, 1994; Knapp *et al*, 1998*b*).
- A study of people with schizophrenia living in the community in two London districts (Beecham *et al*, 1995).
- The evaluation of psychiatric and mental handicap hospital rundown and community care developments (Knapp *et al*, 1992; Cambridge *et al*, 1994; Donnelly *et al*, 1994; Beecham *et al*, 1997).
- A comparison of an experimental case-management-oriented community psychiatric nursing service with a more traditional model (McCrone *et al*, 1991).
- An evaluation of a new intervention to improve compliance with medication (Healey *et al*, 1998).
- Evaluations of children's mental health and social care (Beecham & Knapp, 1995; Knapp *et al*, 1998*c*).
- Studies of community care for older people (Beecham *et al*, 1993; Petch *et al*, 1996).
- Studies of care for people with challenging behaviour (Felce *et al*, 1998).
- Evaluations of new drugs (Drummond *et al*, 1998).
- An evaluation of specialist work schemes (Schneider & Hallam, 1997; Hallam & Schneider, 1999).

---

schedules used in the study. CSRI questions are largely structured but, given the complexity of community care arrangements, a few narrative answers are required. The design of the questionnaire incorporates blank spaces in which to write additional comments or interpret the occasionally confused responses of the interviewee. A series of 'prompt cards' can supplement the CSRI. These may contain indicative lists of accommodation types, different services and social security benefits. For a local evaluation, they may contain lists of named services.

The CSRI collects retrospective information on service utilisation, service-related issues and income in a manner commensurate with estimating care package costs. The retrospective period (prior to the date of the interview) is a compromise between the accuracy that comes from not asking respondents to cast their minds back too far and the comprehensiveness that can only come by allowing sufficient time to elapse for some uncommon, but potentially expensive services to be used. In the hospital rundown evaluations, we divided the service utilisation section (see below) into two parts, one covering the previous month – in the North London reprovision study, this was the twelfth month after discharge from hospital – and the other asking about less regularly received services (such as hospital admissions or GP visits) over the past 12 months. These durations are not fixed and can be varied to fit particular research designs. For example, repeated use of the CSRI – as in the first phase of the Daily Living Programme (Knapp *et al*, 1994) evaluation, when interviews were conducted at 4, 11, and 20 months after entry to the study – allows data to be recorded only for the period between interviews. For this longitudinal study, information gathered at all interviews was recorded on the same schedule, which meant the interviewer could use data from the previous interview to prompt or guide questions.

The first section of the CSRI covers *background and client information*, for example, recording client study number, gender and date of birth. Depending on the availability of information from other instruments, the interviewer could then ask for details of past admissions and discharges from hospital, participation in a special programme, registration with a general practitioner (GP) and medication. This opening section also records the date and place of interview and identifies the interviewer. A useful development of the CSRI has been to incorporate questions on other socio-demographic indicators, such as educational attainment or ethnicity (The Client Socio-Demographic and Service Receipt Inventory (CSSRI–EU); Chisholm *et al*, 1999).

The second section concentrates on describing the study member's *accommodation and living situation*. Accommodation is usually a major component in terms of its contribution to clients' support arrangements and the associated cost. The CSRI records information on: address, partly for the purposes of identifying facility type and budget, and partly because location influences cost (London is more expensive than the rest of the country, for example), and some adjustment may be needed; tenure of accommodation (such as council or privately rented, residential home or owner–occupier); a simple description of the size of the unit (number of rooms and number of other residents); the amount paid by the client or household in rent or other payments; and receipt of housing benefit, if any.

Many clients with severe mental health problems do not live in domestic accommodation but in specialised facilities, such as residential or nursing homes, hostels or group homes. We can impose a standardised categorisation of facilities using information recorded on the CSRI about residents' tenure, facility size, staffing arrangements and managing agency (NHS, local authority, voluntary or for-profit organisations). Where several clients live in the same facility, some of these questions need be completed only once. In our evaluation of domus care, these overarching questions were separated from the main questionnaire (Beecham *et al*, 1993).

Unfortunately, many people with mental health problems (although generally not the former long-stay in-patients moving to planned community care schemes) quite frequently move from one address to another (Slade *et al*, 1999), and the CSRI can record such changes of address, including hospital re-admissions. Instability of accommodation obviously complicates cost calculation, but for clients it can have dire consequences for ability to work, entitlements to social security and indeed mental health itself. In some applications of the CSRI, where study members are more likely to live in domestic accommodation, this section has been more comprehensive, asking about the composition of the household and whether clients themselves have any care responsibilities. More attention is also paid to how household expenses are covered.

Research has shown that concerns about money can have an adverse effect on some mental health conditions (Brugha *et al*, 1985; Granzini *et al*, 1990). Many people with mental health problems have low incomes, owing in part to the heavy reliance on social security benefits and also to problems associated with under-claiming of benefits, low wages if work is found and unstable work patterns (Melzer *et al*, 1995*b*). Information on *employment history, earnings* and *other personal resources* is therefore collected. Former long-stay hospital residents rarely find (open) employment, but for many other groups of people with mental health problems, employment and its loss are important facets of both service effectiveness and cost. More questions, therefore, may be needed on employment history, and a number of questions may be needed on current employment activities. The costs of lost employment resulting from mental ill health or in-patient treatment will fall to clients (lower income) and to society (lost productivity), the actual values to be attached depending on a variety of labour market and individual circumstances.

If employment-related costs are unlikely to be an issue, it is more important to clarify receipt of social security benefits. In strict economic terms, these should be considered as transfer payments, which do not represent an aggregate cost to society, but they are also good proxies for living expenses, since clients usually rely on these benefits as their main (often only) source of income. Data on *changes* in benefit status over the past year may also be important, as they will reflect changes in clients' accommodation or other circumstances, or changes to the entitlement regulations.

The *service receipt* section is at the core of the CSRI and can take up most of the interview time. Community care is delivered and received within a fragmented 'system' in which many agencies and organisations provide a variety of services. There is certainly no standard package of care handed out as people are referred to psychiatric care and so there will be a great deal of variation between clients' packages of care. In this section, the schedule identifies receipt of services that are not funded within the accommodation budget; either health or social care services available to everybody or specialist mental health services. Information is collected on services for which the client leaves the accommodation facility to attend, such as day activity centres, hospital-based services, appointments at the GP surgery or leisure activities. Some professional support or services are provided to the client at home: home-help, community psychiatric nurse or field social worker visits are examples. For most research purposes, the CSRI provides a list of the different service types, such as local authority day care or out-patient appointment, which forms the left-hand column of a table. For each service type, the number of contacts over the chosen retrospective period is requested and the average duration of these contacts. In the final column, in which 'not-applicable' cells are shaded, the interviewer can record whether the contacts are normally made at a clinic or office or at the client's home. For domiciliary services, it is also important to identify whether the professional sees several clients for a group session (as with occupational therapy) or sees them sequentially (as with GP visits). The allocation of service costs to individuals must take into account the scope of the visit.

For services that are likely to absorb a high proportion of care package costs, we advocate collecting more detail. For example, the length of each in-patient admission should be accurately recorded alongside information on the type of hospital and/or ward. (Intensive psychiatric care units have been found to cost nearly three times as much per day as long-stay hospital wards; Netten *et al*, 1998.) Special consideration should also be given to recording relevant details of a new intervention and its comparator.

The final section of the CSRI considers the role of informal carers. The availability of such support for people leaving long-stay psychiatric hospitals appears to be limited (Knapp *et al*, 1992), but if a number of study members are known to be living independently or with other members of their families, more weight would need to be given to this dimension. The CSRI includes questions on the input of informal carers in terms of time spent (frequency and duration of support) and tasks undertaken (personal care, shopping, domestic tasks and social visits). Financial costs borne by family and friends can also be recorded and may include extra food or heating, increased replacement of clothes and equipment, as well as cash gifts. Family members may receive extra income as a consequence of their relative's problems, such as attendance allowance.

These five sections form the framework for the CSRI, within which responses to questions are carefully structured to facilitate cost estimation. It is the emphasis put on different aspects of each section that provides the instrument's flexibility and its adaptability to different research and service contexts. Each CSRI summarises one person's care package (see Boxes 12.3, 12.4 and 12.5), the components of which we would expect to vary given that any individual study member has a different set of characteristics and needs (broadly defined). By aggregating the service receipt across sample members, a list of all services used can be compiled. A unit cost should be estimated for each of these services.

Estimating unit costs for health and social care services

The second major task in measuring the costs of support for people with mental health problems is the costing or pricing of the various services used by clients. Economic theory advocates basing cost measures on *long-run marginal opportunity cost*. In practice, by 'long-run', we mean to move beyond the small-scale and immediate development of community care (for example), which could probably be achieved by using present services more intensively at very low marginal cost. Since national policy intentions are to develop community services, it would hardly be credible to measure only short-run cost implications. By 'marginal', we mean the addition to total cost attributable to the inclusion of one more client (the production of the marginal unit of output in general economic parlance). By 'opportunity cost', we mean that the resource implications should reflect opportunities forgone rather than amounts spent. The opportunity cost measures the true private or social value of a resource or service, based on its value in the best alternative use. In a perfectly informed and frictionless market economy, this 'best alternative use value' would be identical to the price paid in the market. Not everything is marketed, not every market works smoothly, and information is rarely complete, with the result that observed prices and opportunity costs diverge. The recorded depreciation payments on capital equipment or buildings, for example, will not usually reflect the opportunity costs of using these durable resources, nor will the (zero) payments to volunteers and informal carers usually indicate their social value.

In application of these principles, it happens that today's (short-run) average revenue cost, plus appropriate capital and overhead elements, is probably close to the long-run marginal cost for most services we would encounter. In this chapter, we will say no more about the calculation of these average revenue costs or their capital add-ons, for once we open out the description we will need more space than can presently be made available. Moreover, the details are not everyone's cup of tea. We have written about them elsewhere, briefly

Box 12.3
Psychiatric reprovision package, independent living

Mr A is 39 years old, lives alone in a flat rented from the housing association and has no informal care support. He has gastro-intestinal problems, which require monitoring by his GP. He also takes medication (without supervision) for dermatological problems. He presents no behavioural problems.

Services received	Average weekly cost	Description
Social work	£15.45	Social worker and link worker visit once every two weeks for 30 minutes
GP	£1.50	10 surgery appointments during the past year
Chiropodist	£0.36	Two visits during the past year
Hospital out-patients	£14.79	One appointment each month for a check-up and depot injections
Housing officer	£5.41	Visits once very two weeks for 15 minutes
Accommodation	£109.41	Includes taxes forgone by the local authority, and capital, management and maintenance costs borne by the housing association
Living expenses	£102.27	Income support, invalidity benefit and disability allowances
Total weekly cost of care package, 1997/98 prices	**£249.19**	

Source: Hallam, 1998

(Knapp & Beecham, 1990), in more detail in relation to mental health care (Beecham, 1995), and in much greater depth with various health and social care examples (Netten & Beecham, 1993). An annual compendium is also available that pulls together a number of research and other sources to present nationally applicable unit costs for over 70 health and social care services (Netten *et al*, 1998).

In the psychiatric reprovision study, two main procedures were used to cost or price each service. Accommodation facilities, hospital and day care services were expected to account for a large proportion of the total cost of care packages, and their unit costs were carefully and individually calculated by adjusting published or routinely collected facility accounts. Particular attention was paid to services

Box 12.4
Psychiatric reprovision package, assessment centre

Mr B is 51 and lives with seven other residents in an assessment centre managed by the community health services trust. He needs daily medical care for respiratory problems. Mr B becomes verbally aggressive at least once a month and has episodes of extreme agitation, during which he becomes doubly incontinent. He is able to concentrate for short periods only, has poor hygiene habits and tends to be socially isolated. A heavy smoker, he is considered a health risk and has twice been responsible for causing a fire.

Services received	Average weekly cost	Description
Social work	£0.95	Social worker has visited twice during the past year for one hour each time
Depot injection	£5.37	Cost of the drug given by in-house staff
Chiropodist	£1.42	Visits once a month seeing four residents on each occasion
Dentist	£0.15	One check-up during the year
Optician	£0.23	One visit to optician for sight test in past year; glasses were not prescribed
Day centre	£3.54	Drops in for approximately one hour per week
Accommodation	£1225.59	Includes care, hotel and building-related costs of the residential facility
Living expenses	£29.99	Personal expenses and bus pass
Total weekly cost of care package, 1997/98 prices	**£1267.24**	

Source: Hallam, 1998

at Friern and Claybury Hospitals, the costs of which would be required as comparators for community care costs. The planned level of detail to be obtained, and therefore the accuracy of the pricing, was lower where the service was likely to contribute less to total cost, such as input from field social workers, nurses, psychiatrists or chiropodists. For these services, national statistics or data from other studies were used to build up our unit costs. In all cases, prices were calculated to approximate the long-run marginal costs of care, including the opportunity costs of all capital employed.

Box 12.5
Psychiatric reprovision package, staffed group home

Ms C is 57 years old and lives in a small registered care home that has six places. It is one of four units with a central office and waking staff cover at night. She has no particular health or behavioural problems, but is a careless smoker, causing problems on a daily basis.

Services received	Average weekly cost	Description
Social work	£0.11	One visit by field social worker during the past year. Two residents seen during this visit
GP	£1.37	Three visits during the past year
Psychiatrist	£1.70	Two visits during the past year seeing two residents on each occasion
Chiropodist	£1.42	Four 30-minute visits per year
Resource centre	£70.93	Attends five days a week, four hours a day
Accommodation	£897.22	Includes care, hotel and premises costs of residential facility as well as personal expenses
Total weekly cost of care package, 1997/98 prices	**£972.75**	

Source: Hallam, 1998

Costing full care packages

The CSRI is a means to an end, rather than an end in itself. The interview collects the data that enable packages of care to be identified. This information must then be manipulated and joined with information on the costs of those services. This data preparation stage allows service receipt to be allocated at a constant unit over a defined period of time. The unit of measurement for service receipt (per hour, say) should be the same as that used for the calculation of service costs. The period of time is often defined by the research: for the North London reprovision study, the follow-up period was one year after discharge from hospital; for the Care in the Community programme evaluation, the follow-up was nine months; and for the Daily Living Programme, several follow-up periods were used, varying from 4 to 9 months.

Boxes 12.3, 12.4 and 12.5 provide three illustrative case studies, taken from the economic evaluation of psychiatric reprovision in North London. For each person, we describe the components of his or her care packages, that is, the frequency and duration of contact with any services over the year prior to interview. The average weekly costs are listed for each component, estimated using the approach outlined above, and the total weekly cost of the care package calculated. In the next section, we consider some of the ways in which these cost-related data can be used to address policy and practice issues.

Illustrations of costs research

We can illustrate the employment of the resultant economic data by considering some results from the long-running evaluation of psychiatric reprovision in North London. In debates about the rundown of long-stay hospital provision and its replacement by community care, doubts about economic viability are rarely far from the surface. In this chapter, we address three questions. What are the service and cost consequences of moving long-stay patients from the hospital to be supported by community-based services? Can we predict subsequent community costs from information gathered on patients in hospital? Of the many variants of community care, which are the more costly, and which the more cost-effective?

The decision to close two of the largest psychiatric hospitals in North London was taken in 1983, since which date the regional health authority and the Department of Health have funded research to examine the psychiatric reprovision services being established to replace them. In association with the Team for Assessment of Psychiatric Services (TAPS), researchers from the PSSRU at the University of Kent at Canterbury and the London School of Economics, and more recently the Centre for the Economics of Mental Health at the Institute of Psychiatry, have been studying the economics of reprovision (Beecham *et al*, 1997; Knapp *et al*, 1997). The main focus of the economic evaluation has been on in-patients who have been in continuous residence for at least a year, and who, if over 65 years of age, do not have a current diagnosis of dementia. In this chapter, we concentrate on people who left hospital and for whom follow-up data were collected one year after discharge. (Many former hospital residents have also been assessed five years after discharge.) The first reprovision patients moved to the community in 1985.

Describing community care services and costs

By March 1993, when Friern Hospital was closed, a total of 813 people who met the study criteria had left the two hospitals under the rundown plans, most under the reprovision arrangements that carried financial transfers. Baseline information for all patients in the hospitals was collected by the TAPS researchers covering: mental health status, using the Present State Examination (PSE; Wing *et al*, 1974) and the Social Behaviour Schedule (SBS; Sturt & Wykes, 1986)); physical health; personal and historical data; patient attitudes; living skills, using the Basic Everyday Living Skills schedule (BELS; Leff, 1997); information on patients' social networks using the Social Network Schedule; and an assessment of living environments. Altogether, including the 'new long-stay' patients who had accumulated in the two hospitals since the study began, baseline information has been assembled on nearly 1000 in-patients. The TAPS research design compared aspects of the quality of life for patients discharged from the two hospitals with similar patients who remained behind, but also assessed change before and after discharge from hospital (Leff *et al*, 1996*a*; Leff *et al*, 1996*b*; Leff, 1997).

Detailed service utilisation data formed the basis of our cost estimates for 533 people leaving the two hospitals, and community care costs were more broadly estimated for a further 218 people. The remaining 8% of the full sample of leavers died before the interview date, could not be traced or moved out of the region. For 533 people for whom data were collected on the CSRI, community service use and the associated costs are summarised in Table 12.1. These data aggregate the care packages (see the examples in Boxes 12.3, 12.4 and 12.5) for each study member in the sample. The figures illustrate the variety of services used by psychiatric re-provision clients, spanning specialist mental health provision and secondary and primary health care services, as well as social care services provided by public sector agencies (local authority social services departments) and independent sector organisations. The low level of contact with police or probation services is noteworthy – former long-stay patients rarely cause high-support burdens to the criminal justice system.

The final two columns of Table 12.1 show the relative contribution to total costs for each service. Accommodation placements obviously dominate, as most study members live in high-support residential homes or staffed group homes. Hospital-based services also continue to play a major role. In-patient services were used by only 15% of sample members, but absorbed 16% of the costs of support for those who were re-admitted. Day support services, whether provided within or outside the hospital, are also an important source of support,

TABLE 12.1
Distribution of costs by service

Services used in the community	Clients using each service[1] (%)	Average contribution of service to total cost (%)	
		Over all clients using service (%)	*Over all clients (%)*
Accommodation and living expenses	100.0	86.9	86.9
Hospital out-patient services	25.9	1.9	0.5
Hospital in-patient services	14.8	16.1	2.4
Hospital day patient services	22.9	14.7	3.4
Local authority social services day care	17.4	9.7	1.7
Voluntary organisation day care	15.2	8.1	1.2
Social club services	6.6	2.3	0.2
Education classes	4.5	6.9	0.3
Community psychiatric services	57.8	0.9	0.5
Chiropody	41.3	0.1	0.1
Nursing services	29.1	1.5	0.5
Psychology services	14.4	1.0	0.1
Occupational therapy	8.6	2.5	0.2
Drugs (depot injection)	14.3	1.0	0.1
Miscellaneous services[2]	18.6	0.9	0.2
Physiotherapy	2.4	–	–
GP	74.5	0.5	0.3
Dentist	25.3	0.2	–
Optician	19.9	0.2	–
Community pharmacist	5.8	0.7	–
Field social work	23.6	4.3	1.0
Police and probation services	5.8	0.7	–
Client's travel	29.3	0.4	0.1
Volunteer inputs	1.7	4.2	0.1
Case review	9.9	0.5	0.1

1. Data available only for those people for whom a full CSRI was completed (*n*=533).
2. Includes a number of services each used by only a few study members. Examples are finance officer, aids and adaptations, audiology, aromatherapy, employment officer, home-help, job club and reminiscence group.

together accounting for just over 6% of the total costs of support for all clients (final column). In contrast to these quite expensive services, some are used by a much higher proportion of clients, but make a smaller contribution to total cost; community psychiatry services, chiropody, and the GP are examples.

This type of descriptive information begins to reveal where the cost burdens lie. Which services must expand to support former long-stay hospital patients as they move to community-based care? If in hospital all these services (or functions) were provided from within the hospital budget, who now funds these components? These are issues about the distribution of resources in community mental health care provision that can only be addressed by taking a comprehensive approach.

Associations between costs, client characteristics and needs

The average cost of community care for our sample of 751 former long-stay hospital residents was £690 per week (1997/1998 prices), yet the most expensive care package was at least 20 times more costly than the cheapest. Why do care package costs vary?

We would expect a primary source of this variation to be client needs or problems. For example, do people with greater needs or problems get more support? We use the term 'problem' to describe those psychosocial characteristics of clients on which psychiatric and associated support services are expected to have an impact. If costs summarise, albeit imperfectly, the resources expended or services delivered to clients, how well are services tailored to address these problems? Using a cost function approach, ordinary least squares (OLS) regression was employed to explore the causal links between cost and its hypothesised determinants. We summarise the findings here and the methodology, and full results and implications, are considered at greater length in other papers (Knapp *et al*, 1995; Knapp, 1998). The estimated cost functions indicated that community care costs are sensitive to differences in a number of client characteristics as assessed in hospital, explaining 21% of the variation in the total weekly cost of support. Demographic characteristics exert only a limited influence on costs; neither age nor gender proves to be significant, but costs are higher for people who have never married. Three of the reasons for original admission to hospital (transfer from another psychiatric facility, inability to cope and admission to hospital under the Mental Health Act) are associated with the much later community reprovision costs, but their effects are not easy to interpret and the data may have referred to circumstances prevailing many years earlier. Easier to understand, perhaps, is the effect of people's history of hospital care. A greater proportion of life spent in hospital and a greater number of previous admissions to hospital increased the costs of support packages in the community, suggesting that prolonged institutionalisation increases the need for community support services.

The influences of clinical factors on cost are particularly interesting. People with more negative symptoms (a measure constructed from the PSE scores) have higher than average costs. Higher scores on the Social Behaviour Schedule reflect higher staff-reported ratings of abnormal behaviours and, with one exception, imply higher costs. The negative effect of attention-seeking behaviour could be indicative of a therapeutic response, or may be related to social network size and gregarious behaviour. Two indicators of physical health needs (number of areas in which daily nursing care is required and taking medication for physical illness) are both associated with higher costs. Diagnosis had no obvious effect on cost once the above factors had been taken into account.

A third set of analyses on the reprovision study data explored whether particular variants of community care for former long-stay in-patients were more costly, or more cost-effective. Exploring inter-sectoral cost differences has particular policy relevance today. Are public sector services more costly or less efficient than non-public ones? Does the high cost of care in health authority facilities, in contrast to facilities run by other organisations, reflect the creation of environments that encourage client dependency, or at least not encourage independence? Or, alternatively, is high cost the logical corollary of the tendency for health authority facilities to accommodate those former residents with greater needs? To address these questions, analyses were undertaken on data for the 429 former in-patients who were living in specialised accommodation; that is, residential or nursing homes, hostels, staffed group homes or sheltered housing, which were distinguished using standardised definitions. Sectoral responsibility for individuals was defined as that which managed the accommodation facility: NHS, local authority social services department, voluntary (non-profit) organisation, private (for profit) organisation or individual, or consortium arrangements (usually health and voluntary sector organisations working together). Costs were found to be lowest in the private sector and highest in the NHS and consortium sectors. However, quality of care indicators suggested that the lowest-cost sector is performing least well, and higher-cost sectors offer better quality (Knapp *et al*, 1999).

Conclusion

The types of analyses described above begin to address some fundamental issues of efficiency and equity on the allocation of mental health care resources. Who gets what services at what cost? Can scarce mental health resources be better employed in one way than another? Alongside data on clients' needs and characteristics, finding the answers to these questions relies on good-quality costs data. Sensible expectations of any service are that it will respond to the needs of each user and seek to improve their welfare (broadly defined) or at least prevent further deterioration in, say, symptoms. It is also sensible, therefore, to assess the resource inputs (costs) at a similar level, giving research the capacity to evaluate together the costs and the effectiveness of a service.

In this chapter, we suggest that costs summarise the end-product of decisions to commit resources in a particular way: the provision of services and other support. At the client or individual level, such decisions result in the provision of a 'care package', or a set of services that each client uses. Just as mental illness has consequences for individuals in many areas of their life, so too will their care package span many types of different support services. These services often involve several provider agencies and organisations, but management information systems are not yet sufficiently developed to capture a full picture of all the components of the care package. To carry out our research, therefore, we developed a specific instrument for collecting costs-related data for people with mental health problems, the CSRI.

Since its first use in 1986, the CSRI has been developed and modified as the demands for cost information have both increased and broadened in scope. One research-based issue has been to consider whether a shortcut could be found for the CSRI and its attendant methodologies. This would make cost estimation a less daunting and less time-consuming research task and therefore increase the frequency with which cost and cost-effectiveness studies are undertaken. Our re-analysis of five large research databases allowed us to identify the services that contributed most to the total costs of supporting people with mental health problems. Accommodation and living expenses, in-patient hospital stays, NHS and local authority day services, and out-patient appointments were found to account for between 90% and 98% of total costs (Knapp & Beecham, 1993). This 'reduced list' methodology was implemented in a study of residential care services in eight health districts (Chisholm *et al*, 1997).

Building on our work of the 1980s, the CSRI has been adapted to evaluate a variety of service contexts and a wider range of adult and child client groups, and there has also been considerable international interest. Adapting the CSRI for use in cross-national studies has involved careful translation, as well as work to standardise service definitions across different care systems (Drummond *et al*, 1998; Chisholm *et al*, 1999). Local versions for evaluating mental health care in Italy and Spain have been developed (Amaddeo *et al*, 1996; Vásquez-Barquero *et al*, 1997), and work is currently underway to adapt the

CSRI for use alongside a case register (Amaddeo *et al*, 1997) and for use in clinical practice.

In the Foreword to Drummond (1980), Alan Williams suggested that:

> "one cannot but help sympathise with clinicians and other health service professionals who feel that with so many pressures upon them they might at least be spared the distasteful task of having to think about efficiency, and the husbanding of scarce resources, on top of all their other problems." (p. vii)

Two decades later, the pressure to economise has increased markedly. The cost-effectiveness imperative is stronger than ever. The demands for cost information have grown, and requirements for cost information now permeate all levels of decision-making and serve to emphasise the changed context within which mental health services are planned, delivered and received. The supply of (decent) cost information has not kept pace with the demands that techno-logical and practical changes have created, but methodologies have been developed and banks of data and experience are being constructed to bolster the supply response and to aid cost-sensitive decision-making. There will never be answers to each and every cost question, but the distance between what is demanded and what can be supplied appears to be narrowing.

Acknowledgements

Research described in various parts of this chapter has been funded over a number of years by the Department of Health and North East Thames Regional Health Authority, and some has been conducted in collaboration with Angela Hallam, Barry Baines and the TAPS, led by Julian Leff. We record our considerable gratitude for this support and assistance, but we bear the sole responsibility for the chapter.

References

Amaddeo, F., Bonizzato, P., Beecham, J., *et al* (1996) ICAP: un'intervista per la raccolta dei dati necessari per la valutazione dei costi dell'assistenza psichiatrica. *Epidemiologia e Psichiatria Sociale*, **5**, 201–213.

——, Beecham, J., Bonizzato, P., *et al* (1997) The use of a case register for evaluating the costs of psychiatric care. *Acta Psychiatrica Scandinavica*, **95**, 195–198.

Beecham, J. (1995) Collecting and estimating costs. In: *The Economic Evaluation of Mental Health Care* (ed. M. Knapp), pp. 61–82. Aldershot: Arena.

—— & Knapp, M. (1992) Costing psychiatric interventions. In: *Measuring Mental Health Needs* (1st edn) (eds G. Thornicroft, C. Brewin & J. Wing), pp. 163–183. London: Gaskell.

—— & —— (1995) The costs of childcare assessment. In: *Social Work Assessment with Adolescents* (eds R. Sinclair, L. Garnett & D. Berridge). London: National Children's Bureau.

——, Cambridge, P., Hallam, A., *et al* (1993) The costs of domus care. *International Journal of Geriatric Psychiatry*, **8**, 827–831.

——, —— & Allen, C. (1995) Comparative efficiency and equity in community-based care. In: *The Economic Evaluation of Mental Health Care* (ed. M. Knapp). Aldershot: Arena.

——, Hallam, A., Knapp, M., *et al* (1997) Costing care in the hospital and in the community. In: *Care in the Community: Illusion or Reality* (ed. J. Leff). Chichester: John Wiley & Sons.

Brugha, T., Bebbington, P., Tennant, C., *et al* (1985) The list of threatening experiences: a sublist of twelve life event categories with considerable long-term contextual threat. *Psychological Medicine*, **15**, 189–194.

Cambridge, P., Hayes, L. & Knapp, M. (1994) *Care in the Community: Five Years On.* Aldershot: Arena.

Chisholm, D., Knapp, M., Astin, J., *et al* (1997) The Mental Health Residential Care Study: the costs of provision. *Journal of Mental Health*, **6**, 85–99.

——, ——, Knudsen, H. C., *et al* (1999) Client Socio-Demographic and Service Receipt Inventory – European Version: development of an instrument for international research. EPSILON Study 5. *British Journal of Psychiatry*, **177** (Suppl. 39), s28–s33.

Costello, E., Burns, B., Angold, A., *et al* (1993) How can epidemiology improve mental health services for children and adolescents? *Journal of American Academy of Child and Adolescent Psychiatry*, **32**, 1106–1114.

Donnelly, M., McGilloway, S., Perry, S., *et al* (1994) *Opening New Doors: An Evaluation of Community Care for People Discharged from Psychiatric and Mental Handicap Hospitals.* Belfast: HMSO.

Drummond, M. (1980) *Principles of Economic Analysis in Health Care.* Oxford: Oxford University Press.

——, Stoddart, G. & Torrance, G. (1997) *Methods for the Economic Evaluation of Health Care Programmes*, 2nd edition. Oxford: Oxford University Press.

——, Knapp, M., Burns, T., *et al* (1998) Issues in the design of studies for the economic evaluation of new atypical antipsychotics: the ESTO study. *Journal of Mental Health Policy and Economics*, **1**, 15–22.

Felce, D., Lowe, K., Perry, J., *et al* (1998) Service support for people with severe intellectual disability and the most challenging behaviours in Wales: processes, outcomes and costs. *Journal of Intellectual Disability Research*, **42**, 639–652.

Granzini, L., McFarland, B. & Cutler, D. (1990) Prevalence of mental disorders after catastrophic financial loss. *Journal of Nervous and Mental Disease*, **178**, 680–685.

Griffiths, R. (1988) *Community Care: Agenda for Action.* London: HMSO.

Hallam, A. (1998) People with mental health problems leaving long-stay psychiatric hospital. In: *Unit Costs of Health and Social Care 1998* (eds A. Netten, J. Dennett & J. Knight). Canterbury: PSSRU, University of Kent at Canterbury.

—— & Schneider, J. (1999) Sheltered work schemes for people with severe mental health problems: service use and costs. *Journal of Mental Health*, **8**, 163–178.

Healey, A., Knapp, M., Astin, J., *et al* (1998) Cost-effectiveness evaluation of compliance therapy for people with psychosis. *British Journal of Psychiatry*, **172**, 420–424.

House of Commons (1983) *Mental Health Act.* London: HMSO.

Johnson, S., Ramsey, R., Thornicroft, G., *et al* (1997) *London's Mental Health.* London: King's Fund.

Knapp, M. (1984) *The Economics of Social Care.* London: Macmillan.

—— (1995) *The Economic Evaluation of Mental Health Care.* Aldershot: Arena.

—— (1997) Economics and mental health: a concise European history of demand and supply. In: *Making Mental Health Services Rational* (ed. M. Tansella), pp. 157–166. Roma: Il Pensiero Scientifico.

—— (1998) Making music out of noise – the cost function approach to evaluation. *British Journal of Psychiatry*, **173** (Suppl. 36), 7–11.

—— & BEECHAM, J. (1990) Costing mental health services. *Psychological Medicine*, **20**, 893–908.

—— & —— (1993) Reduced-list costings: examination of an informed short cut in mental health research. *Health Economics*, **2**, 313–322.

—— & ROBERTSON, E. (1989) The cost of child care services. In: *Child Care Research, Policy and Practice* (ed. B. Kahan). Milton Keynes: Open University Press.

——, CAMBRIDGE, P., THOMASON, C., *ET AL* (1992) *Care in the Community: Challenge and Demonstration.* Aldershot: Avebury.

——, BEECHAM, J., KOUTSOGEORGOPOULOU, V., *ET AL* (1994) Service use and costs of home-based versus hospital-based care for people with serious mental illness. *British Journal of Psychiatry*, **165**, 195–203.

——, ——, FENYO, A., *ET AL* (1995) Community mental health care for former hospital in-patients. Predicting costs from needs and diagnoses. *British Journal of Psychiatry*, **166** (Suppl. 27), 10–18.

——, —— & HALLAM, A. (1997) The mixed economy of psychiatric provision. In: *Care in the Community: Illusion or Reality* (ed. J. Leff), pp. 37–47. Chichester: John Wiley & Sons.

——, WILKINSON, D. & WIGGLESWORTH, R. (1998*a*) The economic consequences of Alzheimer's disease in the context of new drug developments. *International Journal of Geriatric Psychiatry*, **13**, 531–543.

——, MARKS, I., WOLSTENHOLME, J., *ET AL* (1998*b*) Home-based versus hospital-based care for serious mental health illness. Controlled cost-effectiveness study over four years. *British Journal of Psychiatry*, **172**, 506–512.

——, SCOTT, S. & DAVIES, J. (1998*c*) The cost of anti-social behaviour in younger children. *Clinical Child Psychology and Psychiatry*, **4**, 457–473.

——, HALLAM, A., BEECHAM, J., *ET AL* (1999) Private, voluntary or public? Comparative cost-effectiveness in community mental health care. *Policy and Politics*, **27**, 25–41.

LEFF, J. (1997) *Care in the Community: Illusion or Reality.* Chichester: John Wiley & Sons.

——, DAYSON, D., GOOCH, C., *ET AL* (1996*a*) Quality of life of long-stay patients discharged from two psychiatric hospitals. *Psychiatric Services*, **47**, 62–67.

——, TRIEMAN, N. & GOOCH, C. (1996*b*) Prospective follow-up study of long-stay patients discharged from two psychiatric hospitals. *American Journal of Psychiatry*, **153**, 1318–1324.

MAUGHAN, B. & RUTTER, M. (1998) Continuities and discontinuities in anti-social behaviour from childhood to adult life. *Advances in Clinical Child Psychology*, **20**, 1–47.

McCRONE, P., BEECHAM, J. & KNAPP, M. (1991) Community psychiatric nurse teams: cost-effectiveness of intensive support versus generic care. *British Journal of Psychiatry*, **165**, 218–221.

MELTZER, H., GILL, B., PETTICREW, M., *ET AL* (1995*a*) *Physical Complaints, Service Use and Treatments of Adults with Psychiatric Disorders.* London: OPCS Social Survey Division, HMSO.

——, ——, ——, *ET AL* (1995*b*) *Economic Activity and Social Functioning of Adults with Psychiatric Disorders.* London: OPCS Social Survey Division, HMSO.

NETTEN, A. & BEECHAM, J. (eds) (1993) *Costing Community Care: Theory and Practice.* Aldershot: Avebury.

——, DENNETT, J. & KNIGHT, J. (1998) *Unit Costs of Health and Social Care 1998.* Canterbury: PSSRU, University of Kent at Canterbury.

PETCH, A., CHEETHAM, J., FULLER, R., *ET AL* (1996) *Delivering Community Care: Initial Implementation of Care Management in Scotland.* Edinburgh: The Stationery Office.

SCHNEIDER, J. & HALLAM, A. (1997) Specialist work schemes: user satisfaction and costs. *Psychiatric Bulletin*, **21**, 331–333.

SLADE, M., SCOTT, H., TRUMAN, C., *ET AL* (1999) Risk factors for tenancy breakdown for mentally ill people. *Journal of Mental Health*, **8**, 361–371.

STURT, E. & WYKES, T. (1986) Assessment schedule for chronic psychiatric patients. *Psychological Medicine*, **17**, 485–493.

VÁSQUEZ-BARQUERO, J-L., GAITE, L., CUESTA, M., *ET AL* (1997) Versión española del CSRI: una entrevista para la evaluación costes en salud mental. *Archivos de Neurobiologia*, **2**, 171–184.

WEISBROD, B., STEIN, M. & TEST, L. (1980) Alternatives to mental hospital treatment: economic benefit–cost analysis. *Archives of General Psychiatry*, **37**, 400–405.

WING, J., COOPER, J. & SARTORIUS, N. (1974) *The Measurement and Classification of Psychiatric Symptoms*. Cambridge: Cambridge University Press.

13 Assessing systems of care for the long-term mentally ill in urban settings

M. SUSAN RIDGELY, HOWARD H. GOLDMAN and JOSEPH P. MORRISSEY

Measuring the perceived needs of a community for mental health services can serve as a valuable complement to a direct assessment of the needs of individuals. Often, it is too difficult or too expensive to assess directly the needs of a population, and an indirect survey of the opinion of key informants about the need for services in the community may usefully substitute for a direct assessment. Several indirect approaches are being employed to assess systems of care for the long-term mentally ill in the evaluation of a service demonstration sponsored by The Robert Wood Johnson (RWJ) Foundation in nine large cities in the USA. This chapter describes this demonstration programme and its evaluation, focusing in particular on a key informant survey used to assess changes in the system of care. In the process, we attempt to explain its relevance to mental health services assessment and planning in the USA and the UK.

Background

The organisation and financing of mental health care in the USA is complex, especially when contrasted with the centralised British NHS. In the USA, public mental health care is provided by an array of public and private mental health facilities, financed by an equally perplexing array of funding sources, including federal, state and local government categorical funds and public (Medicaid and Medicare) and private health insurance.

A nationwide system of state mental hospitals, first built in the second decade of the 19th century, long dominated public mental health care.

By the early 20th century, the USA had become the locus of public responsibility for mental health care. Following World War II, with the community mental health centre movement of the 1960s, and the subsequent community support movement of the late 1970s and early 1980s, responsibility for mental health care became more diffuse, as the focus broadened from state mental hospitals to community general hospitals and other community-based facilities, and from the treatment needs to the social welfare needs of severely mentally ill persons in the community. Alarmed by the release of thousands of patients from state mental hospitals to alternative community settings, critics of the policy of de-institutionalisation pointed to the widespread neglect of the needs of severely mentally ill persons. Patients were faced with obtaining care in a highly differentiated system where many critical supportive services were either non-existent or fragmented and poorly funded. Increasingly, then, since the 1980s, the focus in the development of mental health policy has been on the need to coordinate fragmented systems of care in local communities. The focus has been on pushing the locus of public responsibility for mental health care to the most local of geopolitical entities – in the case of the USA, city and county government.

The RJW Foundation Program

In the Autumn of 1985, The RWJ Foundation, the largest private health care philanthropy in the USA, announced the Program on Chronic Mental Illness, one of the foundation's largest health care initiatives and its first initiative in mental health care (Shore & Cohen, 1990). The Program, funded in 1987 for five years, has been contributing $29 million in grants and low-interest loans to nine demonstration sites.[1] The demonstration was designed as a test of comprehensive systemic changes in the organisation, financing and delivery of mental health and other supportive services to individuals with severe mental illness. Nine cities were chosen to participate in the five-year demonstration: three on the east coast (Baltimore, Maryland; Philadelphia, Pennsylvania and Charlotte, North Carolina); three in the mid-west (Columbus, Cincinnati and Toledo, Ohio); and three in the west (Denver, Colorado; Austin, Texas and Honolulu, Hawaii).

---

[1] A 'site' of the demonstration is the city or county recipient of the grant from The RWJ Foundation, the specified benefits from the federal government, and ongoing technical assistance from the Program Office (Miles Shore, MD and Martin Cohen, MSW of the Massachusetts Mental Health Center in Boston).

Earlier reforms of public mental health systems focused on the need to address individuals' social welfare needs as well as their mental health needs by including housing, income support and vocational programmes explicitly. The RWJ Foundation Program on Chronic Mental Illness went beyond advocating a more inclusive view of the mental health system of care by proposing that major organisational and financing changes may be necessary to ensure the delivery of that care. In the 20 years prior to the demonstration, state, federal and local funding sources had allowed localities to develop services, many of which were outside the bounds of the public mental health system. These 'systems' of services included a variety of providers, none of whom bore ultimate responsibility for meeting the needs of severely mentally ill persons. The RWJ Foundation Program focused on the need for coordination and integration of services, and each city in the demonstration was expected to create a local mental health authority, which would constitute an organisational locus of responsibility for the care of severely mentally ill adults in the geographic area.[2] According to the application guidelines and subsequent documents, the authority was described as:

> "an entity combining public accountability with the flexibility of the private sector (public accountability to ensure continuation of the public funding that pays for the greatest part of services and private-sector flexibility to solve the problems created by the civil service, legislative and political constraints on public operation of services)." (Shore & Cohen, 1990)

Thus, the intervention in this demonstration goes beyond the development of a specialised programme and includes governmental and organisational changes in each city/county site, integrating both decision-making and service delivery for severely mentally ill persons, including housing, disability, rehabilitation, financing and crisis management 'interventions'. The local mental health authorities were intended to assume fiscal, clinical and administrative responsibility for meeting the treatment, *housing* and supportive care needs of these persons. Specifically:

> "as a single point of administrative, clinical and fiscal responsibility, the authority was fully accountable for all aspects of the organisation and functioning of the system of care: which services are

---

[2] The approach to managing mental health care proposed by RWJ was built loosely on the experience of public authorities (Walsh & Leighland (1986). For a more complete discussion of the concept of a local mental health authority within the RWJ Program on Chronic Mental Illness, see Shore & Cohen (1990) and Goldman *et al* (1990).

provided, including which were purchased versus which were
provided directly by the authority; which consumers were served
and by which providers; how consumers were served; and finally,
how the available resources, including finances, were allocated to
serve consumers." (Shore & Cohen, 1990)

The development of a local mental health authority was central
to the demonstration. The RWJ Foundation identified the lack of
such an authority as one of the main problems in the delivery of
mental health care in urban areas. During the 1960s, under the
Community Mental Health Centers (CMHCs) Program, *catchment
areas* divided jurisdictions across large cities, and often represented
barriers to access for severely mentally ill people. Some clients simply
were not fortunate enough to live in a catchment area equipped
with the particular service they needed. Others were mobile
across catchment area boundaries with no CMHC or speciality
mental health agency taking responsibility for their care. Issues of
availability and accessibility dominated the discussion of the
shortfalls of this and other federal programmes delivering health
and social services to the poor.

The RWJ Foundation Program represents an important social
reform on behalf of individuals with severe mental illness. It builds
on experimental evidence that cost-effective treatments can be
developed and administered in community settings (Weisbrod *et
al*, 1980; Hoult & Reynolds, 1984) and on quasi-experimental
evidence that governmental intervention can put community
support systems into place in states and local communities (Tessler
& Goldman, 1982). There was considerable evidence, however, that
large metropolitan areas are failing to care adequately for persons
with severe mental illness. The reasons for these historic and
current failures have been enumerated elsewhere (Goldman &
Morrissey, 1985; Mechanic, 1991) and, in the particular case of large
cities, with focus on the effects of bureaucracy, entrenched interests
and 'perverse financial incentives' over a more reasonable approach
to delivering services. This services demonstration not only provides
a test of a remedy to this problem in large urban areas but
also provides an opportunity for a programme of research to be
conducted by a large number of investigators at multiple sites,
integrated into a national evaluation.

Relevance of the RWJ model to the UK situation

The specifics of the national evaluation will be discussed below.
First, however, it seems germane to briefly address the relevance of

the RWJ Program model to the current situation in Britain. Changes in National Health Service (NHS) policy, as a result of the government White Papers, are stimulating variations in the organisation and financing of public health care. With the advent of self-governing trusts, health authorities are now in the position of contracting for, as well as providing, health services. As some health authorities move to a more decentralised system of care, involving multiple providers, including voluntary organisations, the issues of coordination of care will arise.

In addition, the Audit Commission report makes reference to the need for better coordination of services across district health authority and local authority social services boundaries. While much recent discussion has focused on the use of 'keyworkers', analogous to case managers[3] in the US systems, undoubtedly some attempt will be made to address the larger structural and financing barriers that result from the lack of one authority being responsible for the community mental health and social welfare needs of severely mentally ill persons. The development of 'community support systems' (CSS) for severely mentally ill persons may have been an American concept, but it seems clear that district health authorities will need to address the social welfare, housing and vocational, as well as mental health treatment, needs of their mentally ill constituency in local communities. Joint planning has not been a successful mechanism for many communities, raising the possibility that alterations in the organisation of care may be deemed necessary to make the most efficient use of health and welfare dollars. It was precisely the need for one authority for mental health and social services support that produced the RWJ model, although each of the demonstration sites implemented the concept of a centralised mental health authority in their own way, based on local conditions and opportunities.

The design of the national evaluation

The principal objective of the national evaluation was to assess the impact of interventions associated with the development of a local mental health authority in each of the demonstration cities. The evaluation assesses whether organisational and financing changes at the city level result in improved systems of care for persons with

---

[3] For a discussion of the origins and uses of case management in a variety of human services, see Willenbring *et al* (1991).

severe mental illness, and whether mature systems (later in the demonstration) are able to produce greater continuity of care. The evaluation was an agenda of research more than it was an 'evaluation' in the narrowest sense of the word. The national evaluation comprises five interrelated components: a site-level study, a community care study, housing studies, financing studies and disability studies. Table 13.1 characterises the five components and Table 13.2 lists data sources and instruments used in these studies.

It is not possible to discuss each of these studies at length. Therefore, we will focus on the study most germane to the issue of measurement of needs, the key informant survey within the site-level study, and will explain the methodology and the relationship of this aspect of the site-level findings to client outcomes.

Developing the key informant survey

As the view of providing for the needs of chronically mentally ill persons has broadened, beyond 'treatment' to ensuring that basic

TABLE 11.1
Research components of the national evaluation of the RWJ Foundation Program on Chronic Mental Illness

Component	Features
(1) Study of the mental health authority and systems of care	Political and administrative changes Implementation of innovative services Inter-organisational coordination
(2) Community care	Individual client assessment of symptoms, functioning and quality of life Quasi-experimental, pre-post design needs, service use and continuity of care
(3) Housing studies	Site-level assessment of housing development (finance and acquisition) Effect of housing arrangements and residential supportive services on individual outcomes in terms of functioning and quality of life Use of special rental subsidies
(4) Financing studies	Effect of mix of revenue sources and financial incentives on services Patterns of utilisation and costs
(5) Disability and vocational studies	Acquisition of benefits for disabled individuals Effect of vocational rehabilitation on employment

TABLE 11.2

Data sources and instruments for the national evaluation of the RWJ Foundation Program on Chronic Mental Illness

Study component	Data sources	Instruments
Site-level study	Documents Site visits Key informant survey	Assessing local service systems for chronically mentally ill persons
Community care study	Management information system Client interviews Case manager interviews	Community care client questionnaire (baseline and follow-up)[1] Case manager questionnaire[2]
Housing studies Site level	Documents Site visits Housing management information system	
Client level	Client interviews	Community care client questionnaire[1]
Section 8	Client interviews	Section 8 quetionnaire (identical to community care client questionnaire follow-up
Financing studies Site visits	Site visits Financial reports Budgets Management information systems	
Medicaid	State Medicaid plan State Medicaid files	
Disability and vocational rehabilitation studies Site level	Site visits	
Client level	Social Security Adminstration pilot study	

1. Derived from the Quality of Life (Lehman, 1988), Denver Consumer Questionnaire (Demmler *et al*, 1988), Uniform Client Data Instrument (Goldstrom & Manderscheid, 1984), Continuity of Care Provider Questionnaire (Tessler, 1987), Symptom Checklist (SCL–90; Derogatis & Cleary, 1977) and American Housing Survey (US Department of Commerce, 1989).
2. Derived from the Uniform Client Data Instrument (Goldstrom & Manderscheid, 1984) and Continuity of Care Provider Questionnaire (Tessler, 1987).

life needs (such as those for food and shelter) are met, the view of what constitutes the mental health service system has also broadened. Rather than the traditional mental health service delivery system, the concept of a 'community support system' was central to subsequent programme development efforts (Turner & TenHoor, 1978; Tessler & Goldman, 1982). This concept encompasses a much more complex reality owing to the sheer number and types of providers (e.g. mental health, social welfare, employment, housing, rehabilitation and criminal justice) operating in the system of care.

Systems concepts for describing service delivery (such as avail-ability, accessibility, accountability, adequacy, quality, continuity, comprehensiveness and viability) have become well accepted in the health and mental health service arenas. These key service variables taken together define a 'good' service delivery system, as opposed to simply a set of 'good' services. Despite widespread acceptance of these concepts of good system performance, survey methods for assessing the capacity and performance of service systems for severely mentally ill persons are not well developed. After looking for an established instrument without success, a 'key informant survey' was developed to obtain performance ratings of the local service system from knowledgeable persons in each of the demonstration sites.[4]

In addition to the key informant survey, the site-level evaluation team was employing three other methods to collect data pertinent to organisational and service system changes. These include: periodic interviews with local RWJ Program staff to obtain updates on the status of the local mental health authority and other system improve-ments; site visits to obtain assessments of mid-course corrections; and an inter-organisational network study[5] to obtain quantitative measures of the centrality of the local mental health authority and system coordination in five of the nine cities. A variety of contextual information was also available through secondary sources.

Construction of the survey

The key informant survey, Assessing Local Service Delivery Systems for Chronically Mentally Ill Persons, was constructed with five discreet

---

[4] The idea for this type of survey came from prior research on CSS programmes in New York State (Morrissey *et al*, 1986). In that study, respondents were asked to rate the extent of service delivery problems, but the range of items was quite limited.
[5] This separate study, funded by the National Institute for Mental Health, was conducted by Robert Paulson (University of Cincinnati) and Joseph Morrissey (University of North Carolina at Chapel Hill), Co-Principal Investigators. RO1 MH 44839.

parts. The basic building blocks of the instrument allow us to tap respondents' informed judgements about three key areas: client needs, service system performance, and the specific performance of the local mental health authority.

The questionnaire yielded both quantitative and qualitative data. The quantitative data are derived from a series of Likert-type scale items that relate to several distinct constructs. The first section was designed to provide an indication of client needs or the extent to which persons with a severe mental illness were experiencing service delivery problems. This section probes the types of problems encountered with regard to the 11 CSS elements.[6] Respondents were asked to indicate whether certain situations are occurring in their community, and if so, to give their judgement of the severity of the problem. The following examples of items are illustrative.

To what extent are the following problems occurring for chronically mentally ill (CMI) persons in City A:

(a) not having access to in-patient services because there are too few public in-patient beds;
(b) not having access to adequate amounts of food and clean clothing; and
(c) lacking opportunities for vocational training or sheltered work?

In the next section, respondents were asked specifically to rate the adequacy and quality of existing services within each of the 11 service categories. Adequacy was examined by asking how many of those who need each service are getting it (all, most, some, few or none), and quality was measured by asking respondents to consider the technical and interpersonal aspects of care and the physical setting. Respondents were not rating the care given by particular facilities, but rather making global judgements about care in these categories across the city. The next section of the questionnaire was devoted to measuring current service system performance, in terms of availability and accessibility, as well as the level of coordination of services and information. Respondents were asked to assess how well the current service system performs on a number

---

[6] The 11 CSS service elements include the basic services believed to be essential to maintain severely mentally ill persons in the community, and they include: outreach services; emergency services; mental health treatment services; psychosocial rehabilitation services; case management; assistance with basic human needs; vocational and prevocational services; shelter/housing; medical/dental care; substance misuse services; and supportive services (peer and family support).

of dimensions. Some examples of items include: How well does the current service system for chronically mentally ill persons in City A perform on these activities:

    (a) avoiding excessive waiting lists or long delays in scheduling;

    (b) providing services at reasonable cost to CMI persons;

    (c) training staff to work caringly and comfortably with CMI persons; and

    (d) developing agreements among agencies at the direct service delivery level to avoid needless duplication of effort.

The final section focuses on the performance of the mental health authority, with regard to its structure and administrative effectiveness, its role in articulating a clinical plan for services to the target population, and its success in securing and coordinating the flow of fiscal resources to individual service providers.

Qualitative data are obtained in the last section of the questionnaire in the form of several open-ended questions about the major accomplishments and shortcomings of the local RWJ Program. These data are a rich source of detail and observations that are complementary to the numerical data provided in the main body of the questionnaire.

The respondents

The respondent pool was developed in consultation with the RWJ Program staff at each of the nine sites. The process was iterative. We relied upon the concept of a community support system and its associated functions to ascertain the sectors from which knowledgeable respondents could be identified. For most agencies, the key informant was to be the chief executive officer, but for some more centrally involved agencies, multiple points of view were sought.[7] We reviewed the lists created by the Program staff, adding and substituting agencies and informants where appropriate. We sought to apply the same selection criteria and sampling strategy in each city (regardless of the boundaries of the service system as viewed by local participants), so that cross-site comparisons would be meaningful.

Finally, the key informant survey was pre-tested in Rochester, New York, in collaboration with the Monroe-Livingston Demonstration Project. This site was chosen because a capitation financing project,

---

[7] One of the reasons to seek multiple points of view within an agency is the prevailing view that issues may be differentially perceived depending on one's place in the agency (i.e. the 'front-lines' *versus* the 'top floor').

being operated by Integrated Mental Health, Inc., was a demonstration of systems reorganisation in the mental health field, similar to, but not a part of, the RWJ Program. While the focus of the reorganisation in Rochester has to do with a particular financing mechanism, Integrated Mental Health acts as a local mental health authority, managing and coordinating services, much as the authorities in the RWJ sites are doing. The pre-test indicated that the key informant instrument had face validity to participants in the various sectors and could be administered as a mailed questionnaire with an acceptable response rate after two follow-ups.

Findings from the key informant survey

Information concerning analysis of the data from the key informant survey, as well as the specific findings, have been reported elsewhere (Morrissey *et al*, 1994*a*; Morrissey *et al*, 1994*b*). Briefly, the findings from the first wave of data collection (mid-1989) indicated that the key goals of the RWJ Foundation Program were being addressed in the sites. While respondents indicated that dramatic improvements had occurred in specific services, their ratings of service system performance indicated that there continued to be significant problems in service coordination across the demonstration sites, with variability among the sites. Consistent with data from annual site visits, respondents' ratings of the performance of local systems of care sorted the cities into three groupings: a high-functioning group (Toledo, Columbus, Cincinnati and Charlotte); a middle group (Austin, Denver and Honolulu); and a more poorly rated group (Philadelphia and Baltimore). The largest cities in the demonstration were rated most poorly in 1989.

The findings of the key informant survey, together with the data from a companion inter-organisational network analysis, provided clear evidence that most of the RWJ Program sites created a centralised mental health authority that, with the exception of two sites (Honolulu and Denver), was rated highly on its ability to centralise clinical, fiscal and administrative authority. Overall, however, key informants rated the authorities themselves (as discreet organisations) more highly than they rated the performance of the local service systems, suggesting that the development of a new management entity is somewhat easier to accomplish than improving the overall performance of an urban, public system of mental health care.

Caution must be exercised in interpreting these findings. As is true of many evaluations of ongoing systems change, a true baseline measure was not possible in the RWJ Program evaluation. Without a baseline measure, it is possible that the biggest jump in service system performance actually occurred during the first two years of demonstration – before the 'operational phase' and before our initial measurement in 1989. If so, the measurement between 1989 and 1991 underestimated the true impact of the demonstration. It is also possible that expectations for major change during the two-year period between 1989 and 1991 were unrealistic, given that large urban areas have complex governmental and service environments. Finally, there may have also been 'ceiling effects' – suggested by the tendency of some sites to score highly in 1989 and not show improvement in 1991 (e.g. two of the Ohio sites). If there are ceiling effects, this suggests that the level of performance eventually attained, rather than the improvement attained between two points in time, may be the more realistic measure for assessing the success of the demonstration (Morrissey *et al*, 1994*b*).

One of the core assumptions of the RWJ Program was that the development of a centralised mental health authority was the most effective way for large urban areas to organise services. The logic model for the demonstration involved two other assumptions: that the development of a centralised mental health authority would lead to enhancements of the service system; and that enhancements in the performance of the service system would lead to improvement in client outcomes (Goldman *et al*, 1990). The findings of the key informant survey suggest an explanation for the lack of observable effect of the RWJ Program on client outcomes (Lehman *et al*, 1994). Even though the key informant survey demonstrated that, for the most part, local mental health authorities had attained high levels of performance within the demonstration period, overall service system performance lagged behind (Morrissey *et al*, 1994*b*). Another factor that may help to explain the lack of impact on client outcomes was mental health authorities' focus on the development and enhancement of case management programmes, rather than on the development of treatment interventions of known clinical impact (Ridgely *et al*, 1996). Even the best coordination of clinically inadequate services is unlikely to positively affect symptomatology and quality of life of seriously mentally ill individuals (Ridgely *et al*, 1996; Burns *et al*, 1999).

Other methods for assessing needs in the RWJ Program on Chronic Mental Illness

The key informant survey was not the only tool used in the RWJ Program evaluation to measure the need for services, and several of the component studies examine the extent to which the identified needs of individual clients were met. Furthermore, the key informant survey was only one element in the assessment of changes in the system of care in each city. Each element was designed to characterise the implementation of innovation and to predict (or explain) the impact of changes in the system of care on individual client outcomes.

First, each administration of the key informant survey was preceded by a three-day site visit to each city. The visit was conducted by two or three members of the site-level RWJ Program evaluation team, who spoke with stakeholders (e.g. providers, consumers, government officials, etc.) serving analogous roles in each site. Additional visits were made to study special aspects of the demonstration, including the mechanisms for financing services or developing new housing units. The site visits provided more detail than could be gained from a questionnaire and more comprehensive observations of actual services and interactions among individuals. The key informant surveys confirmed a great many observations made during the more subjective site visits. They also suggested aspects of the demonstration that we had not seen, or raised questions that required further inquiry. While believing in the strength of site-visiting as an RWJ Program evaluation tool (Silverman *et al*, 1990), we have noted some problems. For example, the data from the key informant survey in one site indicated that the larger group of respondents in that site were more positive about the demonstration than was evident at the site visit. This discrepancy suggests limits of these data-collection strategies. Civic pride in this community may have artificially inflated responses, while site visits can reach only a limited number of informants. Consequently, we feel strongly that site-visiting and key informant surveys are complementary, rather than alternative, methods for collecting qualitative data on programme implementation.

Second, data from the key informant surveys and site visits are supplemented by documentary evidence (e.g. annual reports, planning reports, government documents and newspaper accounts) used in further assessment of programme implementation. Third, a study of inter-organisational networks and how they may have changed over the course of the demonstration completes our assessment of the development of a system of services.

Our design then calls for us to describe and assess these changes at the system (or site) level and to predict what kind of impact these changes might have on individual client outcomes (in terms of symptoms, functioning and quality of life). Client outcomes are assessed using self-reports in structured interviews. Clients are asked about their needs (what needs they have identified for themselves and what needs have been identified by others), what services they have received to meet these needs, and how they feet about these services. Service utilisation data (e.g. patterns of use) will be analysed to describe *continuity* in episodes of care. The relationships among client outcomes, continuity of care, exposure to particular services and service agencies, and the nature of system coordination (based on data from the site-visits, the key informant survey and the inter-organisational analysis) will be studied. Taken together, these analyses constitute an integrated evaluation of the RWJ Program on Chronic Mental Illness.

The results of these assessments may be used to guide the planning of future mental health services, as well as making mid-course corrections in the current system of services. The key informant survey was constructed to capture information about the 11 elements of a community support system. Data about client needs and system performance in each of these 11 areas can be translated into recommendations for the enhancement of specific service domains. For example, if the needs for housing are being met and the system of residential services is viewed as performing well, then a planner for a local mental health authority might conclude that the current strategy has been working and the approach and level of effort should be maintained. Conversely, if the rehabilitation needs of the population were not being met because of poor performance by the service system in this area, then remedial activity would be indicated. This survey would not identify particular agencies where remedial action might be taken, but would highlight areas of need according to the 11 service elements.

Overall, the key informant survey provides feedback on the performance of the local mental health authority, providing guidance on changes in the structure or process of governance and on administration of mental health and support services in the community. It is hoped that such assessments will encourage a process of ongoing RWJ Program evaluation and quality assurance for mental health service planning.

As this chapter has indicated, the RWJ Program evaluation of the RWJ demonstration has focused on the development of *systems of care*. What this emphasis has overshadowed is the assessment of the *quality* of services at the level of individual service programmes. The demonstration *assumes* that there was an effective technology for treating, rehabilitating and caring for individuals with severe mental illnesses; the RWJ Program evaluation assumes that these demonstration sites will implement the proper technology, *if* they can implement a system to deliver the services. Although these may not be completely reasonable assumptions, they are imbedded in the conceptualisation of the demonstration and its evaluation. The primary focus of the demonstration was on system creation, services integration and continuity of care.

If we set aside the conceptual reasons for avoiding the assessment of quality of care, there are two other reasons for skirting the issue of quality: there was little consensus on operational measures of quality, and it was very difficult to make the observations necessary to evaluate quality. Such observations often require intimate access to the interactions between client and provider – and the very act of observing the interaction probably distorts the interaction. Proxy measures of quality often are not satisfactory substitutes. Because of limitations in the RWJ Program evaluation methods and restricted access to observe clinical interactions, we continue to focus on structural and process measures. We assess individual outcomes without being able to connect these dependent measures to specific service interventions. It is a bit like looking for one's watch beneath the street lamp, even though the watch was lost at the other end of the street, just because the light was better at this end. At some point, we need to bring the light to the assessment of the quality of services and programmes.

Acknowledgements

While this chapter bears the names of three investigators participating in the national evaluation of the RWJ Foundation Program on Chronic Mental Illness, it reflects the work of the larger group. The authors thank Anthony Lehman at the University of Maryland; Sandra Newman, Elizabeth Ann Skinner and Don Steinwachs at the Johns Hopkins University; Richard Frank at Harvard; Catherine Jackson at RAND; and Dee Roth at the Ohio Department of Mental Health.

The national evaluation was supported by grants from the RWJ Foundation, the National Institute of Mental Health, several other US federal agencies, and the State of Ohio Department of Mental Health to the Mental Health Policy Studies Program, Center for Mental Health Services Research (Department of Psychiatry, University of Maryland at Baltimore, 645 W Redwood Street, Baltimore, MD 21201, USA).

References

BURNS, T., CREED, F., FAHY, T., *ET AL* (1999) Intensive versus standard case management for severe psychotic illness: a randomized controlled trial. *The Lancet*, **353**, 2185–2189.

DEMMLER, J., SHERN, D. L., COEN, A. S., *ET AL* (1988) *Denver CMI Initiative Study 3: Client Needs, Life Situation and Satisfaction with Initiative Program. Client and Collateral Survey.* Colorado: Colorado Division of Mental Health.

DEROGATIS, L. R. & CLEARY, P. A. (1977) Confirmation of the dimensional structure of the SCL-90: a study in construct validation. *Journal of Clinical Psychology*, **33**, 981–989.

GOLDMAN, H. & MORRISSEY, J. (1985) The alchemy of mental health policy: homelessness and the fourth cycle of reform. *American Journal of Public Health*, **75**, 727–731.

—, — & RIDGELY, M. S. (1990) Form and function of mental health authorities at RWJ Foundation program sites: Preliminary observations. *Hospital and Community Psychiatry*, **41**, 1222–1230.

GOLDSTROM, I. D. & MANDERSCHEID, R. W. (1984) The chronically mentally ill: a descriptive analysis from the Uniform Client Data Instrument. *Community Support Service Journal*, **2**, 4–9.

HOULT, J. & REYNOLDS, I. (1984) Schizophrenia: A comprehensive trial of community oriented and hospital oriented care. *Acta Psychiatrica Scandinavica*, **69**, 359–372.

LEHMAN, A. F. (1988) A quality of life interview for the chronically mentally ill. *Evaluation and Program Planning*, **11**, 51–62.

—, POSTRADO, L., ROTH, D., ET AL (1994) Continuity of care and client outcomes in the Robert Wood Johnson Foundation Program on Chronic Mental Illness. *The Milbank Quarterly*, **72**, 105–122.

MECHANIC, D. (1991) Strategies for integrating public mental health services. *Hospital and Community Psychiatry*, **42**, 797–801.

MORRISSEY, J. P., Tausig, M. & Lindsey, M. (1986) Interorganizational networks in mental health systems: Assessing community support systems for the chronically mentally ill. In: *The Organization of Mental Health Services: Societal and Community Systems* (eds W. Scott & B. Black), pp. 197–230. Beverly Hills, CA: Sage.

—, CALLOWAY, M., BARTKO, T., ET AL (1994a) Local mental health authorities and service system change: Evidence from the Robert Wood Johnson Foundation Program on Chronic Mental Illness. *The Milbank Quarterly*, **72**, 49–80.

—, RIDGELY, M. S., GOLDMAN, H. H., ET AL (1994b) Assessment of community mental health support systems: a key informant approach. *Community Mental Health Journal*, **30**, 565–579.

PROGRAM FOR THE CHRONICALLY MENTALLY ILL (1995) *Program Announcement*. Princeton, NJ: The RWJ Foundation.

RIDGELY, M. S., MORRISSEY, J. P., PAULSON, R., ET AL (1996) Characteristics and activities of case managers in the RWJ Foundation Program on Chronic Mental Illness. *Psychiatric Services*, **47**, 737–743.

SHORE, M. & COHEN, M. (1990) Creating new systems of care: The Robert Wood Johnson Foundation Program on chronic mental illness. *Hospital and Community Psychiatry*, **41**, 1212–1216.

SILVERMAN, M., RICCI, E. & GUNTER, M. (1990) Strategies for increasing the rigor of qualitative methods in evaluation of health care programs. *Evaluation Review*, **14**, 57–74.

TESSLER, R. C. (1987) Continuity of care and client outcome. *Psychosocial Rehabilitation Journal*, **10**, 39–53.

— & GOLDMAN, H. (EDS) (1982) *The Chronically Mentally Ill: Assessing Community Support Programs*. Cambridge, Massachusetts: Ballinger.

TURNER, J. & TENHOOR, W. (1978) The NIMH community support program: Pilot approach to a needed social reform. *Schizophrenia Bulletin*, **4**, 319–408.

US DEPARTMENT OF COMMERCE (1989) US Bureau of the Census. Current Housing Reports, Series H-150. *General Housing Characteristics for the US and Regions: 1987. Annual Housing Survey*. Washington, DC: US Government Printing Office.

WALSH, A. & LEIGHLAND, J. (1986) *Public Authorities and Mental Health Programs*. New York: Institute for Public Administration.

WEISBROD, B., TEST, M. & STEIN, L. (1980) Alternatives to mental hospital treatment II: Economic benefit–cost analysis. *Archives of General Psychiatry*, **37**, 400–498.

WILLENBRING, M., RIDGELY, M. S., STINCHFIELD, R., ET AL (1991) *Application of Case Management in Alcohol and Drug Dependence: Matching Techniques and Populations*. Rockville, MD: National Institute on Alcohol Abuse and Alcoholism.

14 Auditing the use of psychiatric beds

BERNARD AUDINI and RICHARD DUFFETT

At the beginning of the 20th century, psychiatric hospitals were places for patients with serious mental illnesses to live. The number of patients occupying beds in psychiatric hospitals peaked in 1954 and has since fallen by 74% (Johnson & Lelliott, 1998). At the beginning of the 21st century, psychiatric wards are facilities for treatment, and the average duration of admissions is measured in weeks as opposed to years. As bed requirements have changed in the last century, it is likely that they will continue to do so in the future. Advances in therapeutic treatments, a new mental health act and changes in government policy will all impact on the number of in-patient and dedicated community beds for those with mental illness. As well as national trends and policies, the need for beds will also reflect the needs of the catchment population that a service treats. All residential provision within either the hospital or the community is an expensive resource. The closure of unnecessary beds can bring about cost savings that can then be spent elsewhere, but too few beds can result in poor care and the 'burn-out' of staff both in the hospital and in the community. Tailoring the bed requirement in an ongoing way to the needs of a catchment area population is the role of audit.

What is audit?

Audit involves systematically looking at the procedures used for diagnosis, care and treatment, examining how associated resources are used, and investigating the effect that care has on the outcome and quality of life for the patient (Department of Health, 1996). Audit can be used to examine the structure (availability and organisation of resources), the process (what is done with resources) and the outcome (effect on health of the intervention). While admission to

241

hospital (or discharge from hospital) is an outcome, this chapter will concentrate on the audit of structure (number and type of bed), the process (how those beds are used) and the methods of audit. Audit aims to improve the quality of care for an identified group of patients using the best available knowledge; it also is an ongoing (or cyclical) process whereby the results of previous audits are fed back to inform future audits. Audit differs from research in this regard. Research tests a hypothesis, aims to add to the body of knowledge and importantly should be generalisable (i.e. not only apply to the group that was studied). Both audit and research, however, involve measurement, and tools used in research may be applicable to audit and vice versa. Audit may also be a component of service evaluation. While service evaluation aims at improving patient care, it collects data to compare one service with another or against service standards and is usually a one-off exercise, as applied by the Health Advisory Service (HAS) (Rix *et al*, 1999).

Why audit?

Research does give an indication of the likely bed numbers a service requires. Data obtained from the national census has been used to obtain measures of deprivation (Jarman, 1983) and can be used to compute an expected bed requirement (Glover *et al*, 1997). But the measures used are not perfect and suggest that, for example, Belgrave Square (the address of the Royal College of Psychiatrists) is more deprived than the national average. These indices have been unable to explain the large variation in acute beds per head of population within London (Audini *et al*, 1999). Even if a hospital service has an appropriate number of beds, this does not guarantee that the service is optimally configured. While it would be inappropriate for all services to be conducting research, audit is an essential activity if the expensive resources of hospital and specialised community beds are to be used optimally, both in terms of their absolute numbers and the type of service they provide. Audit may suggest a reconfiguration of catchment areas to reflect local morbidity, or the balance between the genders, or that the number of rehabilitation and acute beds should be altered.

How to audit the use of psychiatric beds

At the outset, when considering how or what to audit, it is essential that the stakeholders, that is, all those who will be involved in the process or affected by the outcome (or their representatives), are consulted. This allows for a more robust methodology to be developed. In addition, this will encourage ownership of the process and results, aiding in data collection and an increased willingness to implement changes based on the findings.

The function of a psychiatric bed

A psychiatric bed has two functions: first to provide accommodation for the patient and second as a location for a package of care. Patients at the point of admission to psychiatric services usually require both, for example a patient who has relapsed and whose family cannot accommodate them while acutely ill. Often, patients remain in a hospital (accommodation only), even though fit for discharge, because no accommodation in the community is available. This relationship is not static. The need for accommodation and the need for care may vary independently over time, for example a patient may still utilise in-patient resources (ward round and keyworker time) when sent on leave overnight, even though they are not physically occupying a bed (hence not requiring accommodation). In addition, service provision is not uniform, that is, in some services patients may require admission to receive a package of care that can be provided by a neighbouring trust as an out-patient through assertive outreach care, without the need for admission.

The Royal College of Psychiatrists recommends that occupancy levels of psychiatric beds should average around 85% (Hirsch, 1988). This will usually ensure that there will be some empty beds, and at times of increased demand, wards will still be able to admit patients. When ward occupancy level reaches 100%, patients may have to be admitted to wards other than those of their catchment area. Consultants and staff become increasingly preoccupied with finding a bed or transferring patients. When operating at 100% occupancy, a hospital is accommodating patients efficiently, but the quality of the package of care is likely to deteriorate. Paradoxically, as staff devote more time trying to accommodate urgent admissions, they may spend less time on preparing patients for discharge, thereby prolonging their admissions.

There are numerous factors involved in defining what constitutes an adequate number of beds for an individual service. There have been some attempts to calculate bed requirements based on characteristics of the catchment area population (Glover *et al*, 1997), but in reality such simplistic measures cannot be taken in isolation, and local characteristics and service provision by a range of providers (local authority social services and housing; health, community and tertiary services; and private and independent agencies) are also important. Within London, there is no demonstrable correlation between measures of deprivation and acute bed provision (Audini *et al*, 1999).

Audits of psychiatric beds may also involve the collection of data about the number of beds in use (accommodation) or the needs of patients who occupy them (package of care required). An example of this first type of audit, which often involves routinely collected data, would be a service examining its bed requirement by reviewing occupancy levels over a given time frame. This type of audit might show that occupancy levels are low indicating that some beds could be closed and the funding transferred elsewhere to other parts of the service. If occupancy levels are high, it may sugest that some additional resources are required, although not necessarily the same type as being audited. Alternative provision may be more appropriate, for example rehabilitation beds or intensive community services.

The second type of audit examines the characteristics of patients or residents and the package of care they require. This might suggest that their needs would be better served if the number of acute beds was decreased and more rehabilitation beds offered. While these two types of audits are not exclusive, they are complementary and in the rest of the chapter they will be considered in turn.

Auditing accommodation needs

MILMIS (Monitoring Inner London Mental Illness Services)

In London and elsewhere, bed occupancy levels often exceed 100%, as patients are sent on leave to create beds for other patients who urgently require admission. Even with this undesirable practice, patients are admitted as extra-contractual referrals (ECRs) to beds outside their catchment area trust (MILMIS Project Group, 1995). In 1994, in response to complaints from many clinicians that they were having difficulty in finding sufficient beds to admit acutely disturbed patients, the Royal College of Psychiatrists' Research Unit set up the MILMIS study. The MILMIS project was designed to see if mental health services were meeting the demand for beds and whether current College guidance about occupancy levels was being adhered to, to quantify the problem of demand for acute beds outstripping supply and to identify the extent of the problem within inner-London.

A survey was designed to quantify the demand for acute beds and identify whether sufficient supply was available. The method had to be practical for trusts of very differing configurations to employ. In addition, as no services were obliged to participate and funding was limited, the project relied on services being willing to collect their own data and supply it to the College Research Unit (CRU). The study, therefore, had to be one which provided data that the local services valued themselves and which were not so sensitive that they were unwilling to share them. Since June 1994, the MILMIS group, coordinated by the CRU, has conducted seven census-based surveys; four at six-month intervals from June 1994 to January 1996, and three at annual intervals from January 1997 to January 1999. These provide information on both the extent of the problem and the number of additional beds required if the recommended 85% occupancy level for catchment area services is to be achieved.

MILMIS surveys have two parts, a census day on which bed use is studied, and a census week during which incidents of violence, sexual harassment and self-harm are recorded. At midnight on the census day, the number of acute psychiatric beds available to each service is recorded, together with the number of people registered as being in-patients on acute wards. Patients registered as being in-patients include those on leave; thus, the number in-patients may exceed the number of available beds. For each in-patient, status under the Mental Health Act, leave status and duration of admission is determined. In addition, a count is made of the number and location of people who are awaiting admission to an acute psychiatric ward. These people might be waiting in a non-acute psychiatric ward, a medical ward, an acute psychiatric ward in another trust, a private psychiatric hospital, a community setting, a police cell or a prison. Efforts are made to ensure that patients are not counted twice within the same trust.

For the purpose of the MILMIS surveys, an 'acute bed' is defined as a bed designated for the admission of general adult psychiatric patients under the age of 65 years. Beds in locked psychiatric wards are included if they provide short-term care for patients, but not if they are primarily for forensic patients. Rehabilitation or continuing care beds are excluded, as such beds are effectively for tertiary referrals and are not usually provided for patients directly from the community. Beds are excluded if they are designated as offering specialist services, for example for drug detoxification or treatment of eating disorders, even if they are located within an acute ward.

For the first census, many more questions were asked than could be addressed within the census time frame; in addition, services interpreted some questions slightly differently. Subsequent surveys therefore concentrated on the core data outlined above and researchers visited all sites to verify data. Immediately prior to MILMIS IV (January 1996), two members of the CRU visited all sites to ensure that data were collected in a standard way. New data collectors were visited and trained prior to MILMIS V (January 1997), and two researchers visited all sites to assess data collection methods following MILMIS VI (January 1998). MILMIS VII (January 1999) involved the same inner-London mental illness services as in previous censuses, with an additional service. All new data collectors were trained in methods of data recording. The full MILMIS group met on 10 occasions to discuss the data collection method and results.

Calculating bed requirement

To quantify the extent of this unmet need for acute beds, occupancy rates were calculated in three different ways using three different numerators, and expressed as a percentage of the total number of acute beds (denominator):

'Ward' occupancy	numerator = the total number registered as in-patients (row 5 in Table 14.1)
''True' occupancy	ward occupancy plus those who are awaiting admission (rows 12–17)
'Minimum' occupancy	true occupancy minus those on leave who were thought not to need a bed kept available (row 19)

Each definition of occupancy makes its own contribution to describing the use of beds. True occupancy provides information about the number of beds required to meet the needs of all patients who should be accommodated on that day. Ward occupancy relates to the number of patients whose care is the responsibility of the ward staff. Ideally, a bed should always be available for each of these patients. Minimum occupancy provides an absolute measure. A minimum occupancy of greater than 100% indicates that care is unsafe and/or unsupportive, because beds are not available to patients who need them that day.

Findings

The results of the seven MILMIS surveys are summarised in Table 14.1.

Bed provision

The 13 services that had returned data had a mean of 45.1 acute beds per 100 000 population at the time of MILMIS VII (range 24–109).

TABLE 14.1

Results of the seven MILMIS censuses conducted between June 1994 and January 1999

	June 1994	January 1995	July 1995	January 1996	January 1997	January 1998	January 1999
Number of services	12	12	12	12	13	13	13
Combined population	2.6	2.9	2.9	2.9	2.9	2.9	2.6
Total admission beds	1109	1235	1250	1328	1296	1369	1175
Beds per 100 000 population	42.6	42.5	43.1	45.7	44.6	47.2	45.1
Patients on in-patient register	1236	1321	1352	1411	1413	1445	1314
% in beds for 3–6 months	27	20	17	20	17	15	19
% in beds for 6–12 months	8	9	8	12	8	7	9
% in beds for >12 months	4	3	4	5	3	4	4
% detained	50	48	48	49	46	53	51
No. on leave, urgent need for bed (incl. AWOL)	54	94	92	79	73	88	123
No. on leave, no urgent need for bed	87	93	86	103	159	193	118
No. in other beds in trust	53	43	30	54	19	49	25
No. in medical beds	5	7	3	9	13	3	7
No. in NHS ECR beds	42	18	28	40	16	73	12
No. in private ECR beds	60	84	68	68	90	57	68
No. at home/in community	30	29	38	38	21	21	52
No. in prison/police cells	14	8	8	25	2	3	4
True occupancy (%)	130	123	122	125	123	121	128
Ward occupancy (%)	111	107	108	106	109	106	112
Minimum occupancy (%)	122	115	115	114	111	107	112
Services with occupancy >100%	11	10	12	9	10	6	13
No. of first-degree assaults	67	84	93	80	77	64	95
No. of second-degree assaults	37	43	29	51	36	24	35
No. of third-degree assaults	1	4	2	3	13	1	2
Incidents of sexual harassment	53	37	66	78	11	30	33
Incidents of sexual assault	8	4	1	1	0	0	0
Self-harm incidents	34	33	21	20	16	12	31

Bed provision did not correlate significantly with the social deprivation levels of participating services, as measured by Jarman UPA–8 Scores (Jarman, 1983).

Use of alternatives to local acute beds

Patients awaiting urgent admission or transfer to an inner-London acute bed were in a variety of settings: some had been admitted elsewhere as ECRs (range for MILMIS I–VII = 80–130); some were in other types of psychiatric ward (range 19–54), general medical wards (range 3–13), at home or in another community setting (range 21–52), or in a prison or police cell (range 2–25).

In most services, at all time points, acute bed provision has been inadequate to meet demand. At the time of MILMIS I, all but one service had minimum occupancy levels above 100% (mean 122%, range 97–153%); at MILMIS VII, five services had minimum occupancy levels below 100% (mean 112%, range 72–157%). Four of five trusts, which had increased acute beds between MILMIS II and VII, also had a fall in minimum occupancy levels between these two census points. Only one of the remaining seven trusts showed a decrease in minimum occupancy levels.

As Table 14.1 shows, between 27% and 39% of acute beds on MILMIS census days were occupied by patients who had been in hospital for more than three months. Another consistent finding is that one-half of patients were detained under sections of the Mental Health Act. Incidents of violence and sexual harassment were very common.

Comment

The MILMIS study is limited in that its focus is on acute bed provision and has ignored other in-patient facilities and community alternatives to admission. Between 1994 and 1999, there were consistently more patients requiring acute in-patient care than there were beds available. The consequences of this are threefold:

    (a) the quality of care is compromised by admitting patients to hospitals distant from their homes, discharging or sending patients on leave prematurely and not admitting others;

    (b) the difficulty of admitting patients when needed puts pressure on community services; and

    (c) the high use of ECRs results in a transfer of funds away from already hard-pressed inner-London services.

This leads to poor quality of care and is not cost-effective. The widespread use of ECR provision diverts funding from community mental health teams (CMHTs) and interrupts continuity of care when patients are admitted to distant services. As a consequence, the demand for beds is paradoxically increased (Tyrer *et al*, 1998).

Other factors, not measured by MILMIS, might have affected bed usage during the period of the censuses. These include a continuation of increasing demand (numbers of patients registered as in-patients have increased) and local service developments that might be alternatives to admission, such as assertive outreach, out-of-hours teams, 24-hour staffed accommodation and respite facilities.

The MILMIS data allow for estimations to be made of the number of additional admission beds, or community alternatives, required to meet a target mean occupancy level of 85%. For MILMIS I, the requirement was 19 beds per 100 000 population; for MILMIS VII it had reduced to 14 beds per 100 000 population.

The MILMIS surveys offer a way of monitoring the impact of policy and service development initiatives at a local and London-wide level. In particular, they give some indication of the extent of alternative or additional services required to reduce pressures on acute beds to acceptable levels. These new developments might be additional beds or community alternatives to hospital care. The latter will include assertive community teams, 24-hour nursed beds and bed management initiatives leading to diversions from admission.

Auditing the characteristics of patients

The National Health Service (NHS) is no longer a virtual monopoly provider of mental health residential care. This makes it difficult to assess the volume, range and adequacy of local provision. In 1983, the NHS managed about 82% of residential provision for the mentally ill (under the age of 65 years); by 1993, this had fallen to about 58%. The private sector in particular is playing a much greater role. This shift in provider agency has almost certainly accentuated the impact of the reduction in overall numbers, by further reducing the availability of residential places with 24-hour cover. Whereas virtually all hospital beds have 24-hour cover by staff awake at night, surveys conducted in 1990 and 1992 suggested that perhaps as little as one-quarter of non-NHS facilities have similar levels of cover, and less than one-half have any staff on the premises at night (Faulkner *et al*, 1992; Lelliott & Wing, 1994). Many non-NHS residential facilities are therefore likely to be unable to accommodate mentally ill people who require close or constant supervision. The relative lack of high-staffed hostel places for medium- or long-term care, means that perhaps as many as 1000 'new long-stay' patients aged 18–64 years remain in hospital despite being 'medically fit' for discharge; these patients occupy about 5% of available hospital beds (Lelliott & Wing, 1994).

Residential care study

A study designed to answer important questions on the range and type of provision and the characteristics of residents (aged 16–64 years) placed within facilities for those with mental health problems was that of Lelliott *et al* (1996). Eight health districts were selected and all facilities within their boundaries were included. This included those managed by a variety of agencies, including the NHS, local authority (social services or housing department), voluntary sector bodies or private companies or individuals. All residents in facilities designated solely for the mentally ill were assessed regardless of whether the person was judged by the keyworker to be mentally ill. NHS facilities were treated differently in that only people who were in hospital were assessed. Patients in hospital were included if on the census day they had remained in hospital for more than six months, or had their discharge delayed during the period of data collection because residential places in the community were unavailable.

Assessment schedules

The schedules used for this study were tailored to examine the characteristics of residents and the facility.

The Resident Profile used was based on a modified version of a schedule used in the national audit of new long-stay psychiatric patients (Lelliott *et al*, 1994), which itself was based on the FACE Profile (Clifford, 1993) and the Community Placement Questionnaire (Clifford *et al*, 1991).

The Facility Profile gathered detailed information about: the managing agent; the fabric of the building(s) (including number and type of rooms and amenities); the categories of residents catered for; the number and qualifications of staff; extent of cover services provided (including at night) to residents and non-residents; and input to the facility from external mental health workers.

Analysis of resident data

The resident profile contained 27 items relating to clinical, behavioural and social functioning, each rated on a scale of 0–3 for severity.

Many of these were inter-correlated. To reduce the number of variables for use in subsequent analyses, some of these items were collapsed into five composite variables. This process was informed by two principal components: analysis of items relating to psychiatric symptoms and risk to self, and of items relating to personal and interpersonal functioning.

These composite variables, and the items that were summed to create them, were:

(a) *mental illness*: hallucinations and delusions, abnormal mood, other mental health problems, memory impairment and over-activity;

(b) *affective symptoms*: mood, suicide risk and other mental health problems;

(c) *vulnerability*: self-neglect, memory impairment and over-activity;

(d) *activities of daily living (ADLs)*: personal appearance and hygiene, housework, cooking, shopping, laundry, use of public transport and budgeting; and

(e) *social interaction*: conversation with staff and conversation with other residents.

Some individual data items were examined separately:

(a) *history of violence*: serious violence, other dangerous/criminal behaviour or admission to special hospital or regional secure unit;

(b) *recent aggression*: aggressive or disruptive behaviour in the past month;

(c) *risk of violence*: in the event of the resident being discharged to independent living;

(d) *recent suicidal behaviour*: in the past month;

(e) *risk of deliberate self-harm*: in the event of the resident being discharged to independent living;

(f) *recent self-neglect*: in the past month;

(g) *risk of non-deliberate self-harm*: in the event of the resident being discharged to independent living; and

(h) *recent alcohol or drug misuse*: in the past month.

Findings

The eight sites differed in population size and density, and in level of social deprivation. Data collectors identified 368 eligible facilities; these accommodated 1951 people who met study criteria on census day. Volume and range of provision differed between districts. Overall, 37% of residential places are managed by the NHS,

14% by the local authority, 17% by the voluntary sector and 32% by the private sector.

Residents' characteristics

Demographic characteristics

Fifty-six per cent of residents were men; women residents (average age 56 years) were older than men (average age 47 years). Eighty-seven per cent of residents were White, 7% were married and only 4% were employed or students at the time of the survey, the remainder being unemployed – 38%, retired – 26% or medically retired/disabled – 33%.

Psychiatric history

As a group, the residents had histories of long-term mental illness. Only 6% had had their first contact with mental health services less than one year before the survey; for 62%, the first contact had been more than 10 years previously. Only 13% had never been admitted to a psychiatric ward, whereas 37% had had five or more previous admissions. About one-third had spent a lifetime total of more than five years in psychiatric hospitals and only 18% had spent less than three months in hospital. Consistent with this history of long-term contact with mental health services, about two-thirds of residents had moved into the facility directly from some other form of residential setting.

Diagnosis

Ninety-two per cent of residents had been assigned a diagnosis by their keyworker; of these, 60% were reported to have schizophrenia or paranoid psychosis, 16% affective psychosis, 12% neurotic disorders, 5% dementia, 5% personality disorder and 2% alcohol- or drug-related disorders.

Symptoms of psychiatric illness

Sixty-four per cent of residents were assessed as having experienced moderate or severe problems in at least one domain of psychiatric symptomatology in the month before assessment (rated as a score of 2 or 3 on a scale of 0–3).

Physical health

Only 56% of residents had been free of any form of physical disability or physical health problems in the month prior to assessment; 27% had experienced moderate or severe problems during this period.

Social, personal and interpersonal functioning

Using a global rating, keyworkers considered that 46% of residents had severely impaired quality of life functioning or were totally reliant on others. A further 24% had only moderate levels of functioning, with large areas of activity significantly affected. As rated by their behaviour in the month before assessment, 74% of residents had moderate or severe problems in at least one specific activity of daily living (ADL).

Dangerousness and risk to self

About one-quarter of residents had a history of violence. More than one-fifth had displayed a moderate or severe level of aggression in the month before assessment. Keyworkers thought that, if discharged, 29% of residents would pose moderate or severe risk of acting violently or dangerously, 21% of committing deliberate self-harm and 61% of harming themselves unintentionally.

Consistent with these assessments, keyworkers thought that 89% of residents would experience some problems if discharged immediately to a less dependent setting and that for 48% of residents these problems would be severe or very severe.

Differences between residents in facilities of different types

The profile of residents in different types of accommodation varied.

Forensic units

Residents had more frequent histories of violence and posed greater risk of acting violently if discharged than any other group. They were less disabled than residents in long-stay wards or high-staffed hostels in terms of mental illness, vulnerability, impairment of ADLs, recent self-neglect and risk of non-deliberate self-harm.

Acute wards

Residents (all of whom had a length of stay of greater than six months and/or delayed discharged because alternative accommodation was unavailable) were less disabled in many respects than those in both long-stay wards and high-staffed hostels. This was true for mental illness, impairment of ADLs, social interaction and risk of non-deliberate self-harm. They had also shown less recent aggression and were assessed as being less at risk of acting violently if discharged to a less dependent setting than residents in long-stay wards. However, they had greater recent problems as a result of drug and alcohol misuse than those in long-stay wards or high-staffed hostels.

Long-stay wards and high-staffed hostels

Residents in these two types of facility were the most disabled in many respects. They were more vulnerable and more impaired in ADLs than other resident groups, had poorer social interaction than all but residents in forensic units, and had displayed greater recent levels of self-neglect and aggression than residents in facilities with lower levels of staffing. The striking differences between residents in these two categories of facility were that those in long-stay wards were more likely to have histories of violence and to be at risk of acting violently if discharged to a less dependent setting than residents in high-staffed hostels.

Staffed care homes

These residents resembled those in high-staffed hostels, except in having less impairment in ADLs and of social interaction. Like those in high-staffed hostels, residents in staffed care homes had histories of violence less often, and had lower risk of violence occurring if discharged to a less dependent setting, than people in long-stay wards.

Low-staffed and medium-staffed hostels

There were few differences between the profiles of residents in low- and mid-staffed hostels. Both groups were less disabled than residents in high-staffed hostels and long-stay wards in terms of vulnerability, impairment of ADLs, social interaction, recent aggression and recent self-neglect.

Group-homes

As can be seen from Table 14.2, residents of group homes scored low on all variables in relation to residents in other categories of accommodation.

TABLE 14.2
Classification of residential provision in the eight districts

Facility type	Resident places/ facility	Night cover	Day cover	Ratio of staff:resident places[1]	% of staff with a care qualification[1]	No. of facilities[2]	No. of residents[3]	Provider agency NHS	LA	Vol.	Priv.[4]
Forensic unit	>6	Waking	Constant	1.33 (1.00–1.65)	62 (54–70)	20	41	83	0	0	17
Acute ward	>6	Waking	Constant	1.27 (0.97–1.58)	63 (58–67)	35	259	100	0	0	0
Long-stay ward	>6	Waking	Constant	0.95 (0.85–1.09)	49 (42–57)	28	287	100	0	0	0
High-staffed hospital	>6	Waking	Constant	0.67 (0.58–0.77)	15 (11–20)	90	452	6	17	7	70
Medium-staffed hospital	>6	Sleep-in	Constant	0.39 (0.31–0.47)	14 (6–21)	47	373	2	17	39	42
Low-staffed hospital	>6	On-call/ none	Regular	0.19 (0.15–0.23)	15 (2–28)	28	181	0	5	39	56
Group home	<6	On-call/ none	Visited	0.16 (0.10–0.22)	33 (19–43)	66	222	1	42	56	1
Staffed care home	<6	Sleep-in	Constant	1.01 (0.83–1.20)	7 (3–12)	50	132	0	36	12	52

NHS, National Health Service; LA, local authority (social services or housing department); Vol., voluntary sector bodies; Priv., private companies or individuals.
1. Means (95% CIs for the mean) for facilities in category. Thirteen facilities had incomplete data for staffing variables.
2. Four facilities (accommodating four residents) had missing data.
3. No. of residents who met study criteria.
4. % of residents in facilities managed by each of the four provider agencies.

Comment

In combining details of facility and resident characteristics (Fig. 14.1), this study presents a 'snapshot' of the use of residential accommodation by mentally ill people. It provides a much more detailed, and probably accurate, picture than do Department of Health data returns, because it includes residents in facilities managed by all agency registers.

The scope of the study also meant that data collection was devolved to a relatively large number of people. Also, although local data collectors were trained in the use of the schedules, they had to rely on the judgements of the many keyworkers they interviewed. These keyworkers would have known the resident best, but would have varied considerably in the nature and level of their training. Many of the individual clinical and social items in the resident profile have been demonstrated to have acceptable reliability under test conditions. The items on social functioning, taken from the Community Placement Questionnaire (Clifford *et al*, 1991), had highly significant κ coefficients when tested for interrater reliability. Similarly, the measures of psychiatric symptoms in the resident profile are a version of the Health of the Nation Outcome Scales (HoNOS), whose items have been shown to have good interrater reliability (Wing *et al*, 1996). Less confidence can be placed in some of the other items rated. Few of the keyworkers would have had a medical qualification, and so opinions as to diagnosis were likely to be based on the records kept by the facilities.

Classification of facilities

Inconsistency in local terminology and criteria used to define residential facilities hinders service planning and makes comparisons between districts difficult to interpret. When comparisons are made in this study between facilities in different districts or managed by different provider agencies, like is compared with like in terms of size, extent of day and night cover and staffing levels (see Table 14.2).

Who receives residential care?

The great majority of patients occupying residential accommodation have long-term, severe mental illness. About two-thirds have active psychiatric symptoms, three-quarters significant impairment in carrying out functions essential for independent living and more than one-quarter moderate or severe physical disability or ill health. About one-third are judged to pose a moderate or severe risk of acting violently if discharged and twice this number to pose a risk to themselves from self-neglect.

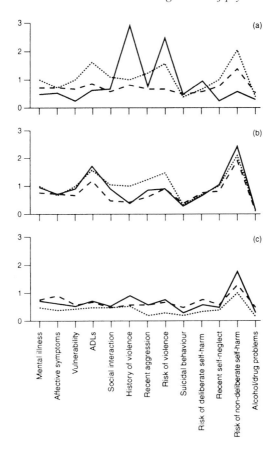

Fig. 14.1 Clinical, social and behavioural profiles of residents in eight categories of accommodation. (a) Forensic units (—— , 20 facilities, 41 residents), acute wards (--- , 35 facilities, 259 residents), long-stay wards (•••• , 28 facilities, 287 residents); (b) long-stay wards (••••), staffed care homes (--- , 50 facilities, 132 residents), high-staffed hostels (—— , 90 facilities, 452 residents); (c) mid-staffed hostels (—— , 47 facilities, 373 residents), low-staffed hostels (--- , 28 facilities, 181 residents), group homes (•••• , 66 facilities, 222 residents).
Reproduced with permission from Lelliott et al (1996).

Differences between resident groups and the implications

Those on acute wards were an exception in that they were less disabled in some respects than those on long-stay wards or high-staffed hostels. Since only patients who had been in hospital more than six months and those who should have been discharged were included, it is likely that the acute ward sample includes many patients who were ready for discharge to less dependent settings.

The finding of a gradient of severity of resident disability between facilities with the highest and lowest levels of staffing (see Fig. 14.1) confirms and quantifies what is perhaps obvious; that the more ill, vulnerable and less competent people with mental illness are, the more dependent and in greater need of care they are. The only other possible explanation, which could not be ruled out by this study, is that people in lower-staffed facilities have better outcomes. Only a little more than one-half of residents are in facilities with 24-hour cover and staff awake at night.

History and risk of violence are the only variables that distinguish the residents of long-stay wards from residents of high-dependency non-hospital facilities. Perhaps this partly explains why people who pose a risk of violence form a large proportion of new long-stay hospital patients whose discharge is delayed because no suitable accommodation is available in the community (Lelliott & Wing, 1994).

Three related factors may mitigate against people who are potentially violent entering non-hospital, high-dependency accommodation: local workers might have decided overtly that people who pose the highest risk of violence should be cared for in the local facilities with the highest staff:bed ratios; or the policies and procedures (either overt or covert) of non-NHS facilities exclude people with histories of violence (Wykes *et al*, 1982); or the relative lack of staff with nursing qualifications in non-hospital facilities.

The training of mental health nurses equips them to care for people with severe mental illness and gives them experience of working with very disabled people and with those who pose serious risk to themselves or others. The finding that only 21% of workers in non-hospital facilities have any care qualification is of particular interest and, perhaps, concern. One consequence of the continuing shift away from NHS management of long-term facilities appears to have been a reduction in the role played by mental health nurses in residential settings. This is an issue that commissioners of residential services might consider. Further study is needed to replicate, and explore the implications of, these findings on staff levels and staff mix; future work might explore in more detail the training of residential care staff.

Discussion

The audit cycle should result in changes that improve patient care. The two studies/audits described have been influential in identifying deficits in mental health service provision. Since the start of the MILMIS study, the number of acute beds in London has increased, the phenomenon of over-occupancy is now well recognised and has informed the London commission report (Johnson *et al*, 1998) and the London-wide bed management strategy (Strathdee *et al*, 1997). The audit of characteristics of people with mental illness in residential accommodation highlighted the need for 24-hour nursed bed accommodation for those with enduring mental illness and a lack of provision for patients with a history of violence. Following this report, the Department of Health issued guidance (Department of Health, 1996) on the provision of 24-hour staffed placements.

The methodology of both studies, while coordinated centrally, involved local personnel in the study design, and they were responsible for data collection. Services do not need to rely on highly experienced researchers to conduct useful local audits. The audits also highlight the changing nature of health services, in particular, the changing nature of acute wards and the changing provision for those with mental illness, much of which is now outside the NHS.

References

AUDINI, B., DUFFETT, R., LELLIOTT, P., *ET AL* (1999) Over-occupancy in London's acute psychiatric units – fact or fiction? *Psychiatric Bulletin*, **23**, 590–594.

CLIFFORD, P. (1993) *FACE Profile*. Available from the Quality Development Unit, Abbey Orchard House, 4 Abbey Orchard Street, London SW1P 2JJ.

——, CHARMAN, A., WEBB, Y., *ET AL* (1991) Planning for community care: The Community Placement Questionnaire. *British Journal of Clinical Psychology*, **30**, 193–211.

DEPARTMENT OF HEALTH (1996) *24-hour Nursed Care for People with Severe and Enduring Mental Illness*. Leeds: NHS Executive.

FAULKNER, A., FIELD, V. & LINDESAY, J. (1992) *Who is Providing What? Information about UK Residential Care Provision for People with Mental Health Problems*. London: Research and Development for Psychiatry (134–138 Borough High Street, London SE1 1LB).

GLOVER, G. R., ROBIN EMANI, J. & ARABSCHEIBANI, G. R. (1997) A need index for mental health care. *Social Psychiatry and Psychiatric Epidemiology*, **33**, 89–96.

HIRSCH, S. R. (1988) *Psychiatric Beds and Resources: Factors Influencing Bed Use and Service Planning. Report of a Working Party of the Section for Social and Community Psychiatry of the Royal College of Psychiatrists*. London: Gaskell.

HOUSE OF COMMONS HEALTH COMMITTEE (1994) *Memorandum from the Department of Health on Public Expenditure on Health and Personal Social Services*. London: HMSO.

JARMAN, B. (1983) Identification of under privileged areas. *British Medical Journal*, **286**, 1705–1709.

JOHNSON, S. & LELLIOTT, P. (1998) Mental health services in London: evidence from research and routine data. In: *London's Mental Health* (eds S. Johnson, R. Ramsay, G. Thornicroft, *et al*), pp. 167–192. London: King's Fund.

——, RAMSAY, R., THORNICROFT, G., *ET AL* (1998) *London's Mental Health*. London: King's Fund.

LELLIOTT, P. & WING, J. (1994) A national audit of new long-stay psychiatric patients. II: Impact on services. *British Journal of Psychiatry*, **165**, 170–178.

—, — & CLIFFORD, P. (1994) A national audit of new long-stay psychiatric patients. I: Method and description of the cohort. *British Journal of Psychiatry,* **165**, 160–169.

—, AUDINI, B., KNAPP, M., *ET AL* (1996) The mental health residential care study: Classification of facilities and description of residents. *British Journal of Psychiatry,* **169**, 139–147.

MILMIS PROJECT GROUP (1995) Monitoring inner London mental illness services. *Psychiatric Bulletin,* **19**, 276–280.

RITCHIE, J., DICK, D. & LINGHAM, R. (1994) *The Report of the Enquiry into the Care and Treatment of Christopher Clunis.* London: HMSO.

RIX, S., BEADSMORE, A., SHEPHARD, G., *ET AL* (1999) *Standards for Adult Mental Health Services.* Brighton: HAS 2000 & Pavilion Publishing Ltd.

STRATHDEE, G., CARR, S., THOMPSON, K., *ET AL* (1997) *The London Bed Management: A Modular Bed Management Set Programme for Purchasers and Providers.* London: Sainsbury Centre for Mental Health.

TYRER, P., EVANS, K., GANDHI, N., *ET AL* (1998) Randomised controlled trial of two models of care for discharged psychiatric patients. *British Medical Journal,* **316**, 106–109.

WING. J. K., CURTIS, R. H. & BEEVOR, A. S. (1996) *HoNOS: Health of the Nation Outcome Scales. Report on Research and Development: July 1993–December 1995.* London: Royal College of Psychiatrists.

WYKES, T., STURT, E. & CREER, C. (1982) Practices of day and residential units in relation to the social behaviour of attenders. *Psychological Medicine Monograph Supplement,* pp. 15–27.

15 The Cardinal Needs Schedule: a standardised research instrument for measuring individual needs

AUSTIN LOCKWOOD and MAX MARSHALL

The Medical Research Council's Needs for Care Assessment (MRC NCA) was a groundbreaking advance, which gave rise to the whole field of psychiatric needs assessment (Brewin *et al*, 1987, 1988). Like all new advances, however, the MRC NCA was not without its problems. In our work using the schedule to assess the needs of homeless people (Hogg & Marshall, 1992), we encountered four key problems – one of a philosophical nature and three of a psychometric nature.

To overcome these problems we developed the Cardinal Needs Schedule (CNS; Marshall 1994; Marshall *et al*, 1995*a*), which is effectively a highly modified version of the MRC NCA. In the sections that follow, we will describe: (a) the problems encountered with the MRC NCA; (b) the modifications made to create the CNS; (c) a description of the CNS and its psychometric properties; (d) applications of the CNS; and (e) alternative versions of the CNS for use with other patient groups.

Problems with the MRC NCA

The MRC NCA measures need in three stages. In stage one, standardised rating scales are used to rate psychiatric symptoms and social functioning. In stage two, scores on these instruments are used to identify problems in 20 areas of psychiatric and social functioning. In stage three, a panel of raters uses clinical judgement to decide whether a need was present in each of these areas. We will consider the problems with this approach under two headings: philosophical and psychometric.

Philosophical problems

The MRC NCA is described as adopting a 'normative' approach to assessing need – that is to say, 'need' is assessed from the perspective of the clinician. While not denying the validity of other perspectives on need (for example, the patient's perspective), the creators of the schedule have argued that the normative approach most closely reflects everyday clinical practice. In our work with the homeless mentally ill, we concluded that this was an oversimplification of clinical reality. For example, using the MRC NCA, we frequently found ourselves in situations where we had to use 'clinical judgement' to assess whether a patient would accept help or to estimate how much a patient's behaviour was causing problems to carers. We reached the conclusion that clinical judgement is a process that actually involves the integration of carers' and patients' perspectives on need with those of the clinician. We therefore proposed a new four-stage model of needs assessment. Stages one, two and four of this model are similar to those followed by the MRC NCA (i.e. measuring functioning, identifying problems and deciding if a need was present), but we proposed an additional stage in the assessment procedure, which involved deciding whether identified problems were worthy of action. This stage involved explicitly considering the perspective of the patient and the carer. Problems were then judged worthy of action if: (a) they were particularly severe or serious; (b) the patient wanted help with the problem; or (c) the problem was causing substantial distress to carers. Under this new model, problems meeting our criteria for being 'worthy of action' were called 'cardinal problems', and only cardinal problems could become needs.

Psychometric problems

We found three key psychometric problems with the MRC NCA. The first problem was related to the philosophical problem described above; while the creators of the MRC NCA recommend that patients and carers be taken into account, the MRC NCA did not offer any mechanism of systematically eliciting or utilising these views. The second problem was that we ourselves and other users (Holloway, 1991) had found the MRC NCA a time-consuming assessment, partly because of the large number of standardised instruments required to complete it, and partly because of the recommendation that ratings of need be made by a full multi-disciplinary team. The third problem was that the output from the MRC NCA was complex and difficult to interpret. For example, there are nine different possible categories of need for each area of functioning in the Schedule ('no need', 'no meetable need', 'unmet need', 'met need', 'need for assessment', 'not applicable', 'future need', 'possible need' and 'over-provision'). While such a meticulous and detailed approach was necessary in the early stages of needs assessment, we concluded that, for practical research purposes, most of these needs categories were redundant and occasionally confusing. We therefore set out to modify the MRC NCA to make it consistent with our new model of needs assessment and to overcome the three key psychometric problems outlined above.

Modifications to the MRC NCA

Our first modification to the MRC NCA was to introduce an extra stage to the rating process to make it consistent with our new four-stage model of needs assessment (as described above). In this stage, we applied criteria for acting on a problem, based on severity and the views of clients and carers. Our second modification was to develop two short semi-structured interviews to elicit the views of the patient and the main carer in a systematic way. Our third modification was to simplify the information collection process by: (a) using fewer and more efficient standardised instruments; (b) automating the process as far as possible by using a custom-built computer program; and (c) reducing the number of persons required to make the rating of need (one psychiatrist and one person from another discipline). Finally, we restructured the output of the MRC NCA to make it simpler and more clinically relevant. The CNS allows for only three outcomes for each area of functioning: (a) 'no cardinal problem', indicating that the patient did not have a problem severe enough to require intervention; (b) 'need', indicating that the patient had a problem, which was severe enough to require intervention, but for which a suitable intervention had not yet been offered to the patient; and (c) 'persists despite intervention' (PDI), indicating that the patient had a problem that was severe enough to require intervention, but for which all suitable interventions had already been offered. Our new instrument, the CNS, is described below.

The CNS

The CNS rates need in four stages.

Stage 1: Measuring functioning

Standardised instruments are used to measure the patient's performance in 15 areas of psychiatric and social functioning. The main instruments used are:

- *The Manchester Scale* (Krawiecka *et al*, 1977), which is a brief rating of psychotic symptoms, symptoms of anxiety and depression and the side-effects of psychiatric medication.
- *REHAB* (Baker & Hall, 1988), which is a scale for measuring socially unacceptable behaviour (seven items) and general behaviour (16 items).
- *The Additional Information Questionnaire* (Marshall *et al*, 1995*a*), which was constructed specifically for the CNS and records items such as employment, substance misuse or history of violence or self-harm.

Stage 2: Identifying problems

During this stage, data scores on the standardised instruments are entered into a computer program, 'Autoneed', which compares them with pre-set criteria for having a problem in each area of functioning. If a patient's rating in an area of functioning is unsatisfactory according to these criteria, Autoneed identifies the patient as having a problem in that area.

Stage 3: Identifying cardinal problems

During this stage, criteria are applied to determine whether problems identified at Stage 2 are 'cardinal problems' (i.e. problems worth acting on). These criteria are: (a) the *cooperation criterion*, which takes account the patient's view of the problem and willingness to accept help with the problem; (b) the *carer stress criterion*, which takes account of the level of stress the patient's problem is causing for carers; and (c) the *severity criterion*, which takes account of the severity of the problem. Data for the cooperation and the carer stress criteria are obtained from semi-structured interviews with the patient and the main carer.

It is important to note that not all criteria are applied for each area of functioning. The cooperation criterion is applied in areas where interventions are unlikely to be successful without the client's consent (for example, areas where some skills-based training might be offered).

The Carer Stress Criterion is applied in areas where interventions would be likely to reduce the stress experienced by carers, regardless of whether or not the client consented (for example, socially embarrassing behaviour). The severity criterion is applied in areas where the problem may pose a risk to the safety of the patient or others (for example, self-harm or violence).

Stage 4: Identifying needs

For each area of functioning in the CNS, a list of suitable interventions is provided. For example, under the area of functioning 'psychotic symptoms', the relevant interventions are: 'psychiatric assessment'; 'standard neuroleptic'; 'atypical neuroleptic'; 'monitoring medication'; 'support and reassurance'; and 'family intervention'. Each intervention is precisely defined. Whenever a cardinal problem is identified at Stage 3, a panel of two clinicians (one psychiatrist and one other person – usually a psychiatric nurse) is required to rate each of the relevant interventions according to whether it has been 'offered' or 'not offered' within the past year. Where interventions have been offered more than one year previously, but not in the past year, the rating panel must use their judgement to decide whether it is worth trying again with the intervention. In certain circumstances, interventions may also be rated 'inappropriate' (for example, family therapy in a patient who does not have a family). If one or more interventions in an area of functioning have been rated as 'not offered', then the patient is said to have a 'need' in that area of functioning. In the case of more than one intervention being rated 'not offered', the rating panel must choose which intervention is most likely to meet the need, and Autoneed records the patient as having a 'need' for that intervention. If all interventions in an area of functioning have been rated 'offered' or 'inappropriate', then Autoneed records the patient as having a PDI problem.

Reliability of the CNS

The reliability of the CNS was investigated in two studies conducted on a psychiatric rehabilitation unit. These studies exploited the fact that it was the ward's practice to allocate each patient a 'primary' nurse and an 'associate' nurse, who would work on opposite shifts. This practice allowed us to investigate how far the Schedule would be sensitive to different responses from two carers who knew the patient equally well.

Interrater reliability

This study was designed to take into account all possible sources of unreliability that might arise during a needs assessment using the CNS. These areas were: (a) disagreement in rating problems, arising from differences in data collected from standardised instruments; (b) disagreement in rating cardinal problems, arising from different responses from the patient to different interviewers on the Client Opinion Interview, and different responses from different carers to different interviewers on the Carer Stress Interview; and (c) disagreement in rating need. For the purposes of the study, two investigators independently completed the Manchester Scale, Client Opinion Interview and Additional Information Questionnaire with each of the 15 patients on the unit. Separate REHAB assessments were completed for each of these patients by his or her primary nurse and associate nurse. The Carer Stress Interview was also conducted independently, with the first investigator interviewing the primary nurse and the second investigator interviewing the associate nurse. The final stage in the ratings (deciding whether suitable interventions had been offered) was also carried out independently for each patient, on the basis of the two independently collected data-sets. Thus, it was possible to make two, completely independent sets of ratings using the CNS on the same population of 15 patients.

The κ statistic was calculated for each area of functioning, according to whether a need was rated in the area. The value of κ was greater than 0.75 for five areas of functioning (indicating 'excellent agreement'; Landis & Koch, 1977) and greater than 0.6 ('good agreement') in four areas. Agreement was 'fair' in two areas and 'poor' in two areas. Kappa could not be calculated for the remaining two areas (where agreement was 100% but there were no needs). The two unreliable areas were 'hygiene and dressing' and 'under-activity'.

Test–retest reliability

One week following the interrater reliability study described above, one of the investigators conducted a second needs assessment on each of the 15 patients involved. For the test–retest reliability study, the same nurse that had been interviewed for the original ratings was interviewed again. The mean κ score for this study was 0.8.

Validity of the CNS

Studies conducted to investigate the construct validity and concurrent validity of the CNS are described below.

Construct validity

The construct validity of the CNS was examined during a randomised controlled trial of social services case management for people with severe mental disorder (Marshall *et al*, 1995*b*). During this trial, 80 patients in the treatment and control groups had their needs assessed using the CNS. Interventions offered to these patients were monitored for 14 months following this assessment. Neither the patients themselves nor the professionals involved in caring for them were made aware of the initial needs assessment.

At the end of the trial, for each of the 15 areas of functioning rated by the Schedule, we randomly selected two subjects who were rated as having a need in the area and two subjects who were not (making a total of 60 selections). A rating was then made of the interventions that each patient had received over the 14 months of the trial, blind to the baseline needs assessment. We found that if the CNS rated a patient as having a need for a particular intervention, then that patient was much more likely to receive that intervention in the next 14 months (odds ratio 7.50, 95% CI 2.24–25.06) than a patient who was rated as not having a need for that intervention. Thus, judgements of need made by the CNS predicted the judgements of the clinicians caring for the patients in the trial, even though those clinicians were unaware of the findings of the needs assessment.

In a second validity study, conducted during the same case management trial, we asked the case managers of patients in the treatment condition ($n=40$) to record in a daily diary how much time they spent with the patients. We then investigated the hypothesis that over the study period case managers would spend more time with patients who had more needs. This hypothesis was confirmed, as there was a significant positive correlation between number of needs and amount of time allocated by case manager ($r=0.34$, $P<0.05$).

Concurrent validity

The concurrent validity of the CNS was also tested during the same case management study. Our hypothesis was that patients with more needs would rate themselves as having a lower quality of life (on a scale of subjective quality of life). To investigate this, patients at baseline were asked to rate their quality of life on Lehman's QOL scale (Lehman, 1983). Subsequent analysis confirmed the hypothesis, as there was a significant negative correlation between number of needs and quality of life – in other words, the more needs patients had, the lower they tended to rate their quality of life ($r=-0.36$, $P<0.001$).

Autoneed

Although it is possible to use the CNS in 'pen and paper' format, this is discouraged. Ratings involve comparing a large number of data points with an equally large number of thresholds; undertaken manually, this would take at least an hour for each patient and there would inevitably be errors made. Such a task is ideally suited for a computer program. As stated above, a computerised version of the schedule has been developed (known as Autoneed). Autoneed was written using Microsoft Visual Basic; it is a stand-alone program running under Microsoft Windows 95/98/NT and does not require any other software to run.

Autoneed allows data from the standardised instruments used by the CNS to be entered into an industry-standard database format (Microsoft SQL Server). Once these data are entered, the decisions involved in rating problems and cardinal problems (Stages 1–3 described above) are automatic. User intervention is required at Stage 4. At this point, Autoneed presents the user with a list of suitable interventions for each area of functioning where a cardinal problem was rated. The user is then asked to rate each of these interventions as 'offered', 'not offered' or 'inappropriate'. Once these data have been entered, the program then goes on to rate each of the cardinal problem areas as a 'need' or a 'PDI'. Data can be then printed or exported in a number of standard spreadsheet and database formats.

Autoneed was designed to be highly configurable. Although the logical processes involved in rating problems, cardinal problems and needs are 'hard-coded' into the program, the actual data are stored in a flexible database format. It is therefore possible to alter: (a) the areas of functioning rated; (b) the standardised instruments used to collect data; (c) the thresholds used to rate problems and cardinal problems; and (d) the interventions rated for each cardinal problem. This flexibility has meant that it is has been possible to reconfigure Autoneed to suit a number of different versions of the CNS (see below).

Applications of the CNS

The main applications of the CNS are described below.

As an outcome measure

The CNS can be used as an outcome measure in clinical trials, and it is particularly useful in evaluating interventions, such as case management or assertive community treatment, where an important goal of treatment is to identify and meet patients' needs. For example, the CNS was used an outcome measure in the randomised controlled trial of case management described above (Marshall *et al*, 1995*b*), in which it was shown that after 14 months, there were no significant differences in numbers of needs between case-managed patients ($n=40$) and controls ($n=40$).

As a survey instrument

The CNS can also be used as a survey instrument, to determine the needs and/or quality of care of populations of severely mentally ill patients. For example, Murray *et al* (1996) surveyed a representative sample of patients treated for a psychotic disorder in the past five years in Hamilton, a socially deprived area of Scotland. Of 71 patients interviewed, they found that 42% had one or more clinical needs and 49% had one or more social needs. Typically, for such surveys, they found that the commonest clinical needs were in the areas of psychotic symptoms, side-effects and depression/anxiety; and the most common social needs were for employment, accommodation and improving social life. They concluded that systematic assessment of needs with research instruments can give valuable insights into the successes and failures of community care and that that it is possible to plan services for the area on the basis of the findings of such a survey.

As an intervention

The CNS cannot be used without training and basic computer skills. These requirements make it impractical for everyday clinical work. However, we considered it possible that some clinical benefit might be gained if patients were to have their needs assessed by an independent rater, who then 'fed back' the results of the assessment to the patient's keyworker. This approach would address the problem of training keyworkers, because less people would need to be trained, and would also reduce the potential for bias in making ratings, because the person making the ratings would not be directly involved in caring for the patient.

With the introduction of the CPA (Kingdon, 1994) in England, we had an opportunity to test this theory, as under the CPA all severely mentally ill patients are allocated a keyworker who is responsible for assessing their needs and formulating a care plan to meet these needs. In a small pilot study (Lockwood & Marshall, 1999), we employed a research nurse to carry out needs assessments using the CNS on a group of 20 patients with severe mental disorders. The findings of the assessment were then fed back to the CPA keyworkers responsible for the patients' care. As well as feeding back the identified needs, we also provided some suggestions on how to obtain the interventions identified by the assessment by linking Autoneed to a database of local voluntary and statutory organisations offering services to the severely mentally ill. This database was indexed by the interventions offered by the organisations concerned, so that it was possible to easily cross-reference a client's needs with organisations providing suitable interventions.

The results of this pilot study were encouraging, in that significant reductions in the number of needs were seen over the six months following the intervention. Significant reductions were also seen in the level of anxious and depressive symptoms. As a result, we have begun investigating the efficacy of 'needs feedback' in a multi-centre randomised-controlled trial, funded by the Wellcome Trust.

Versions of Autoneed for use with other patient groups

The flexibility of the computer program Autoneed means that new versions of the CNS can easily be developed for populations other than the severely mentally ill. So far, four versions of the CNS have been developed, based around the original Autoneed skeleton. Thus, versions of the CNS are available for: people with learning difficulties; families of people with schizophrenia; mentally ill adolescents; and mentally disordered offenders.

People with learning difficulties

The CNS has been modified to assess the needs of patients with learning difficulties (further details available from the author upon request). This version of the schedule uses REHAB and the Manchester Scale, as well as a modified version of the Additional Information Questionnaire, to rate problems in 22 areas of functioning. Cardinal problems are rated in a similar way to the original version, using modified versions of the Carer Stress and Client Opinion interviews. A specialised list of interventions, based on a survey of experts in learning difficulties, is available for each area of functioning.

Relatives of patients with severe mental disorder

The Relatives' Cardinal Needs Schedule (RCNS; Barrowclough *et al*, 1998) is an adaptation of the CNS, which can be used to assess the needs of relatives of people with severe mental disorders for psycho-social interventions. The RCNS rates need in 14 areas of functioning, covering five categories (support, information and liaison; coping with symptoms; relationships; hardship; and negative emotions). Problems are rated on the basis of responses to two questionnaires: the Knowledge about Schizophrenia Interview (Barrowclough *et al*, 1987) and the Family Questionnaire (Barrowclough & Parle, 1997). A relative's interview, which was designed for the needs schedule, is used to obtain thresholds for cardinal problems.

Mentally ill adolescents

Kroll *et al* (1999) have developed a version of the CNS to assess the needs of mentally ill adolescents. This version of the schedule uses interviews with both clients and their main carer to rate problems in 19 areas of functioning, including social, psychiatric, educational and life skills. Cardinal problems are rated on the basis of further interviews to elicit carer stress, client cooperation and problem severity.

Mentally disordered offenders

The CNS has also been modified to predict the risk of re-offence in adult patients with a forensic history (further details available from the author upon request). Ratings are based on interviews with patients, a nurse involved in their care, their responsible clinician and a number of standardised instruments specifically designed for use in forensic psychiatry.

Conclusion

The CNS stands somewhere between the MRC NCA and the Camberwell Assessment of Need (CAN; Slade *et al*, 1999; described elsewhere in this book). It resembles the MRC NCA in being primarily a research instrument that is designed to produce a highly systematic and precise judgement of the particular types of intervention that are required to meet patients' needs. It also resembles the CAN in its efforts to elicit patients' views and to explicitly include them in the decision-making process. The CNS is a briefer instrument than the MRC NCA, but longer then the CAN, and unlike the CAN it is not suitable for routine clinical use. The CNS is a valid and reliable instrument that has been shown to be of value in clinical trials and surveys. As yet, it is unclear whether the CNS will be shown to have any value as a clinical intervention in its own right. The flexible design of the Autoneed computer program has meant that it has been relatively easy to adapt the Schedule for use in a number of study populations.

References

BAKER, R. & HALL, J. N. (1988) REHAB: A new assessment instrument for chronic psychiatric patients. *Schizophrenia Bulletin*, **14**, 97–111.

BARROWCLOUGH, C. & PARLE, M. (1997) Appraisal, psychological adjustment and expressed emotion in relatives of patients suffering from schizophrenia. *British Journal of Psychiatry*, **171**, 26–30.

——, TARRIER, N., WATTS, S., *ET AL* (1987) Assessing the functional value of relatives' knowledge about schizophrenia: a preliminary report. *British Journal of Psychiatry*, **151**, 1–8.

——, MARSHALL, M., LOCKWOOD, A., *ET AL* (1998) Assessing relatives' needs for psychosocial interventions in schizophrenia: a relatives' version of the Cardinal Needs Schedule (RCNS). *Psychological Medicine*, **28**, 531–542.

BREWIN C. R., WING, J. K., MANGEN, S. P., *ET AL* (1987) Principles and practice of measuring need in the long-term mentally ill: the MRC Needs For Care Assessment. *Psychological Medicine*, **17**, 971–982.

——, ——, ——, *ET AL* (1988) Needs for care among the long-term mentally ill: a report from the Camberwell High Contact Survey. *Psychological Medicine*, **18**, 457–468.

HOGG, L. I. & MARSHALL, M. (1992) Can we measure needs in the homeless mentally ill? Using the MRC Needs for Care Assessment in hostels for the homeless. *Psychological Medicine*, **22**, 1027–1034.

HOLLOWAY, F. (1991) Day care in an inner city. II. Quality of the services. *British Journal of Psychiatry*, **158**, 810–816.

KINGDON, D. (1994) Care programme approach. Recent government policy and legislation. *Psychiatric Bulletin*, **18**, 68–70.

KRAWIECKA, M., GOLDBERG, D. & VAUGHN, M. (1977) A standardised psychiatric assessment scale for rating chronic psychotic patients. *Acta Psychiatrica Scandinavica*, **55**, 299–308.

KROLL, L., WOODHAM, A., ROTHWELL, J., *ET AL* (1999) Reliabilty of the Salford Needs Assessment Schedule for Adolescents. *Psychological Medicine*, **29**, 891–902.

LANDIS, J. R. & KOCH, G. G. (1977) The measurement of observer agreement for categorical data. *Biometrics*, **33**, 159–174.

LEHMAN, A. (1983) The well being of chronic mental patients: assessing their quality of life. *Archives of General Psychiatry*, **40**, 369–373.

LOCKWOOD, A. & MARSHALL, M. (1999) Can a standardised needs assessment be used to improve the care of people with severe mental disorders? A pilot study of 'Needs Feedback'. *Journal of Advanced Nursing*, **30**, 1408–1415.

MARSHALL, M. (1994) How should we measure need? Concept and practice in the development of a standardised assessment of need. *Philosophy, Psychology, Psychiatry*, **1**, 27–40.

——, HOGG, L. I., GATH, D. H., *ET AL* (1995*a*) The Cardinal Needs Schedule – a modified version of the MRC Needs for Care Assessment Schedule. *Psychological Medicine*, **25**, 605–617.

——, LOCKWOOD, A. & GATH, D. H. (1995*b*) Social services case management for long-term mental disorders: a randomised controlled trial. *Lancet*, **345**, 409–412.

MURRAY, V., WALKER, H. W., MITCHELL, C., *ET AL* (1996) Needs for care from a demand led community psychiatric service: a study of patients with major mental illness. *British Medical Journal*, **312**, 1582–1586.

SLADE, M., THORNICROFT, G., LOFTUS, L., *ET AL* (1999) *CAN: Camberwell Assessment of Need. A Comprehensvie Needs Assessment Tool for People with Severe Mental Illness.* London: Gaskell.

16 Measuring individual needs for care and services

CHRIS R. BREWIN

The concept of need, currently so topical, has a long and controversial history within the social sciences. In the psychological literature, for example, needs have frequently been invoked as explanations for human behaviour. An early usage of the term was as a drive towards specific behaviour patterns (e.g. needs for achievement or dominance), but this has fallen into disfavour, owing to the lack of explanatory power. Needs have also been seen as objective human requirements for physical and mental health (e.g. needs for warmth or security or self-actualisation), and as subjective expressions of want or desire (Tracy, 1986). Because of these varying meanings, subjective wants are often referred to as 'felt' or 'perceived' needs to distinguish them from needs that are considered to have a more objective basis.

Individuals lacking these objective requirements are often described as being 'in need', and hence needs are for some writers synonymous with the presence of objective lacks. Thus, for Mallman & Marcus (1980) need is "an objective requirement to avoid a state of illness" (p. 165), and for Tracy (1986) "a need of a living system is a lack of a specific resource which is useful for or required by the purposes of that system" (p. 212).

Mental health professionals are not primarily interested in needs as explanations of behaviour, but as grounds for professional intervention, and the concept of need as an objective lack has been interpreted in three ways. One interpretation is as a lack of health or well-being, and needs have been defined in terms of ameliorating symptoms, distress, behavioural problems, skills deficits, poverty, poor housing, and so on. In this usage, needs are in effect assessed failures to attain general goals of health and well-being (e.g. Leighton *et al*, 1963; Stein & Test, 1980). Or, again, "need is seen as a shortfall compared with a state of being which is generally acceptable" (Davies

273

& Challis, 1986, p. 562). Some studies of needs consist largely of descriptive accounts of a set of clinical problems (e.g. Falloon & Marshall, 1983). Such failures or shortfalls must in principle fall within the domain of professional expertise, although where the boundaries are drawn, for example, between social and medical expertise, varies from study to study.

The second interpretation is as a lack of access to particular forms of institutionalised care targeted at these objective lacks. For example, Lehtinen *et al* (1990) interpret needs as reflecting an inadequate level of service for the severity of the problem. Thus, patients with severe disorders receiving primary rather than specialised psychiatric care would be rated as having unmet need. Similarly, for Shapiro *et al* (1985), unmet needs are defined as the combination of definite morbidity and lack of mental health service utilisation. The Community Placement Questionnaire (Clifford *et al*, 1991) is a survey instrument designed to assess the varying types of institutionalised care required by long-stay patients resident in hospitals scheduled for closure.

The third interpretation of the term 'need' is as a lack of specific activities by (professional or lay) mental health workers. These may include both treatment-oriented activities such as medication and individual therapy, and support-oriented activities such as ensuring access to leisure facilities and arranging for a home help. Thus, in the terminology developed at the MRC Social and Community Psychiatry Unit, 'needs for care' have been defined as requirements for specific activities or interventions that have the potential to ameliorate disabling symptoms or reactions. In contrast, 'needs for services' reflect institutional requirements and are defined as needs for specific agents or agencies to deliver those interventions (Brewin *et al*, 1987). Mangen & Brewin (1991) outline a procedure for deriving estimates of needs for services from individuals' needs for specific items of care.

Typically, the distinction between need as a lack of health or well-being and need as a lack of a specific intervention is not made – to cite only one of many examples, Birchwood & Smith (1988) include among the needs of families caring for a relative with schizophrenia both the amelioration of adverse emotional reactions (an objective lack) and specific items of care such as providing information and practical advice. That the distinction is nevertheless an important one is illustrated by the existence of certain objective lacks, such as intractable treatment-resistant symptoms, for which no specific interventions are effective. Such situations, which would qualify as needs according to one usage of the term but not according to the other usage, have been explicitly described as 'problems without needs' (Brewin *et al*, 1987) and as constituting 'no meetable need' (Brewin & Wing, 1989). Similarly, there are examples of individuals who have unmet needs for specific items of care, but no unmet need for access to agents or agencies other than those currently provided.

These three usages of the term 'need' within the psychiatric literature reflect in part the different concerns of the various investigations that have been carried out. When studying populations with inadequate provision or low contact with services, such as random community samples, the families of the mentally ill or the mentally ill living in greatly under-resourced environments, it has generally been considered sufficient to establish lack of health or well-being in order to establish the presence of need. Similarly, unmet need has been equated with the combination of a lack of health or well-being and a lack of access to institutionalised care. This assumes a low probability that in such samples: (a) all available treatment avenues would have been exhausted, so that individuals receiving services were not actually in need; and (b) individuals in contact with services might still have unmet needs owing to inappropriate treatment.

However, studies of groups already in high contact with services, such as the long-term mentally ill, have frequently found it necessary to go further and assess the lack of the specific items of care or services that appear most appropriate to the individual's circumstances. For these groups, the equating of receiving care with having one's needs met is even more unwarranted than it is in the populations described in the previous paragraph, in part because of the lack of well-validated treatment methods and the requirement for an active and highly flexible approach to treatment. In these groups, the existence of unmet need will not only reflect the absence of any care at all, but will also, in some cases, reflect an absence of appropriate care as measured against some ideal template.

Measuring need in low-contact groups

A number of studies, mostly community psychiatric surveys, have attempted to assess need from the presence of morbidity and/or from service utilisation. In the Stirling County study (Leighton *et al*, 1963), need for psychiatric attention was rated on a five-point scale: 'most abnormal', 'psychiatric disorder with significant impairment', 'probable psychiatric disorder', 'doubtful' and 'probably well'. Individuals considered to have a definite need for psychiatric help fell into the first two categories, these judgements being based on the presence of clear psychiatric disorder, the presence of significant impairment, and the nature of the symptoms, including conditions that needed attention for diagnostic and prognostic purposes, whether or not treatment was possible.

Shapiro *et al* (1985) presented operational definitions of need employed in the 1981 Eastern Baltimore Mental Health Survey, one of the sites participating in the National Institute for Mental Health (NIMH) Epidemiologic Catchment Area Program. In this survey, the presence of need for care or services (no distinction was made between the two) was defined in a number of ways, either: (a) specialist mental health service utilisation or general health service utilisation for a mental health problem in the past six months (7.1% of the sample); or (b) the presence of two or more manifestations of a mental health problem (a further 6.4% of the sample). These manifestations consisted of a diagnosable disorder on a standardised psychiatric interview, or a high score on a mental health screening instrument, or social role impairment owing to mental health problems for at least one entire day during the past three months. Individuals who had at least two manifestations of emotional disorder, but had not used mental health services, were defined as having an unmet need.

Clearly, the use of multiple criteria for establishing the presence of need means that comparable data are unlikely to be obtained elsewhere, unless a specific attempt at replication is made. From a purely practical point of view, the criteria used have reasonable face validity, but the conflation of need, demand and utilisation is likely to prolong the conceptual confusion already characteristic of this area. The assumptions that people who visit mental health centres have a need for treatment that is then met remain untested. It is also hard to tell from this study the length of the psychiatric episodes that individuals experienced and the degree of disability: it was neither an incidence study, since current morbidity was not required, nor a prevalence study, since the critical periods for the occurrence of a diagnosable disorder and for the occurrence of disability were not the same.

A different approach to measuring needs for mental health treatment was taken by Lehtinen *et al* (1990) in their epidemiological survey in Finland. This decision was primarily based on whether or not subjects reached case criteria for a recognised psychiatric disorder using the PSE–ID–CATEGO system (Wing & Sturt, 1978). Subjects were rated as having a need for care at a specialist or at a primary level, depending on the severity of the disorder, and then categorised as: (a) having an unmet need for care, by which it was meant that the subject was not under care although it was needed; (b) being under inadequate care – receiving care from a general practitioner (GP), although the involvement of specialist services was warranted; or (c) being under adequate care – the agent was appropriate to the severity of the disorder. Virtually all individuals reaching case criteria were adjudged to be in need of mental health services – half of them for specialist services – but over 50% were not receiving any treatment at all.

Although these authors referred to the measurement of needs for care, it should be noted that according to the distinction made earlier they were measuring needs for services. That is, they were mainly concerned with whether the individual was receiving treatment from an appropriate agent rather than with the appropriateness of the treatment itself. It appears that the judgement of appropriateness of services was made *a priori*, rather than reflecting any specific inadequacy or breakdown in the care being provided by the GP. Another point to note is the reliance on the PSE: there were no explicit requirements concerning the duration of the illness episode or the amount of social impairment. In this respect, it is interesting to note that only about a third of those who had a psychiatric diagnosis mentioned some degree of need for mental health care themselves.

In conclusion, there are problems in equating 'objective' estimates of need with perceived need, demand or service utilisation, all of which will almost certainly result in an under-estimate. Morbidity surveys are likely to yield better estimates, but specific rules must be formulated to exclude brief transient disorders that will clear up of their own accord and to take proper account of social impairment independently of the amount of morbidity. Even these data will tend to be under-estimates, because no allowance is made for the adequacy of the specific treatment being received (for further discussion of community surveys, see the chapter by Bebbington in this volume).

Measuring need in high-contact groups

Citing their dissatisfaction with morbidity and service utilisation surveys, and with the method of asking consumers – who as a group are probably ill-informed about the range of potential items of care and service to define their own needs, Levin *et al* (1978) had intake workers in community mental health centres (CMHCs) rate their patients' needs for 13 types of service. They devised an instrument called SNAPOR (Services Needed, Available, Planned, Offered and Rendered) that enquired about the need for and provision of services, such as individual sessions, group sessions, family sessions, medication, hospitalisation, etc. When rating services needed, workers were to ignore their actual availability. Even allowing mental health workers to define patients' needs themselves, and taking no account of the effectiveness of services actually provided, Levin *et al* found that the centres were only delivering about half the services that their own workers thought were required.

Most of the research on high-contact groups has been concerned with the long-term mentally ill. According to Stein & Test (1980), the needs of these patients can be summarised in terms of material resources, coping skills, motivation, freedom from pathologically dependent relationships, support and education of the community members who are involved with them, and a supportive system that assertively helps patients to achieve their goals. These needs, as we have seen, are a mixture of individual goals for health and well-being and specific requirements for interventions and services. The original intention appears to have been to describe a treatment philosophy that would underpin intervention, rather than to enumerate variables that would be specifically targeted in pre- and post-treatment assessments.

Some studies that have attempted to assess the needs of this group directly have relied on questionnaires or interviews completed by key informants. For example, Wasylenki *et al* (1981) simply asked staff members responsible for discharge planning to identify patient after-care needs in the medical/therapeutic, housing, vocational/ educational and social/recreational areas. In the latter three areas, Wasylenki *et al* found strikingly low rates of referral, even in response to after-care needs identified by staff themselves.

Solomon & Davis (1985) had social workers in two state-receiving hospitals in Cleveland, Ohio, complete a Service Needs Assessment Form for each patient. Services required were collapsed into seven categories – socialisation, individual therapy, group therapy, chemotherapy, vocational rehabilitation, residential treatment and financial assistance – and social workers' recommendations were compared with records of all relevant public agencies to determine whether or not corresponding services had been delivered. Even when it is considered that the authors, like Wasylenki *et al*, took no account of the effectiveness of those services that were delivered (a serious limitation), this study too revealed high levels of unmet need, particularly for rehabilitative services. Although needs for individual counselling, chemotherapy and financial assistance were apparently met for a high proportion of patients, the majority of the sample had either none or between one-quarter and one-half of their needs met. The authors note that of the group that did receive services 11% utilised services that did not match any of their assessed needs.

Wykes *et al* (1985) reported a similar procedure, in which for each patient a member of staff was asked to assess the presence of need for 13 types of care: assessment, administration of medication, personal counselling, relative counselling, training in domestic skills, occupational therapy, industrial training or therapy, sheltered work, hotel services, behaviour modification, self-care, security and social activities. The four possible ratings were: (a) no need, no service provided; (b) over-provision, service provided but no need; (c) need for and utilisation of service; and (d) unmet need for service. These judgements were then compared with the judgements of the research team, who had collected a large amount of additional information on each patient. Kappa coefficients measuring agreement on the presence or absence of need between day staff and the research team were significantly greater than chance for 10 out of the 13 items of care, but there were fewer agreements about whether particular needs were being met by services. The authors comment that "the staff's judgement of specific needs did not have a very close correspondence with the team judgements" (p. 83).

One obvious problem with having care staff assess the needs of their own patients is that their judgements may be excessively conservative, and constrained by their knowledge of current practice and the treatment resources available. It has also frequently been noted that information about any particular patient tends to be dispersed among members of a clinical team, so that no one individual is in full possession of the facts. In Mann & Cree's study (1976) of new long-stay patients, they found that staff agreed with the research team about the overall proportion of patients that were suitable for discharge into the community, but that there was little agreement on specific individuals (personal communication cited in Wykes *et al*, 1985).

The alternative approach to is to employ specially trained researchers. The method of team judgement used in the Wykes *et al* (1985) study and the results obtained with it have been described in more detail by Wykes *et al* (1982). The team first elicited information from patients, staff, relatives and case records, one of their tasks being to reconcile conflicting reports. They then rated the needs for different types of care and judged whether the needs were met or unmet, or whether there was over-provision. On the whole, they did not try to assess the adequacy of interventions being offered, and the need was generally regarded as being met if an identified problem was being addressed by a suitable intervention.

A similar technique has been reported by Cormier *et al* (1987), who had trained raters collect information from patients, staff and medical notes. They then rated the need for 20 different items of care over the past six months, assuming an ideal system of care in which there were no constraints owing to resources, staff training, etc. This proviso was made in order to avoid excessively conservative ratings that simply serve to reflect the status quo. Types of care included therapeutic interventions, such as medication and family therapy, and psychosocial interventions, such as vocational rehabilitation and financial advice. In their study of patients with a diagnosis of schizophrenia discharged from the psychiatric units of general hospitals, Cormier *et al* reported a poor fit between needs for and utilisation of most rehabilitation and psychosocial services. Over-provision was not rated, and once again there was no explicit assessment of whether interventions were or were not effective.

Putting together the best of the needs assessments described above, one would end up with a procedure that had the following character-istics: (a) standardised assessment by trained raters; (b) measurement of over- as well as under-provision; (c) assumption of ideal conditions rather than accepting current service limitations; and (d) information drawn from patients, staff, medical notes and relatives. The importance of including relatives in assessments has been recently supported in a study by Brewin *et al* (1990). Relatives in their sample, compared with both the patients themselves and day staff, reported that patients had significantly greater numbers of problems. Interestingly, relatives' ratings did not differ from those of professional hostel staff who also knew the patients in a residential setting, suggesting that relatives' perceptions reflected different opportunities for observation and were not being coloured by a more intimate relationship to the patient.

All of the above methods of assessment suffer from one important limitation, namely that it is far from clear on what basis patients were rated as having needs for the various forms of care. For example, what set of clinical or social problems did raters have in mind when they made these judgements? What forms of care did they judge to be appropriate to which kinds of problem? And what did they do when patients were already in receipt of treatment or intervention aimed at a particular problem? In these respects, judgements of needs have tended typically to be opaque and difficult to question.

One of the main contentions expressed in our previous work (e.g. Brewin *et al*, 1987) was that needs cannot be properly assessed and compared between settings without an explicit model of care that states the assumptions behind the development of the instrument. Such an explicit model permits both the ideology of an instrument and the logic of individual judgements to be freely inspected. In other words, one cannot realistically measure the needs of specific groups without clear views about the therapeutic and rehabilitative process. These principles have been built into the MRC Needs for Care Assessment (MRC NCA; Brewin *et al*, 1987; Brewin & Wing,

1989; Mangen & Brewin, 1991), which was designed for use with the mentally ill living in the community and in high contact with psychiatric services. Data on the reliability and validity of the instrument are encouraging, and are discussed in more detail by Mangen & Brewin (1991).

The MRC Needs for Care Assessment

Model of care and definition of need

The care model on which the assessment is based attempts to reflect the clinical reality of working with individuals with chronic mental health problems. It is well documented that this group tends to have a low tolerance for stress, difficulty in forming stable social relationships and high levels of dependency (e.g. Stein & Test, 1980; Lamb, 1982; Shepherd, 1983). The intractable nature of their problems and consequent feelings of helplessness frequently result in demoralisation, effort withdrawal and lack of initiative in overcoming difficulties. Few treatments have demonstrable efficacy, and providing care typically involves a great deal of flexibility and persistence on the part of staff. Multiple clinical symptoms and problems in social functioning are the norm. Relatives who support patients often labour under a considerable burden and have numerous problems themselves (MacCarthy, 1988; MacCarthy *et al*, 1989).

This clinical picture leads naturally to a (much simplified) model of care. The aims of care are to reduce symptoms and distress to the maximum possible extent and to equip patients with the skills required to live independently in the community. This should have beneficial effects on patients' self-esteem and level of dependence, and make them less vulnerable to changes in their support network, while at the same time minimising the burden on their relatives or on those who are charged with caring for them. To achieve this, a wide range of potential problems must first be assessed at regular intervals. Second, for each problem, a range of possible interventions should be specified to ensure that all therapeutic options are considered. Third, to maintain an appropriately assertive approach to therapy, provision must be made for the case where interventions are initially refused or are (either wholly or partly) ineffective.

Our definition of need is therefore, as indicated above, based on the principle that some specific intervention must be identified that might reduce or ameliorate an objective lack. In this case, the objective lack is social disablement, by which we mean lowered physical, psychological and social functioning, compared with societal norms (Wing, 1978, 1986). In other words, actions by care staff are not assumed to be meeting a need simply because social disablement exists, but must also satisfy additional criteria indicating whether those actions are appropriate or inappropriate. This leads to the following formal definition of need for care:

- Need is present when: (a) a patient's functioning (social disablement) falls below or threatens to fall below some minimum specified level; and (b) this is owing to a remediable, or potentially remediable, cause.
- A need (as defined above) is met when it has attracted some at least partly effective item of care, and when no other items of care of greater potential effectiveness exist.
- A need (as defined above) is unmet when it has attracted only partly effective or no item of care and when other items of care of greater potential effectiveness exist.

Measurement principles

These definitions are represented in Table 16.1, which specifies how assessments of social disablement and assessments of items of care are combined to yield judgements concerning need. Twenty separate areas of functioning, both clinical and social, are assessed to determine the patient's specific problems. Because of the likely dispersal of information about patients, already noted, the investigator is charged with consulting a number of informants, and particularly relatives with whom the patient lives. Reliance on a single source of information is to be avoided. For each area of functioning in which

TABLE 16.1
Assessment of functioning, assessment of interventions and need status

Assessment of functioning	Assessment of interventions	Need status
No problem or mild problem	None employed	No need
Significant current or recent problem	None even partly effective	No meetable need
	Some potentially effective	Met need
	None fully effective: no alternatives	Met need
	None fully effective: alternatives available	Unmet need for treatment
Level of functioning not known		Unmet need for assessment

there is a problem, the assessment then specifies a set of potential interventions agreed upon by a cohort of rehabilitation workers (Brewin *et al*, 1987). Each intervention is given a rating by the investigator that reflects whether it is appropriate, whether it has been tried, how effective it has been and, where known, whether it has proven acceptable to the patient. Ratings of problems in functioning and of interventions are then combined algorithmically to generate a set of 20 needs ratings per patient. In each area of functioning, the patient can be rated as having no problem and no need, a met need, a problem but no meetable need, an unmet need for intervention, or an unmet need for assessment. The rationale for our definitions of social disablement are given in more detail in Brewin *et al* (1987). The intention was to set down minimal acceptable levels of health and social functioning. Thus, health was defined in terms of the absence of various kinds of symptoms, rather than in terms of the achievement of positive health goals. Similarly, acceptable social functioning was defined in terms of possession of the minimum skills required to function independently in the community, rather than in terms of higher level skills that might maximise the individual's autonomy and quality of life.

The symptoms and competencies covered in the most recent version (version Two/2) of the MRC NCA are shown in Box 16.1. Ratings reflect whether symptoms are current (i.e. were present in the past month), absent in the past month but recently present, or completely absent. The distinction between 'current' and 'recent' symptoms is necessary in order that items of care offered for purely preventative purposes can be rated appropriately.

In each area of social disablement, the MRC NCA specifies a list of between two and eight appropriate items of care, covering such diverse types of care as medication, counselling, behaviour pro-grammes, remedial education and the provision of a sheltered environment. A total of 34 different types of intervention are included. Our aim was to be over- rather than under-inclusive, and this meant including items of care not necessarily in widespread use, although we judged them to be generally acceptable to professionals. The original list of items of care was also validated against the judgements of rehabilitation care staff (Brewin *et al*, 1987), and has been slightly amended in the light of subsequent empirical work. In each area of social disablement, there is the facility to add a specific item of care that seems appropriate but does not figure on the standard list.

The principle that problems can only be considered as needs if there are currently feasible or appropriate interventions deserves further comment. This principle follows logically from our definition

Box 16.1
*Areas of functioning covered in Version Two/2 of the MRC Needs for Care Assessment
(Brewin & Wing, 1989)*

Section A: Symptoms and behavioural problems
Positive psychotic symptoms
Retardation (slowness and under-activity)
Side-effects of medication
Neurotic symptoms
Organic brain disorder
Physical disease and disorders
Violence or threats to self/others
Socially embarrassing behaviour
Distress about social circumstances

Section 2: Personal and social skills
Personal cleanliness
Household shopping
Cooking or buying meals
Household chores
Use of public transport
Use of public amenities
Basic literacy and arithmetic skills
Occupational skills
Social interaction skills
Management of money
Management of household affairs

of need as a requirement for some specifiable form of care. Hence, if all forms of care are inappropriate, have proven to be ineffective, or have been refused by the patient, need cannot be said to exist. Instead, the individual will be rated by our methods as having a problem but no meetable need. Mangen & Brewin (1991) cite the example of a patient with terminal cancer who, from the perspective of service providers, does not have a meetable *need* for a cure, so long as the cancer is untreatable by currently available methods. The same patient may, on the other hand, have meetable needs for pain relief and for counselling.

Problems with no associated meetable needs do occur from time to time with the long-term mentally ill, and were found to account for approximately 6% of identified problems in the Camberwell High Contact Survey (Brewin *et al*, 1988). It seems to us essential to be able to distinguish in this way those problems for which no effective care can realistically be offered *at the time of the assessment*. While recognising the limitations of current forms of care, this in no way lessens the obligation on agents to develop new and more effective interventions, or to persevere in the future with interventions that may have been unacceptable or ineffective in the past. Indeed, future repetitions of the MRC NCA would make this duty explicit, and might well result in problems without needs being reclassified as met or unmet needs. The concept of a problem with no meetable need highlights the very important fact that professional knowledge and practice are sometimes inadequate to meet all our patients' problems.

In addition to the primary need status, the assessment permits three secondary judgements to be made in each area of disablement. *Over-provision* is rated whenever one or more items of care are rated as being superfluous. In some cases, this will be because an item of care continues to be given even though it is not targeted at a specific problem or appears to be completely ineffective. In other cases, the rating reflects that the patient is in receipt of an item of care even though there has been no disablement for a considerable period of time, and there is no apparent danger of relapse. *Future need* can be rated when a patient is currently socially disabled, but cannot receive the appropriate item of care because of incapacitating symptoms or other priorities for intervention. *Lack of performance* is rated when a patient is known to be socially competent in some area of functioning and is not receiving any care, but is not currently exercising that skill. The intention here is to draw attention to a possible area in which action might be required. In the Camberwell High Contact Survey (Brewin *et al*, 1988), instances of over-provision were found to be as common as unmet needs for treatment, but future needs and 'lack of performance' were relatively rare.

Training and manpower requirements

The judgements required of assessors involve familiarity both with long-term patients and their characteristic problems and with the specific items of care that are considered. Thus, the assessment is not suitable for investigators who have not had clinical experience of this patient group, unless considerable extra training is provided. The conclusion of those who have used it is that it is best completed by a clinical team or by a research team that includes members with varying professional backgrounds. Psychiatric and psychological expertise is of prime importance. All users of the instrument should first attend an authorised training programme to familiarise themselves with the instrument. At present, this consists of two half-day workshops, with an intervening period in which users gain first-hand experience of carrying out assessments.

Data collection need not be lengthy if the instrument is used to shape the initial assessments conducted by a clinical team. Almost all the information is of the kind that should be routinely collected on admission, and this should be adequate for most clinical purposes. Additional manpower becomes necessary where comparability with other units or clinical teams is required for research purposes. This may well involve the addition of standardised assessments of functioning such as the Social Behaviour Schedule (Wykes & Sturt, 1986). Data collection will take considerably longer when the instrument is used by external investigators, as in the Camberwell High Contact Survey. Interviewing patients, day staff, relatives and other involved persons where appropriate, summarising the medical records and combining inconsistent information all require substantial resources.

Applying the MRC Needs for Care Assessment to other populations

The fact that the assessment was designed for chronic but potentially remediable difficulties within a British community setting has a number of consequences for its application to other populations. While the principles of assessment may transfer with little modification to some other chronic patient groups, such as those with diabetes mellitus (Brewin *et al*, 1991), other potential applications raise important issues concerning the goals of and the constraints on measurement. Below, we briefly discuss some of the issues raised by applications of the instrument to acute populations, the elderly mentally ill, individuals out of contact with services, long-stay hospital in-patients and patients from other cultures. All these examples illustrate the central theme of this chapter, namely that the design of assessment instruments is intimately bound up with the model of care being provided.

Acute psychiatric crises

The model of care on which the assessment is based assumes that the *order* in which interventions for a given problem are tried is not critical – the important thing is to persist with a range of possible options. This pragmatic approach appears acceptable for stable conditions that do not pose any immediate threat, but is less suitable for crises and other acute problems where it may be vital to intervene immediately in a particular way. At present, the assessment does not include any facility for prioritising interventions, and indeed it is hard to imagine how this could be achieved without the collection of extremely detailed clinical information. Extension of the instrument in this direction would also presuppose that there existed a reasonable degree of clinical consensus concerning crisis management.

The elderly mentally ill

The main issues raised by this group concern the applicability of the interventions specified in the assessment. For example, the active rehabilitative focus of Section B may not be perceived as appropriate for elderly and infirm persons permanently housed in residential units providing cooking, cleaning, leisure and other services. Similarly, remedial education may not be perceived as appropriate for literacy problems in this group. As discussed by Brewin & Wing (1989), it is important to take age, aptitude and residential placement into account, in order not to generate unnecessary unmet needs. But, equally, raters should take into account individual wishes to develop skills in a particular area, and whether such skills would lead to an increase in quality of life. Age alone is not sufficient grounds for ignoring unmet needs generated by our assessment.

Finally, adaptation of the instrument for this group might also benefit from incorporating new sections corresponding to particularly common problems, such as incontinence, and from incorporating additional interventions, such as reminiscence therapy or reality orientation.

Individuals out of contact with services

Many individuals with severe psychiatric problems are out of contact with services, and sometimes homeless. Assessing their objective lacks is not without difficulty, but assessing their needs for specific items of care is considerably more problematic. The instrument is predicated on the assumption that individuals are in contact with services and that the various forms of care can simply be offered. There are therefore major issues concerning the acceptability of items of care, individuals' willingness to visit health service or local authority facilities, and what alternative methods can be devised for delivering care in an effective way. It is likely that in many cases the goal of needs assessment should initially be simply that of establishing: (a) objective lacks; and (b) acceptable channels of service delivery. These might take the form of a lunch club or drop-in centre in preference to more traditional service settings.

Long-stay hospital in-patients

There is perhaps just one part of the assessment that is completely inappropriate for this group, and that is the section on management of household affairs. This section involves estimating the individual's ability to pay rent and bills, arrange repairs and join in the running of the ordinary household. It is hard to see how information of this kind could ever be obtained for long-stay in-patients, since the opportunities for observing them are most unlikely to exist. This section should therefore be rated as not applicable in long-stay samples.

Assessment problems may arise in other sections, for example those involving cooking and shopping, when hospital policy is to provide these services for all, regardless of their specific disabilities. Two choices are available here to the user of the instrument faced with a complete absence of any opportunities to observe patients' skills and abilities. The first option, which should normally be chosen when discharge from hospital is possible or inevitable, or when the patients are in an explicitly rehabilitative setting, is to rate all such examples as needs for assessment. The second option is to rate the level of functioning as unknown but the need as being met, on the pragmatic grounds that one cannot realistically train someone to develop a skill that he or she is then prevented from using. Once again, the model of care being employed constrains the nature of possible assessment.

Patients from other cultures

Note must be taken of cultural constraints when using the instrument on ethnic minorities within Britain, or on patient groups outside Britain. For example, in Verona (and presumably in other parts of Italy), it appears to be inappropriate to expect men to have demonstrated competence in cooking and other household chores. These are not part of the accepted male role, and hence were not accepted as needs either by professionals using our procedure or by service users (Lesage *et al*, 1991). Once again, specific subsections of the assessment may be rated as not applicable in order to cope with this contingency.

Summary

Methods of assessing individual needs for care and services will depend primarily on the nature of the population to be surveyed and on whether they are in high or low contact with psychiatric services. For populations in low contact, service needs have sometimes been estimated from morbidity and existing service utilisation rates. These data are inevitably crude, however, and do not furnish answers to important questions concerning whether individuals are in fact receiving appropriate and acceptable treatment. Such methods, although they may indicate substantial quantities of unmet need, say little about the quality of the unmet need and the factors that might improve service take-up. They also tend not to challenge the therapeutic status quo and are unlikely to result in a radical reappraisal of the adequacy of services.

For patients in high contact, brief assessments of needs for different kinds of service are sometimes made by care staff themselves. Although these methods have often demonstrated large amounts of unmet need, little is known about their validity. On the whole, what is known is not reassuring. With training, however, staff can make reasonably reliable brief assessments about needs for different kinds of day and residential placement (Clifford *et al*, 1991).

Any attempt to specify in more detail how staff should intervene is a relatively time-consuming matter. The MRC NCA is at present the most comprehensive instrument available to assess the needs of the long-term mentally ill. It is also the only instrument to be based on an explicit model of patient care and, repeated at regular intervals, could form the basis of clinical management. Although this model may not find universal favour, we believe that progress in individual needs assessment is only likely to follow attempts to articulate principles of care and open up evaluation methods to public scrutiny.

References

BIRCHWOOD, M. & SMITH, J. (1988) The needs of families caring for a schizophrenic relative: developing a comprehensive service. In: *Current Issues in Clinical Psychology 1986* (eds N. Eisenberg & D. Glasgow), pp. 186–200. Aldershot: Gower Press.

BREWIN, C. R. & WING, J. K. (1989) *MRC Needs for Care Assessment: Manual for version Two/2*. Unpublished manuscript. London: Institute of Psychiatry.

——, ——, MANGEN, S. P., *ET AL* (1987) Principles and practice of measuring need in the long-term mentally ill: The MRC Needs for Care Assessment. *Psychological Medicine*, **17**, 971–982.

——, ——, ——, *ET AL* (1988) Needs for care among the long-term mentally ill: A report from the Camberwell High Contact Survey. *Psychological Medicine*, **18**, 457–468.

——, VELTRO, F., WING, J. K., *ET AL* (1990) The assessment of psychiatric disability in the community: A comparison of clinical, staff, and family interviews. *British Journal of Psychiatry*, **157**, 671–674.

——, BRADLEY, C. & HOME, P. (1991) Measuring needs in patients with diabetes. In: *The Technology of Diabetes Care* (eds C. Bradley, P. Home & M. Christie), pp. 142–155. Reading: Harwood.

CLIFFORD, P, CHARMAN, A., WEBB, Y., *ET AL* (1991) Planning for community care: The Community Placement Questionnaire. *British Journal of Clinical Psychology*, **30**, 193–211.

CORMIER, H., BORUS, J. F., REED, R. B., *ET AL* (1987) Combler les besoins de service de sante mentale des personnes atteintes de schizophrenie. *Canadian Journal of Psychiatry*, **32**, 454–458.

DAVIES, B. & CHALLIS, D. (1986) *Matching Resources to Needs in Community Care*. London: Gower.

FALLOON, I. R. H. & MARSHALL, G. N. (1983) Residential care and social behaviour: A study of rehabilitation needs. *Psychological Medicine*, **13**, 341–347.

LAMB, H. R. (1982) *Treating the Long-term Mentally Ill*. San Francisco, CA: Jossey-Bass.

LEHTINEN, V., JOUKAMAA, M., JYRKINEN, E., *ET AL* (1990) Need for mental health services of the adult population in Finland: Results from the Mini Finland Health Survey. *Acta Psychiatrica Scandinavica*, **81**, 426–431.

LEIGHTON, D. C., HARDING, J. S., MACKLIN, D. B., *ET AL* (1963) Psychiatric findings of the Stirling County Study. *American Journal of Psychiatry*, **119**, 1021–1026.

LESAGE, A. D., MIGNOLLI, G., FACCINCANI, C., *ET AL* (1991) Standardised assessment of the needs for care in a cohort of patients with schizophrenic psychoses. In: *Community-based Psychiatry: Long-term Patterns of Care in South-Verona* (ed. M. Tansella), pp. 27–33. Psychological Medicine Monograph Supplement 19.

LEVIN, G., WILDER, J. F. & GILBERT, J. (1978) Identifying and meeting clients' needs in six community mental health centers. *Hospital and Community Psychiatry*, **29**, 185–188.

MACCARTHY, B. (1988) The role of relatives. In: *Community Care in Practice: Services for the Continuing Care Client* (eds A. Lavender & F. Holloway), pp. 207–227. Chichester: Wiley.

——, LESAGE, A., BREWIN, C. R., *ET AL* (1989) Needs for care among the relatives of long-term users of day care. *Psychological Medicine*, **19**, 725–736.

MALLMAN, C. A. & MARCUS, S. (1980) Logical clarifications in the study of needs. In: *Human Needs* (ed. K. Lederer), pp.163–185. Cambridge, MA: Oelgeschlager, Gunn, & Hain.

MANGEN, S. & BREWIN, C. R. (1991) The measurement of need. In: *Social Psychiatry: Theory, Methodology and Practice* (ed. P. E. Bebbington). Brunswick, NJ: Transaction Press.

MANN, S. & CREE, W. (1976) 'New' long-stay psychiatric patients: A national survey of fifteen mental hospitals in England and Wales 1972/3. *Psychological Medicine*, **6**, 603–616.

SHAPIRO, S., SKINNER, E. A., KRAMER, M., *ET AL* (1985) Measuring need for mental health services in a general population. *Medical Care*, **23**, 1033–1043.

SHEPHERD, G. (1983) Planning the rehabilitation of the individual. In: *Theory and Practice of Psychiatric Rehabilitation* (eds F. N.Watts & D. H. Bennett), pp. 329–348. Chichester: Wiley.

SOLOMON, P. & DAVIS, J. (1985) Meeting community service needs of discharged psychiatric patients. *Psychiatric Quarterly*, **57**, 11–17.

STEIN, L. I. & TEST, M. A. (1980) Alternative to mental hospital treatment: I. Conceptual model, treatment program, and clinical evaluation. *Archives of General Psychiatry*, **37**, 392–399.

TRACY, L. (1986) Toward an improved need theory: In response to legitimate criticism. *Behavioral Science*, **31**, 205–218.

WASYLENKI, D. A., GOERING, P., LANCEE, W., *ET AL* (1981) Psychiatric aftercare: Identified needs versus referral patterns. *American Journal of Psychiatry*, **138**, 1228–1231.

WING, J. K. (1978) Medical and social science and medical and social care. In: *Social Care Research* (eds J. Barnes & N. Connelly), pp. 123–137. London: Bedford Square Press.

—— (1986) The cycle of planning and evaluation. In: *The Provision of Mental Health Services in Britain: The Way Ahead* (eds G. Wilkinson & H. Freeman), pp. 35–48. London: Gaskell.

—— & STURT, E. (1978) *The PSE-ID-CATEGO System: Supplementary Manual.* Mimeo. London: Institute of Psychiatry.

WYKES, T. & STURT, E. (1986) The measurement of social behaviour in psychiatric patients: an assessment of the reliability and validity of the SBS schedule. *British Journal of Psychiatry*, **148**, 1–11.

——, CREER, C. & STURT, E. (1982) Needs and the deployment of services. In: *Long-Term Community Care: Experience in a London Borough* (ed. J. K.Wing), pp. 41–55. Psychological Medicine Monograph Supplement No. 2.

——, STURT, E. & CREER, C. (1985) The assessment of patients' needs for community care. *Social Psychiatry*, **20**, 76–85.

17 The Camberwell Assessment of Need (CAN)

MIKE SLADE and PAUL McCRONE

A *needs-led* approach to the provision of mental health care has been one of the most consistent themes to emerge from evolving community mental health care services during the 1990s. This finds expression in the provisions of the NHS and Community Care Act (1990), and the Care Programme Approach (CPA; Department of Health, 1990). The central tenet of a needs-led approach is that assessment of the needs of patients should be on the basis of their individual circumstances, problems and personal goals. Assessment should not be undertaken in terms of or on the basis of existing services, that is, assessment should not be *service-based*. This means that assessment of need is a separate process from decisions about what care or treatment to provide.

Needs-led assessment means, for example, that assessment should look at whether individuals have access to enough activities that are meaningful (to them) each day, rather than whether they need to attend a day centre. If the assessment indicates that there is a problem with daytime activities, one service response might be to provide a place at a day centre. Another, however, might be support in undertaking voluntary work. Needs-led assessments have two advantages over service-based assessments. First, they point to the most appropriate form of service response (in terms of treatment or care) for the individual's difficulties. Second, they have the potential to indicate needs for which there is currently no service provision, which a service-based assessment by definition would not identify.

What is a need?

Despite the wide recognition that people with severe mental illness usually have a wide range of clinical and social needs, there is continuing confusion and debate about how such needs should be defined and assessed (Holloway, 1993).

A variety of approaches to defining need have been proposed. The American psychologist Maslow established a hierarchy of need when attempting to formulate a theory of human motivation (Maslow, 1954). In Maslow's model, fundamental physiological needs (such as the need for food) underpin the higher needs of safety, love, self-esteem and self-actualisation. He proposed that people are motivated by the requirement to meet these needs, and that higher needs can only be met once the lower and more fundamental needs are met. This approach can be illustrated by the example of a homeless man, who is not concerned about his lack of friends while he is cold and hungry. However, once these physiological needs have been met, he may express more interest in having the company of other people.

Since the work of Maslow, other approaches have been developed to defining need with respect to health care. In the MRC Needs for Care Assessment (MRC NCA; Brewin *et al*, 1987), a need is defined as being present when a person's level of functioning falls below, or threatens to fall below, some specified level, and when there is some remediable, or potentially remediable, cause. The sociologist Bradshaw (1972) proposed a taxonomy of four types of need: need which is either 'felt' or 'expressed' by the patient; 'normative' need, which is assessed by an expert; and 'comparative' need, which arises from comparison with other groups or individuals. Such an approach helps to emphasise that need is a subjective concept, and that judgement of whether a need is present or not will, in part, depend on whose viewpoint is being taken. Slade (1994) has discussed this issue with respect to differences in perception between the patients of mental health services and the involved professionals, and he has argued that once differences are identified, then negotiation between staff and patient can take place to agree a care plan.

Stevens & Gabbay (1991) have distinguished between need (the ability to benefit in some way from health care), demand (wish expressed by the service patient) and supply of services. These concepts can be illustrated by different components of mental health services. For instance, mental health services for homeless mentally ill people are rarely demanded by homeless people, but most professionals would agree that a need exists. In contrast, the demand for counselling services frequently outstrips supply.

Clearly, the need, demand and supply of services will never be perfectly matched. If mismatch is to be minimised, then two principles need to underpin mental health service development. First, services must try to address the identified problems and difficulties of local patients (i.e. local services should be shaped by the specific needs of the population), rather than being provided in line with any national template or historical patterns. Second, a continued effort to demonstrate what is, and is not, effective with different groups is required, so that resources are provided for effective interventions, and not driven by demand or short-term political pressures.

How are needs to be assessed?

There is no perfect individual needs assessment tool. The requirements of different patients vary, and there is inevitable conflict between factors such as brevity and comprehensiveness. Johnson and colleagues (1996) summarised the features of an ideal needs assessment for use in clinical settings as brief, easily learned, quickly administered by clinical staff, valid and reliable. Numerous instruments have been developed by individual teams around the country to aid care planning and reviews. There is little consistency in the information that is collected, with a tendency to concentrate on qualitative, rather than quantitative, data. Psychometric properties are frequently ignored. Although such instruments help to focus a team's approach, they do not provide valid or accurate information to service planners.

One established needs assessment tool is the Camberwell Assessment of Need (CAN; Phelan *et al*, 1995), which is described in this chapter. Other carefully designed needs assessment instruments include the following.

MRC Needs for Care Assessment

The MRC NCA (Brewin *et al*, 1987) was designed to identify areas of remediable need. Need is defined as being present when: (a) a patient's functioning (social disablement) falls below or threatens to fall below some minimum specified level; and (b) this is owing to a remediable, or potentially remediable, cause. A need is defined as being met when it has attracted an item of care that is at least partly effective, and when no other item of care of greater potential effectiveness exists. A need is said to be unmet when it has attracted only a partly effective or no item of care, and when other items of care of greater potential effectiveness exist. The MRC NCA has proved itself to be a robust research instrument, and there is a substantial body of research describing its use (Brewin *et al*, 1988; Lesage *et al*, 1991; Van Haaster *et al*, 1994; O'Leary & Webb, 1996). However, it is probably too complex and time-consuming for routine clinical use, and difficulties have arisen when it was used among long-term in-patients (Pryce *et al*, 1993) and homeless mentally ill (Hogg & Marshall, 1992).

Cardinal Needs Schedule

The Cardinal Needs Schedule (CNS; Marshall, 1994) is a modification of the MRC NCA. It identifies cardinal problems which satisfy three criteria: (a) the 'cooperation criterion' (the patient is willing to accept help for the problem); (b) the 'co-stress criterion' (the problem causes considerable anxiety, frustration or inconvenience to people caring for the patient); and (c) the 'severity criterion' (the problem endangers the health or safety of the patient, or the safety of other people). The instrument involves the use of the Manchester Scale (Baker & Hall, 1988) for mental state assessment, and the REHAB scale (Krawiecka *et al*, 1977), as well as a specially designed additional information questionnaire. A computerised version known as Autoneed is also available. Again, given the detail of this instrument, it is probably more suited to experienced researchers.

Bangor Assessment of Need Profile

The Bangor Assessment of Need Profile (BAN–P; Carter *et al*, 1996) comprises a self-report schedule designed to give a brief and simple indication of the expressed need of people with a long-term mental illness, and a schedule to assess need as perceived by a key informant. Need is present when an item falls below that which the respondent (user or key informant) perceives to be normal or ordinary functioning, and absent when the respondent perceives normal and independent functioning. Reliability is explored, and the instrument is primarily intended for research use.

The Camberwell Assessment of Need

The Camberwell Assessment of Need (CAN; Phelan *et al*, 1995) is an individual needs assessment instrument for use with adults with severe mental illness. It was published in 1994, and is intended to meet the requirements of the NHS and Community Care Act (1990). Four broad principles governed the development of the CAN:

   (a) Everyone has needs, and although people with mental health problems have some specific needs, the majority of their needs are similar to those of people who do not have a mental illness, such as having somewhere to live, something to do and enough money.

(b) The majority of people with a severe mental illness have multiple needs, and it is vital that all of them are identified by those caring for them. Therefore, a priority of the CAN is to identify, rather than describe in detail, serious needs. Specialist assessments can be conducted in specific areas if required, once the need has been identified.

(c) Needs assessment should be both an integral part of routine clinical practice and a component of service evaluation, so the CAN should be useable by a wide range of staff.

(d) Need is a subjective concept, and there will frequently be differing but equally valid perceptions about the presence or absence of a specific need. The CAN therefore records the views of staff and patients separately.

The specific criteria that were established for the CAN are that it:

(a) has adequate psychometric properties;
(b) can be completed within 30 minutes;
(c) can be used by a wide range of professionals;
(d) is suitable for both routine clinical practice and research;
(e) can be learnt and used, without formal training;
(f) incorporates the views of both patients and staff about needs;
(g) measures both met and unmet need; and
(h) measures the level of help received from friends and relatives as well as from statutory services.

The CAN has been developed incrementally, and CAN 3.0 is now in use. The original version was developed for research use, and called CAN–R. Two variants have also been developed: a short version (CANSAS) and a long clinical version (CAN–C). Two elements are common to all three versions. First, all versions assess need in the same 22 domains of health and social needs:

(a) accommodation
(b) food
(c) looking after the home
(d) self-care
(e) daytime activities
(f) physical health
(g) psychotic symptoms
(h) information
(i) psychological distress
(j) safety to self
(k) safety to others
(l) alcohol
(m) drugs
(n) company

(o)   intimate relationships
(p)   sexual expression
(q)   child care
(r)   basic education
(s)   telephone
(t)   transport
(u)   money
(v)   benefits.

Second, all CAN assessments record multiple perspectives. Staff and patient perspectives of need differ (MacCarthy *et al*, 1986; Slade *et al*, 1996, 1998), and need to be assessed separately.

A full description of the CAN family has been published (Slade *et al*, 1999), including copies of each assessment in a format intended for photocopying. The three versions of the CAN are now briefly described.

Camberwell Assessment of Need Short Appraisal

CANSAS is a short (single-page) summary of the needs of a mental health service patient. CANSAS can be used in clinical settings, since it is short enough to be used for review purposes on a routine basis. It can also be used as an outcome measure in research studies, especially when a number of assessment schedules are being used. CANSAS records the views of the patient, carers and staff about the needs of the patient in the 22 domains of health and social needs.

An assessment using CANSAS involves an interviewer asking an interviewee questions about each of 22 domains. The interviewer should be a professional with some knowledge of the difficulties which can be involved in interviewing people with mental health problems, such as impaired concentration, disorganisation and psychotic symptoms. The interviewer should also be familiar with issues relating to safety and confidentiality, as discussed by Parkman & Bixby (1996). The interviewee may be the patient, the carer (e.g. a friend or family member) or a member of staff (e.g. the key-worker). If the patient or carer is being interviewed, administration involves the interviewer going through the CANSAS and asking the patient about each domain in turn. If a member of staff is the interviewee, this normally involves the member of staff filling in the CAN.

Questions are asked about each domain, to identify: (a) whether a need or problem is present in that domain; and (b) whether the need is met or unmet. On the basis of the interviewee's responses, a *need rating* is made:

0 = no serious problem	(no need)
1 = no/moderate problem owing to help given	(met need)
2 = serious problem	(unmet need)
9 = not known	

The need rating is made using the following algorithm:

> If the interviewee does not know or does not want to answer questions on this domain then rate 9 (not known)
>> *otherwise*
>
> If a serious problem is present (regardless of cause, or whether any help is being given or not) then rate 2 (unmet need)
>> *otherwise*
>
> If there is no serious problem because of help given then rate 1 (met need)
>> *otherwise*
>
> Rate 0 (no need).

In other words, a need is *met* if there is not currently a problem in the domain but a problem would exist were it not for the help provided (i.e. the patient is getting effective help). A need is *unmet* if there is currently a problem in the domain (whether or not any help is currently being provided).

Note that just because there is currently no problem, the need rating is not automatically 0. For example, a person with diabetes who is physically well because of his or her prescribed insulin would be rated as 1 (met need) for physical health. Similarly, a need can exist for a variety of reasons. For example, a person with a psychotic illness may currently be unable to do his or her shopping because of a sprained ankle. He or she should be rated as having a need (i.e. need rating 1 or 2) in the 'food' domain, even though this need is not related to the psychiatric condition.

Whoever is being interviewed, it is important that it is his or her views that are assessed. Specifically, there are no 'right' or 'wrong' answers. So, for example, the staff member should give his or her own views about the patient's needs, rather than what he or she thinks the patient's views are. The difference between met and unmet need can be a matter of judgement. The goal is to differentiate between problems that are current and severe and those that are ameliorated by help, but there may still be a blurred boundary where the patient is receiving help which only partly addresses his or her difficulties. Be guided by the interviewee's response – does he or she see the problem as current and severe (need rating 2), or under control with the help the patient is getting (need rating 1)?

A typical CANSAS assessment should take less than 10 minutes, but this will be affected by the number of needs identified and the characteristics of the interviewee. For example, if the patient has difficulties with concentration, then a break may be needed during the interview.

At the end of an assessment, it will be possible to say how many needs the patient has from these 22 domains, and how many of these needs are unmet. A CANSAS assessment by itself is wide-ranging ('comprehensive'), but not thorough, since a person can have needs in a particular domain for a variety of reasons. CANSAS is therefore not an adequate assessment on which to decide whether to offer help, but should be used to identify domains in which more assessment is needed.

Each CANSAS sheet can be used to make up to four assessments. One use would be to record staff and patient assessments of need before and after an intervention. Another use would be to record the perceptions of a range of people at a specific point in time, such as the patient, informal caregiver, keyworker and general practitioner. A third use would be to review changes in needs over time.

CANSAS assessment information can be used in at least three ways:

(a) CANSAS data can be used at the level of the individual patient, by providing a baseline measure of level of need, or for charting changes in the patient over time. For example, one approach would be to use the CANSAS routinely in initial assessments of new service patients, to identify the range of domains in which they are likely to require further assessment and (possibly) help or treatment.

(b) CANSAS data can be used for auditing and developing an individual service. For example, to investigate:

- the impact on needs of providing an intervention for a group of service patients, by looking at changes across this group;
- caseload dependency for different workers; and
- whether enough patients have unmet needs in the domain of benefits to make it worthwhile for a community mental health team to employ a welfare benefits advisor.

(c) CANSAS can be used as an outcome measure for research purposes, such as the impact on needs of two different types of mental health services, or the reasons why staff and service patient perceptions differ.

The Camberwell Assessment of Need – Clinical and Research versions

The CAN–C is intended for clinical use and the CAN–R for research use. Each has four sections for each domain and is completed separately by the staff and patient. Section 1 is the same as in CANSAS, and assesses the need rating (no need, met need, unmet need or not known) for the domain. The purpose of Section 1 is twofold: first, to assess whether there is a need in the domain, and whether effective help is already being given; and second, to decide whether further questions about this domain are necessary. Section 2 assesses the amount of help being received from informal sources (friends, relatives, etc.). Section 3 assesses the amount of help given by and needed from formal services. For all ratings, anchor points and rating guidelines are provided. Section 4 in CAN–C records the patient's perceptions about the domain, and the care plan. Section 4 in CAN–R records whether patients are getting the right type of help for their problem and, in the patient interview only, whether they are satisfied with the amount of help that they are receiving.

Each CAN–C or CAN–R assessment records the perceptions of both staff and patient. To avoid bulky notes, one-page summary sheets have been developed. A typical CAN–C or CAN–R assessment should take 15–20 minutes, but this will be affected by the number of needs identified and characteristics of the interviewee. As with the CANSAS, a break may be needed during the interview.

The CAN–C serves similar purposes to the CANSAS. There are additional benefits:

(a) The CAN–C can serve as an indicator of where the level of care can change. By recording the amount of care received by informal and formal services, staff will be better placed to determine whether more can be done in meeting the needs of patients.

(b) The inclusion of a section where details of a care plan can be recorded enables the preceding quantitative data to be supplemented by staff and patient views as to the importance of particular areas of need, the service response to need and the way forward in addressing need.

(c) The CAN–R assessment information can be employed as an outcome measure in research evaluations, such as its use in the PRiSM Psychosis Study of community mental health services (Leese *et al*, 1998). As with the CANSAS, the CAN–R can also aid research concerning different perceptions of need (Slade *et al*, 1998).

Psychometric properties

The reliability and validity of the CAN have been described in detail elsewhere (Phelan *et al*, 1995). In brief, the selection of items to be included in the CAN was guided by validity, studies including surveys of people with severe mental health problems and mental health professionals. In a study of patients with a diagnosis of psychosis attending an inner-city mental health service, the mean number of needs identified by staff was 7.55, and by patients 8.64 (out of a possible 22). Correlations of the interrater and test–retest reliability of the total number of needs identified by staff were 0.99 and 0.78 respectively. The percentage complete agreement on individual items ranged from 100–81.6% (interrater) and 100–58.1% (test–retest).

CAN resources

A number of resources and variants of the CAN have been developed. These are briefly summarised.

Training for the CAN

The CAN–R, CAN–C and CANSAS are intended for use by mental health professionals without any formal training. Each version contains a page outlining how to rate responses, and in the CAN–R and CAN–C every rating has anchor points for guidance. There will, however, be times when some training in the use of the CAN is appropriate. This might be for several reasons. The length (of the CAN–R or CAN–C) or complexity (of the CANSAS) may appear daunting, particularly if staff are not familiar with using assessment schedules. If the CANSAS or CAN–C is being introduced into routine clinical practice, there may be some resistance from staff, in which case training may serve to reduce apprehension, increase motivation and generate commitment. Alternatively, it may be important to maximise interrater reliability from the outset, for example, in a research project.

A half-day training session has been developed, which is described in full (Slade *et al*, 1999). The goal of the training is both to educate participants about the approach taken to assessing need and to give practice in undertaking a CAN–R assessment. It can be easily modified to provide training for the CANSAS or CAN–C. In brief, the training comprises an introduction to the concept of need and to the CAN–R, use of a short practice vignette to demonstrate assessing staff and patient, and then five full vignettes to rate.

CAN for other patient groups

The CAN versions described in this chapter are intended for assessing the needs of adults with severe mental illness. Versions of the CAN are being developed for use with forensic populations (Xenitidis *et al*, 2000), older adults (Reynolds *et al*, 2000) and adults with both learning disabilities and severe mental illness.

CAN translations

The CAN–R and the CAN–C have been used extensively in the UK. In addition, there are 10 translations of the CAN–R. The different language editions are:

- Cantonese
- Danish
- Dutch
- French
- Greek
- Italian
- Norwegian
- Spanish
- Swedish
- Turkish.

The CAN–R has also been adapted for use with young people in South Africa. This version has been translated into Afrikaans and Xhosa.

The process by which the CAN has been translated has been varied, because the initiative has generally come from the centre requiring the translated version. Some translations have been checked by 'back-translating' into English to ensure that the meaning has not been lost. Furthermore, a five-nation (UK, Italy, The Netherlands, Denmark and Spain) study of care for people with schizophrenia used the CAN–R as an outcome measure. A key part of the study was to develop standardised instruments with demonstrated reliability. The Italian, Dutch, Danish and Spanish versions of the CAN–R were scrutinised by focus groups in each relevant country. This resulted in a number of refinements to the wording of the instrument to make it more contextually and culturally specific. In addition, the existing CAN manual was amended to improve the application of the CAN in different countries. The final versions of the CAN–R were then tested for reliability in each of the five countries and the results indicated acceptable reliability (McCrone *et al*, 2000).

Conclusion

The CAN offers an approach to assessing the needs of patients with mental health problems. A wide range of health and social needs is assessed from different perspectives. Versions are available for different patient groups and in different languages. The CAN is being used routinely in clinical settings, and in local and international research studies. It offers the prospect of becoming the standard approach to needs assessment.

Acknowledgements

This chapter uses material from the CAN book (Slade *et al*, 1999), for which the other authors are Linda Loftus, Michael Phelan, Graham Thornicroft and Til Wykes. Other contributors to the development and dissemination of the CAN include the PRiSM Psychosis Study interviewers, Thomas Becker, Liz Brooks, Graham Dunn, Frank Holloway, Sonia Johnson, Morven Leese, Sue Parkman, Geraldine Strathdee, George Szmukler and Ruth Taylor.

References

BAKER, R. & HALL, J. N. (1988) REHAB: A new assessment instrument for chronic psychiatric patients. *Schizophrenia Bulletin*, **14**, 97–111.

BRADSHAW, J. (1972) A taxonomy of social need. In: *Problems and Progress in Medical Care: Essays on Current Research: 7th Series* (ed. G. McLachlan). London: Oxford University Press.

BREWIN, C., WING, J., MANGEN, S., *ET AL* (1987) Principles and practice of measuring needs in the long-term mentally ill: the MRC Needs for Care Assessment. *Psychological Medicine*, **17**, 971–981.

—, —, —, *ET AL* (1988) Needs for care among the long-term mentally ill: a report from the Camberwell High Contact Survey. *Psychological Medicine*, **18**, 457–468.

CAMPBELL, M. J. & MACHIN, D. (1993) *Medical Statistics: a Commonsense Approach.* New York: Wiley.

CARTER, M., CROSBY, C., GEERTHUIS, S., *ET AL* (1996) Developing reliability in client-centred mental health needs assessment. *Journal of Mental Health*, **5**, 233–243.

DEPARTMENT OF HEALTH (1990) *The Care Programme Approach for People with a Mental Illness Referred to the Specialist Psychiatric Services.* (HC90)23/HASSL(90)11). London: HMSO.

GLOVER, G., ROBIN, E., EMAMI, J., *ET AL* (2000) A needs index for mental health care. *Social Psychiatry and Psychiatric Epidemiology*, **33**, 89–96.

HOGG, L. & MARSHALL, M. (1992) Can we measure need in the homeless mentally ill? Using the MRC Needs for Care Assessment in hostels for the homeless. *Psychological Medicine*, **22**, 1027–1034.

HOLLOWAY, F. (1993) Need in community psychiatry: a consensus is required. *Psychiatric Bulletin*, **18**, 321–323.

HOUSE OF COMMONS (1990) *National Health Service and Community Care Act.* London: HMSO.

JOHNSON, S., THORNICROFT, G., PHELAN, M., *ET AL* (1996) Assessing needs for mental health services. In: *Mental Health Outcome Measures* (eds G. Thornicroft & M. Tansella), pp. 217–226. Berlin: Springer-Verlag.

KRAWIECKA, M., GOLDBERG, D. & VAUGHN, M. (1977) A standardised psychiatric assessment scale for rating chronic psychotic patients. *Acta Psychiatrica Scandinavica*, **55**, 299–308.

LEESE, M., JOHNSON, S., SLADE, M., *ET AL* (1998) User perspective on needs and satisfaction with mental health services: the PRiSM Psychosis Study. 8. *British Journal of Psychiatry*, **173**, 409–415.

LESAGE, A., MIGNOLLI, G., FACCINCANI, C., *ET AL* (1991) Standardised assessment of the needs for care in a cohort of patients with schizophrenic psychoses. *Psychological Medicine*, Suppl. 19, 426–431.

MACCARTHY, B., BENSON, J. & BREWIN, C. (1986) Task motivation and problem appraisal in long-term psychiatric patients. *Psychological Medicine*, **16**, 431–438.

MARSHALL, M. (1994) How should we measure need? *Philosophy, Psychiatry and Psychology*, **1**, 27–36.

MASLOW, A. (1954) *Motivation and Personality*. New York: Harper & Row.

MCCRONE, P., LEESE, M., THORNICROFT, G., *ET AL* (2000) Reliability of the Camberwell Assessment of Need – European Version. EPSILON Study 6. *British Journal of Psychiatry*, **177** (Suppl. 39), s34–s40.

O'LEARY, D. & WEBB, M. (1996) The needs for care assessment – a longitudinal approach. *Psychiatric Bulletin*, **20**, 134–136.

PARKMAN, S. & BIXBY, S. (1996) Community interviewing: experiences and recommendations. *Psychiatric Bulletin*, **20**, 72–74.

PHELAN, M., SLADE, M., THORNICROFT, G., *ET AL* (1995) The Camberwell Assessment of Need: the validity and reliability of an instrument to assess the needs of people with severe mental illness. *British Journal of Psychiatry*, **167**, 589–595.

PRYCE, I. G., GRIFFITHS, R. D., GENTRY, R. M., *ET AL* (1993) How important is the assessment of social skills in current long-stay patients? An evaluation of clinical response to needs for assessment, treatment and care in a long-stay psychiatric in-patient population. *British Journal of Psychiatry*, **162**, 498–502.

REYNOLDS, T., THORNICROFT, G. ABAS, M., *ET AL* (2000) Camberwell Assessment of Need for the Elderly (CANE). Development, validity and reliability. *British Journal of Psychiatry*, **176**, 444–452.

SLADE, M. (1994) Needs assessment. Involvement of staff and users will help to meet needs. *British Journal of Psychiatry*, **165**, 293–296.

——, PHELAN, M., THORNICROFT, G., *ET AL* (1996) The Camberwell Assessment of Need (CAN): comparison of assessments by staff and patients of the needs of the severely mentally ill. *Social Psychiatry and Psychiatric Epidemiology*, **31**, 109–113.

——, —— & —— (1998) A comparison of needs assessed by staff and an epidemiologically representative sample of patients with psychosis. *Psychological Medicine*, **28**, 543–550.

——, THORNICROFT, G., LOFTUS, L., *ET AL* (1999) *CAN: Camberwell Assessment of Need. A Comprehensvie Needs Assessment Tool for People with Severe Mental Illness*. London: Gaskell.

STEVENS, A. & GABBAY, J. (1991) Needs assessment needs assessment. *Health Trends*, **23**, 20–23.

THORNICROFT, G. (1991) Social deprivation and rates of treated mental disorder. Developing statistical models to predict psychiatric service utilisation. *British Journal of Psychiatry*, **158**, 475–484.

VAN HAASTER, I., LESAGE, A., CYR, M., *ET AL* (1994) Problems and needs for care of patients suffering from severe mental illness. *Social Psychiatry and Psychiatric Epidemiology*, **29**, 141–148.

XENITIDIS, K., THORNICROFT, G., LEESE, M., *ET AL* (2000) Reliability and validity of the CANDID – a needs assessment instrument for adults with learning disabilities and mental health problems. *British Journal of Psychiatry*, **176**, 473–478.

18 Mental health services for homeless people

WILLIAM R. BREAKEY, EZRA SUSSER and PHILIP TIMMS

The issues of homelessness and mental illness are not new. Homelessness has been a feature of European and American society at least since Victorian times, and probably longer. In the heyday of the asylums in Britain, 14% of the pauper lunatics in England and Wales outside London, who would otherwise have been wandering the streets, were accommodated in workhouses – the established provision for the indigent (Timms, 1996). The increased visibility of the problem in recent years has revealed a state of affairs that has always existed. We deplore the fact of homelessness in the midst of affluence, particularly as it most harshly affects the most vulnerable citizens. However, experience indicates that the enterprise of providing good-quality assessment and services for the homeless mentally ill should seen as part of the permanent landscape of psychiatry, not just a response to a contemporary crisis.

More than 30 years ago, research on both sides of the Atlantic demonstrated the high prevalence of mental illness in homeless men (Whiteley, 1955; Bogue, 1963; Edwards *et al*, 1968; Spitzer *et al*, 1969; Lodge-Patch, 1970). In the UK, USA and other countries, homeless people in general, and homeless mentally ill people in particular, had become much more visible on the streets of major cities by the end of the 1980s. Critics have linked high prevalence of mental disorder in homeless people to the phasing out of mental hospitals as the primary locus of care for the severely mentally ill (Wyatt & De Renzo, 1986; Lamb, 1992; McHugh, 1992). There are few, if any, empirical data to support these criticisms in the USA, where they were made, and they are not supported by data from the UK. Evidence from the TAPS study of the closure of a North London mental hospital suggested that discharging patients from hospitals was not the immediate cause: very few of the patients they studied became homeless after resettlement in the community, when good discharge plans had been made (Dayson, 1993). A three-year follow-up of long-stay patients discharged from hospitals in Northern Ireland found that none had become homeless (Donnelly *et al*, 1997). Craig & Timms (1992) argued that the increased visibility of homeless mentally ill people was more closely connected to the unplanned closures of hostels for homeless people during the 1980s: in London, there were nearly 10 000 direct access hostel spaces in 1980, declining to just over 2000 in 1989. Similar problems arose in the USA during the same period, when many single-room occupancy hotels in New York, for example, were converted to apartments and condominiums. Whatever mental health service changes may have contributed to the current situation, it is clear that many other factors have had a role: low-cost housing availability, education and employment opportunities, evolving patterns of family life, social security entitlements and so forth (Cohen & Thompson, 1992). None the less, the high prevalence of mental disorders in homeless people and their presumed need for mental health services are readily apparent. A special target population for mental health services has emerged. This is a new area of specialisation, but with increasing experience consensus is developing about the best methods for addressing the health service needs of homeless people in general (McMurray-Avila, 1997), and in particular those who are mentally ill. This chapter describes briefly what has been learned, particularly in the British Isles and North America, about the psychiatric problems of homeless people, their needs for services and strategies for meeting them.

The problem of definition

There is a major problem with the notion of treating homeless people as a homogeneous group. Other special groups such as women, children or the elderly have clear and relatively immutable definitions. By contrast, definitions of homelessness can be broad or narrow. There is evidence, at least in the USA, that much greater numbers of people have experienced homelessness than is generally supposed. Link *et al* (1994), in a telephone survey of a national sample of the US population, found that more than 7% reported having been homeless at some time. Homelessness, to these respondents, probably encompasses a wide range of experiences.

At one end of the spectrum of definitions, a recent political initiative in the UK has resulted in the establishment of a unitary Central London homelessness body (Social Exclusion Unit, 1998). This political creation has been set up to abolish street homelessness, and its effectiveness will be judged by a reduction in the numbers of people sleeping out. At the other end of the spectrum, organisations campaigning for better housing regard as homeless anyone living in accommodation where they do not have the right of permanent residence. The populations described in the psychiatric literature have most commonly been users of hostels or emergency shelters for single homeless people, or family shelters catering mostly to single mothers and their children. These groups are relatively easy to study, compared with people living on the street or families dispersed in temporary accommodation. Meanwhile, teams providing psychiatric services to homeless people report seeing people who live in permanent accommodation, with tenancy rights, but who still spend their days living in the milieu of day centres and soup runs provided for homeless people.

Homelessness has also been defined in terms of 'rootlessness', 'marginalisation' and 'social exclusion' (Social Exclusion Unit, 1998). Homeless people in the UK, although often registered with general practitioners (GPs), still tend to use special health facilities for the homeless rather than mainstream services. Health Care for the Homeless programmes in the USA report the same phenomenon. This provides a concrete example of social marginalisation, or social exclusion, where a person is denied (or denies him- or herself) access to those services and opportunities used by the bulk of the populace. The concept of social exclusion encompasses both people who are excluded by virtue of their long-term mental illness and those who are excluded as a result of their lack of permanent accommodation. It also includes people excluded from the mainstream by virtue of colour, culture, citizenship difficulties or poverty – in the case of refugees, all of these. The fact that asylum-seekers and refugees are increasingly presenting to homeless agencies in London provides some validation of the social exclusion/marginalisation concept. *Criminalisation* is another form of social exclusion. The passage of laws against loitering or vagrancy transforms those who are socially displaced into lawbreakers. The mentally ill, in particular, are vulnerable to committing, or being accused of, offences such as shoplifting, public inebriation, disturbing the peace, trespassing, breaking and entering in abandoned buildings, etc. Lacking social support, and the ability to make bail, they often are incarcerated. Detention centres, jails and prisons have become new asylums, removing mentally ill people from the mainstream of society and also, in many cases, from appropriate services for treatment and rehabilitation (Gunn, 1974; Brooke *et al*, 1996; Lamb & Weinberger, 1998).

Addressing issues of homelessness is complicated by another definitional problem: the great variation in patterns. Some individuals may be homeless for a brief period, others for a lifetime. Some may experience cyclical patterns of living 'rough', residing in a hostel, living with friends and so forth. Thus, the concept of a 'continuum of residential stability' has been used (Breakey & Fischer, 1995). This reminds service providers that homeless people's needs may vary greatly depending on the type of homelessness they are experiencing and their histories of residential instability in the past. It also draws attention to the fact that people in poverty, particularly people disabled by mental illness, may to varying degrees be unstable in their living arrangements and at risk of literal homelessness, either briefly or chronically.

Psychiatric morbidity

Planning psychiatric services requires information on the nature, frequency and severity of specific mental disorders. There are now several studies that have collected such information, using careful sampling strategies and standardised diagnostic methods. These studies demonstrate that a wide range of psychiatric disorders are present in excess among homeless people, including schizophrenia, major affective disorders, post-traumatic stress disorder, substance use disorders, personality disorders and others. Moreover, the disorders are often severe and disabling.

In collecting data on homeless mentally ill people, a number of issues must be considered. First is defining the target population (Bachrach, 1984; Fischer & Breakey, 1986). Definitions and sampling strategies used in epidemiological research have most often focused on those persons residing in shelters, hostels or reception centres (e.g. Tidmarsh & Wood, 1972; Bassuk *et al*, 1984; Fischer *et al*, 1986; Susser *et al*, 1989; Scott, 1991; Herman & Susser, 1998; Barrow *et al*, 1999). However, there are obvious dangers in generalising from these data to homeless people as a whole. Thus, some investigators have reported findings on special sub-populations of homeless people, such as homeless families (Bassuk *et al*, 1986; Buckner & Bassuk, 1997; Vostanis *et al*, 1998), youths (Craig *et al*, 1996; Robertson, 1996; Craig & Hodson, 1998; Ringwalt *et al*, 1998), older people (Cohen & Sokolowsky, 1983; Cohen & Thompson, 1992; Crane, 1993) or military veterans (Rosenheck *et al*, 1991; Rosenheck & Koegel, 1993). Other studies of the homeless mentally ill have been based on clinical samples, in hospitals or other treatment programmes, of individuals who have been selected because they were identified as mentally disabled – which, however, introduces additional sources of bias, if the purpose is to get a measure of the needs of homeless people as a whole. Because of the heterogeneity of the homeless population, findings from one setting can only be applied in another with caution. For this reason, several surveys have attempted to obtain more widely representative samples by drawing subjects from a range of settings (e.g. Roth & Bean, 1986; Koegel *et al*, 1988; Vernez *et al*, 1988; Breakey *et al*, 1989; Smith *et al*, 1992; Robertson *et al*, 1997). Another approach has been to obtain retrospective histories of homelessness from a representative sample of the entire US population (Link *et al*, 1995).

Schizophrenia and affective disorders

A series of US studies in the 1980s were the first to employ standardised diagnostic methods and to draw large representative samples of subjects from non-treatment settings (Susser *et al*, 1993*a*). Their results provide a useful benchmark, because there has been no effort on the same scale in either the USA or Britain since that time. In spite of differences in sampling and diagnostic methods, there is a considerable degree of agreement in their findings. Generally, one-third to one-half of homeless people were diagnosed with a major mental illness; schizophrenia in 10–15% and major affective illnesses, unipolar or bipolar, in 20–30%. In Table 18.1, the prevalence rates for psychiatric disorders are compared with general population rates obtained in the US Epidemiological Catchment Area in the 1980s (Regier *et al*, 1988).

Later well-designed studies in the USA produced results that were in many ways similar (Smith *et al*, 1992, 1993; Herman & Susser, 1998; Phelan & Link, 1999). One difference was that the prevalence of schizophrenia was somewhat lower. The most important contribution of these later studies, however, was to extend this research to other disorders and to in-depth assessments of specific subgroups, such as homeless families and their children.

Prevalence data from four British studies conducted in the 1970s and 1980s are shown in Table 18.2. In general, compared with the American studies, prevalence rates of schizophrenia were higher, 15–30%, and rates of affective and substance use disorders were lower. This may reflect true differences between the homeless populations in the two countries, owing to differences in the services available for mentally ill people. It is also possible that the differences between the US and British studies are due in part to the methods used. The American studies quoted here used standardised diagnostic methods and reported lifetime prevalence rates, whereas British studies generally used less rigorous diagnostic methods and focused on current disorders. What is more, the DSM–III criteria (American

TABLE 18.1

Percentage lifetime prevalence rates of selected DSM–III mental disorders in homeless populations compared with the Epidemiological Catchment Area Combined Five-Site Household Survey Population

Reference	Male (%)	Schizo-phrenia	Affective disorder	Dementia	Substance misuse disorder
Los Angeles Koegel *et al* (1988) (*n*=328)	95.0	13.1	29.5	3.4	69.2
California Vernez *et al* (1988) (*n*=315)	71.0	11.0	22.0	NR	69.0
Baltimore Breakey *et al* (1989) (*n*=125M, 78W)	0.0 100.0	17.1 12.1	23.7 18.6	0.0 3.3	38.2 75.4
New York Susser *et al* (1989) (*n*=177)	100.0	11.0	NR	NR	NR
USA: ECA (5 cities) Regier *et al* (1988) (*n*=18 571)	41.0	1.3	8.3	1.3	16.4

NR, not reported.

Psychiatric Association (APA), 1980) for major depression used in American studies of the 1980s may have included some cases that would not have been classified as major affective disorders by British psychiatrists.

There have been a number of studies of homeless people in other European countries. In general, they have involved smaller samples and a variety of diagnostic approaches. However, their findings are not dissimilar from those in most British studies (Bento & Marmeleiro, 1989; Nordentoft *et al*, 1992; Vasquez *et al*, 1997). Munoz *et al* (1998) published a comparison of data from Madrid with data from Los Angeles. In general, the prevalence rates of mental disorders in the two samples of homeless people were very similar, with only a few differences, which the authors attributed to cultural factors.

Substance use disorders

Very high prevalence rates of substance use disorders are reported in homeless populations, although there is great variability, possibly

Table 18.2

Percentage lifetime prevalence rates of selected psychiatric disorders in hostels, lodging houses and resettlement units in England and Scotland

		n	*Schizo-phrenia*	*Affective disorders*	*Addiction*
Hostels Lodge-Patch, 1970 (men)		123	14.6	8.1	21.1
Common lodging houses Priest, 1976 (men)[*]		77	32.5	5.2	18.2
Resettlement units Scott, 1991 (women)	Age <31 Age >30	24 25	8.3 28.0	20.8 36.0	20.8 48.0
Direct access hotel Timms & Fry, 1989 (men)	New arrivals Residents	65 58	24.6 38.0	6.2 0	15.3 1.7

* 'Definite' and 'probable' cases combined.

related to differences in sampling strategies, differences in methods of diagnosis, including confusion between lifetime and point prevalence rates, or real differences between homeless populations in different places (Fischer, 1991). In Baltimore in the mid-1980s, alcohol misuse and dependence were found to be much more prevalent among homeless people than misuse and dependence on other substances (Breakey *et al*, 1989). In the same period in New York, drug misuse was remarkably widespread among homeless men in the shelter system, with cocaine being the most commonly used drug (Susser *et al*, 1989). Overall, in American studies, median rates for alcoholism of 47% in homeless men and 17% in homeless women can be estimated by compiling data from the many studies published in the 1980s; equivalent median rates for drug use disorders are 23% in men and 26% in women (Fischer, 1991). Among later studies, two (Smith *et al*, 1993; Robertson *et al*, 1997) are notable for representative sampling and thorough assessments. The data suggest, if anything, an increasing prevalence of substance use disorders among the homeless; Robertson and her colleagues (1997) reported that two-thirds of their sample had a history of a substance use disorder.

In Britain, likewise, there is great variation between studies. Stark *et al* (1989) reported that 42% of the long-stay male residents of reception centres in England had a definite drinking problem; Timms & Fry (1989), on the other hand, reported a rate of 2% in residents of a Salvation Army hostel in London. In at least some British studies, the observed prevalence of substance misuse may be low because misusers were explicitly excluded from some hostels that served as sampling sites. More recent British surveys suggest higher prevalence of alcohol disorders. The 1993 census (Gill *et al*, 1996) estimated that 14% of hostel residents and 40% of those using night shelters or sleeping rough were very heavy drinkers (>50 units of alcohol per week for men, >35 units per week for women). Twenty-five per cent of hostel dwellers, 37% of those sleeping out and 46% of those using night shelters were using one or more illegal drugs.

Mental illness–substance misuse comorbidity

The importance of 'dual diagnosis' in the homeless, the co-occurrence of major mental illnesses and substance use disorders, is increasingly apparent (Drake *et al*, 1991). Substance misuse occurs as frequently in the homeless mentally ill as in homeless people in general, and more frequently in the most disabled of the mentally ill. In Baltimore, 80% of severely mentally ill men also had a substance misuse diagnosis, and in severely mentally ill women the rate was close to 40% (Breakey *et al*, 1989). A similar picture is seen in England: 30 out of 81 male shelter users in Nottingham who had been in contact with psychiatric services had a primary diagnosis of alcohol use or dependence (Roy & Read, 1992). A psychiatric outreach team in Birmingham (Commander *et al*, 1997) noted that 23% of those referred to them were diagnosed as having a substance misuse problem.

The co-occurrence of mental illness and substance misuse increases the likelihood that a mentally ill person will become homeless (Belcher, 1989; Drake *et al*, 1989; Susser *et al*, 1991*a*) and poses considerable problems for service providers (Ridgely *et al*, 1986; Drake & Wallach, 1989). The treatment of the mental illness and rehabilitation of the mentally ill person are compromised by the effects of the substance use. Conversely, participation in substance misuse treatment programmes that cater to the general population of substance misusers is difficult for persons with mental illness.

An especially serious kind of comorbidity is the co-occurrence of mental illness and injection drug use. A study of homeless mentally ill people in three US cities documented an alarming frequency of injecting both cocaine and heroin (Susser *et al*, 1997*a*). This practice is associated with a high risk of infectious diseases, including human immunodeficiency virus (HIV), hepatitis B, and hepatitis C. The most common but least studied of these is hepatitis C, which has already been acquired by the great majority of injection drug users in some regions of the USA. There is no effective treatment for this disease; it often leads to chronic disability and is sometimes fatal (Booth, 1998).

Other psychiatric disorders

Already by the 1980s, a wide variety of other psychiatric conditions were documented in addition to the major groups of mental illnesses and substance use disorders. Depressed mood and demoralisation were found to be common, and often disabling, even in those people whose disorder did not meet criteria for affective illness. Reports of suicide attempts were quite frequent (Susser *et al*, 1989). Anxiety disorders, including disorders in the phobic and obsessive–compulsive categories, were also common, often occurring in association with substance misuse. Assessment of personality disorders in a cross-sectional interview is hazardous (North & Spitznagel, 1993). None the less, several investigators have attempted to get a measure of them in homeless populations. Personality disorders were reported in 40% of homeless men and women in Baltimore (Breakey *et al*, 1989) and in 70% of young homeless mothers in Massachusetts (Bassuk *et al*, 1986). The personality disorders that occurred most frequently in the Baltimore sample were those that interfere with a person's capacity to establish helpful and supportive relationships; the schizoid, anti-social and avoidant types (Nestadt *et al*, 1989).

More recent studies have demonstrated how wide the range is of potentially disabling psychiatric disorders that afflict homeless people. An especially notable finding is the high prevalence of post-traumatic stress disorder (PTSD). It appears that at least three different origins of PTSD may be important: experiences prior to homelessness, victimisation while homeless, and the condition of homelessness itself. The possibility of homelessness causing PTSD is entirely plausible but has only recently been studied in depth, in a highly original study by Bresnahan (1999). Her findings suggest that homelessness is indeed a traumatic experience that can give rise to chronic and potentially disabling PTSD. This study is one of the few instances in which the contribution of homelessness to a psychiatric disorder has been examined (Herman & Susser, 1998; Phelan & Link, 1999).

Psychiatric disability

The presence of a mental illness *per se* is not the most critical factor in determining a person's capacity to survive in the community. Many mentally ill individuals cope reasonably well with the demands of everyday life in the community. It is, rather, the level of functional impairment that determines the level of service that a given individual may require, and some investigators have focused their attention on estimation of functional capacity rather than diagnosis. The assessment of functional capacity in the homeless, however, is problematical for several reasons. First, making such a determination generally requires a reliable observer and a period of observation in which the person's performance can be assessed. This may be costly, and is not feasible in a mobile population. Second, most standard instruments for assessing functional capacity are designed for in-patients or persons residing in residential settings. They rely upon the rating of skills in areas where a homeless person may have no opportunity to perform, such as food preparation, performing one's own laundry or managing money.

Notwithstanding the methodological difficulties, several research teams have attempted to assess functional capacity. Barrow *et al* (1989) devised an instrument specifically for use in homeless people. Marshall (1989) used the REHAB scale (Baker & Hall, 1988), first developed for hospital patients. Hamid *et al* (1995*a,b*) found that the Social Behaviour Schedule (Wykes & Sturt, 1986) was a useful tool with homeless people in a London hostel, and Breakey and colleagues (1989) used Axis V of DSM–III (APA, 1980) to rate psychiatrists' observations. All of these groups concluded that many homeless mentally ill persons are quite severely impaired, and may be judged to be in need of an extensive array of rehabilitative and supportive services.

Psychiatric disorders of homeless women

In most places where homeless people congregate, men predominate. Shelters, missions, reception centres and hostels have in the past catered mostly to the needs of men. Until quite recently, homelessness among women was considered rare and an indication of severe social disorder (Caplow *et al*, 1968). Research, therefore, has focused more on homeless men than on women. In recent decades, however, homelessness among women has risen dramatically in the USA, especially among single mothers (Bassuk *et al*, 1997).

Two distinct groups of homeless women, with somewhat different characteristics, have been described. One is the group of mothers of homeless families. Families with children are reported to account for more than 40% of the homeless population in many major cities, including New York, Los Angeles and Philadelphia (US Conference of Mayors, 1989). The mothers are generally younger women, with prevalence rates of mental illness and substance use disorders that are little different from the general population, but who may have higher rates of personality disorder (Bassuk *et al*, 1986; North *et al*, 1993) The other group is composed of women who are older on average, are not accompanied by children and are to be found in places frequented by single homeless people. In this group, the prevalence of substance use and mental illness is considerably higher than in the general population. However, their rates of substance use disorders are generally lower than those in homeless men. A number of studies of homeless women have been reported (Bassuk & Rosenberg, 1988; Shinn *et al*, 1991; Smith *et al*, 1993). Only a few permit comparisons between men and women (Fernandez, 1984; Herzberg, 1987; Breakey *et al*, 1989; Scott, 1991; Robertson *et al*, 1997).

Several studies have suggested that women are generally less socially isolated than men, for example in that they maintain closer contacts with their families (North & Smith, 1993). They are also somewhat more successful than men in obtaining financial entitlements and housing. There is an impression among many investigators that the prevalence of psychiatric disorders and level of disability in women on their own in the shelter system is higher than in men, but this has not been clearly supported by empirical research.

Psychiatric disorders of homeless children

Children living with their families in a homeless condition, most often with a single parent, are a group of great concern. These children have high prevalence rates of anxiety and depressive disorders and, equally importantly, often exhibit developmental delays, cognitive and learning difficulties and are behind in school (Bassuk *et al*, 1986; Fierman *et al*, 1991; Zima *et al*, 1994, 1997). Lack of access to regular schooling and frequent moves create particularly difficult environments for these children during their developmental years (Eddins, 1993).

Psychiatric disorders of homeless youth

Older adolescents who have run away from or been extruded from their homes present a separate set of problems. Adolescent homelessness is more frequent than is generally realised (Ringwalt *et al*, 1998). Homeless youths suffer from illnesses directly related to a lifestyle on the streets that is characterised by violence and deprivation (Kennedy *et al*, 1990; Robertson, 1996). They have often been victims of physical and sexual abuse and family chaos, and have been found to have a greater number of psychological and physical problems than the general adolescent population (Sherman, 1992). They are particularly vulnerable to sexually transmitted diseases, including hepatitis and HIV/acquired immunodeficiency syndrome, as well as unintended pregnancies, violent and traumatic injury and substance misuse (Kennedy *et al*, 1990).

In London, Craig and his colleagues (Craig *et al*, 1996; Craig & Hodson, 1998) found that 53% of homeless youths had a lifetime diagnosis of mental illness (with or without accompanying substance misuse or addiction) compared with 25% of a domiciled control group. For substance misuse disorders, the rates were 23% in the homeless group *v.* 20% in the domiciled group. Forty per cent of the homeless subjects were diagnosed with psychiatric disorder active in the preceding month. The majority (70%) of the homeless subjects' psychiatric disorders had started before they became homeless. The homeless group were slightly less likely to have used a primary care health service in the preceding year, although only 44% of the homeless group had seen a mainstream GP, compared with 82% of the domiciled group. For those with a psychiatric diagnosis, contact during the preceding year with psychiatric services was low in both groups – 22% for the homeless group and 26% for the domiciled group. An American study of homeless and poor housed youths found that approximately 32% had a current mental disorder accompanied by impairment in function, but use of mental health services was low (Buckner & Bassuk, 1997).

Physical illness

The living conditions of homeless people pose a direct threat to health (Bresnahan, 1999). Winkleby (1990) compared homeless with non-homeless poor individuals and documented that the homeless had less access to heated rooms, running water, bathing facilities and cooking facilities. Gelberg and colleagues (1997)found that 40% of the homeless reported that they did not 'wash up' daily. As a consequence of the poor nutrition, lack of adequate hygiene, exposure to violence and to the elements, increased contact with communicable diseases and fatigue that accompany the conditions of homelessness, people without homes suffer from ill health at much higher rates than people living in stable housing. Substance misuse increases the risk, as does chronic mental disability. Mentally ill people often have difficulty with maintaining hygiene and health, even when housed.

American studies of adults have found that one-third to one-half have some form of physical illness (Morse & Calsyn, 1986; Roth & Bean, 1986; Bassuk & Rosenberg, 1988; Gelberg *et al*, 1988). In England, Whynes *et al* (1992) found that overall rates of reported health problems were lower in homeless respondents than in those found in the 1988 General Household Survey. They attribute this to the fact that their homeless sample was relatively young. Westlake & George (1994) found that homeless people with a self-reported history of psychiatric illness had a significantly worse perceived health status on all dimensions than those without such a history, and that the whole sample was worse in its perceived health status than a standard London population. Mortality rates are several times higher than in the general population, and a part of the excess can reasonably be attributed to the homeless condition (Morbidity and Mortality Weekly Report, 1991; Hanzlick & Parrish, 1993; Hibbs *et al*, 1994; Hwang *et al*, 1997).

The most common physical illnesses among homeless persons include upper respiratory tract infections, trauma, female genito-urinary problems, hypertension, skin and ear disorders, gastrointestinal diseases, peripheral vascular disease, musculoskeletal problems, dental problems and vision problems (Reuler *et al*, 1986; Wright & Weber, 1987; Miller & Lin, 1988; Wood *et al*, 1990). American studies reveal that many serious infectious diseases are associated with homelessness. HIV infections, hepatitis B and C, tuberculosis, trench fever and others are frequent (Zolopa *et al*, 1994; McMurray-Avila *et al*, 1999). Seriously mentally ill homeless people have been found to be at higher risk for tuberculosis (Sakai *et al*, 1998) and HIV infections (Susser *et al*, 1997*a*).

Despite their young age (mean age in the mid-30s), half of homeless adults state that they are limited in performing vigorous physical activities (Gelberg *et al*, 1990). Further, many are limited in moderate physical activities (21%), walking several blocks (28%), bending, lifting, or stooping (28%), type or amount of work (43%) or all types of work (29%).

Trauma and victimisation

Numerous studies have documented that homeless individuals are vulnerable to assault and rape (Burroughs *et al*, 1990; D'Ercole & Struening, 1990; Padgett & Struening, 1992; North *et al*, 1994; Goodman *et al*, 1995). An English study of 100 homeless juveniles found that 40% had been beaten up, 23% had been robbed, 25% (43% of females) had been sexually assaulted and 30% had been assaulted with a weapon (Whitbeck & Simons, 1990). In the 1993

English Census hostel sample, 19% had had valuable possessions lost or stolen in the previous six months (Gill *et al*, 1996).

Assessing the needs of homeless populations

Practical problems in collecting data

Certain characteristics of homeless people and aspects of their lifestyles pose problems for data collection (Susser *et al*, 1993*a*).

Geographic mobility

Both hostel and street populations can be relatively static. However, there are segments of these populations that have a high turnover. In a 1986 survey of a Salvation Army hostel in London (Timms & Fry, 1989), about 25% of the hostel's residents had been there for more than 12 months. However, each month there was a turnover of at least 25% of the hostel population. People on the street may need to move around in response to closure of public spaces, police harassment or violence or intimidation from the general public or from other street people. It is difficult to construct a truly representative sampling frame or to collect longitudinal or follow-up data.

Sampling biases

Most studies of homeless people make use of point prevalence data, based on individuals sampled in shelters or other locations where homeless people gather. This method tends to over-sample those individuals who have longer durations of homelessness, including, for example, those with chronic disabling mental illnesses. Conversely, those individuals whose homelessness is of shorter duration are underrepresented. If the intent is to estimate needs of the most severely impaired, this may present no problem; if the intent is to estimate the needs of homeless people as a whole, the needs of certain less chronic groups may be underestimated (Phelan & Link, 1999).

Mobility between different types of accommodation

People move from the streets to night shelters and on to hostels and back again. An individual captured in one homeless setting may be categorised as a 'street' person or as a 'hostel' person when, in fact, this is just one point on his or her accommodation trajectory. This notion has been addressed by roughly categorising homeless people as 'street', 'episodic' or 'situational' (Arce *et al*, 1983), although most surveys still define individuals according to their current geographic location.

Distrust of authority

Individuals in the most marginalised street populations, who presumably have greatest needs, may be extremely difficult to engage in data collection efforts (Smith *et al*, 1991; Crane, 1993). However, many hostel surveys report low refusal rates, perhaps owing to the careful preparatory work that is done within hostels, where interviewers spend some time making themselves known in the milieu (Snow *et al*, 1986; Marshall & Reed, 1992). Payment may be helpful, but low refusal rates have been reported in hostel surveys where payment was not offered (Timms & Fry, 1989).

Unsuitable research instruments

There are many instruments to measure mental state or social functioning. These have almost entirely been designed either in ward settings or for out-patient clinic populations, who are prepared to tolerate lengthy interviews and intrusive questions, and where there are adequate facilities both for practising activities of daily living and for testing them. Homeless populations, whether residents of shelters or hostels, street sleepers or residents of bed-and-breakfast hotels, usually lack any appropriate setting for assessment of practical functioning. Instruments that have established their value in other settings, such as the MRC Needs for Care Assessment (Brewin *et al*, 1987), may have limited applicability (Hogg & Marshall, 1992). Fischer *et al* (1986) commented that the Diagnostic Interview Schedule (DIS; Robins *et al*, 1981), an interview schedule used in many surveys of homeless people, "may not have a high level of sensitivity for chronic disorders in populations of this type". Vasquez *et al* (1997) made a similar comment regarding the use of the Composite International Diagnostic Interview (CIDI; World Health Organization, 1989). Experience with other diagnostic instruments suggests that the problem is more general and may only be counteracted by more prolonged contact with subjects, use of expert clinicians and investigation of old hospital records, where they exist.

Lack of collateral informants

Rating a person's ability to function in everyday life often requires a family or staff member who knows the individual well. In the context of a shelter, although relationships may have been built up over a number of years, the amount of information about someone's background is often extremely scanty.

Poor tolerance of lengthy interviews or questionnaires

Many large surveys have had to use truncated versions of standard questionnaires or have ended up devising their own short screening instruments to try to identify particular sub-populations. The 1993 UK census, for example, had to devise its own psychosis screening instrument and was unable to use the full version of its interview schedule in night shelters and day centres.

Intoxication

In some settings, interviews are likely to be compromised by intoxication, resulting in either failure or only partial completion.

Quantitative and qualitative descriptions of need

Estimates of service need in special populations such as homeless people may be quantitative or qualitative. Quantitative estimates are ideal; they enable rational planning, allocation of resources and accountability. In most cases, however, planners must make do with qualitative estimates. In either case, two issues must be clarified; how is the target population defined, and who makes the determination of need?

The difficulty of defining homelessness has been discussed above. This issue is clearly of as much importance for service providers and planners as it is for epidemiologists. Who should be considered homeless and in need of services? In assessing needs, are we only considering those with major mental illnesses who are 'literally homeless' – that is, living on the streets or in an abandoned building, or in a temporary shelter – or is our target population much broader, including a wider range of marginalised people?

In addition to determining the target population, it must be decided whose perspective to take into account in making a determination of mental health service need. Psychiatric patients' views of what they need may be quite opposed to the views of their treating psychiatrists, and their families may have a third perspective. Many homeless mentally ill people strenuously maintain that they do not need any psychiatric intervention, while professionals involved in the case and other observers are agreed that the person has a clear need for treatment. This is frequently a major issue in providing services for homeless people, who in many cases give low priority to mental health care (Ball & Havassy, 1984). Maslow (1954) emphasises the importance of recognising a 'hierarchy of needs'. In discussions of the needs of homeless mentally ill people in general, there are widely differing opinions, even among professionals. Some believe that a return to more institution-centred models of care is needed and some believe that compulsory treatment is appropriate; others believe strongly in community-based, voluntary approaches. In the absence of consensus, statements of need are thus based on the particular clinical philosophy of the person or groups making the estimate (Breakey, 2001).

Quantitative estimates of need

Need is related to morbidity, but is strongly affected by many other characteristics of the person and the situation in which he or she is placed. Morbidity data are thus helpful, but do not give a full picture of the extent of need or the areas in which need exists. Better estimates of the service needs of homeless people can be derived if the degree of disability experienced by these individuals, their patterns of comorbidity, including co-occurring substance use disorders and physical diseases, their social support networks and other factors are also considered.

To collect such data, it is necessary to delineate the population of concern, select a representative sample, assess the prevalence of psychiatric disorders and disabilities in the sample, determine the individual treatment needs of the people in the sample and extrapolate to the population as a whole. The Baltimore Homeless Study (Breakey *et al*, 1989) adopted a method of this sort. For the purposes of the study, the homeless population was defined as those people who used the shelters in the city or were incarcerated in the city jail. The scope of the study did not permit the investigators to consider other segments of the homeless population. The first step was to obtain an estimate of the size of the population of interest. Because the records maintained by shelters did not permit an unduplicated count, the number of shelter users in the city was estimated using a capture–recapture method (Cowan *et al*, 1988). This provided an estimate of the size of the pool of people from which the shelters in Baltimore drew their clients. The second stage involved a morbidity survey to provide data on the prevalence of mental disorders (and physical disorders), along with an estimate of functional impairment of each person in the sample. Based on these findings, a determination was made by a psychiatrist of the treatment needs of each person examined. Thus, the overall treatment needs of the sample could be determined and by extrapolation the treatment needs of the population of shelter-using people for the entire city could be estimated. The statements of need developed by the psychiatrists in the Baltimore Homeless Study reflected the opinions of that group of examining psychiatrists. For example, they determined that very few of the subjects (2%) needed long-term hospital care. A different group of experts, with a less developed community psychiatry orientation, might have judged differently. Performing a study of this sort is costly and time-consuming, and not practical in most localities.

The other principal approach to estimating health service need in general populations uses proxy indicators, such as the UPA–8 (Jarman & Hirsch, 1992). This method bases estimates of need for services on a measure of the social disadvantage of the community of concern, based on the finding that mental health service utilisation is positively correlated with the level of social disadvantage of the community. However, this method is not suitable for estimating needs in special populations such as homeless people. Homeless people are by definition among the most disadvantaged, but they may be found in surroundings that would not necessarily be described as disadvantaged communities. Also, the barriers to obtaining care that have existed for these individuals are such that their past utilisation patterns provide no indication of the true level of need. Any statement about the needs of homeless people must be based on knowledge of the particular characteristics and circumstances of this population subgroup.

Qualitative descriptions of need

In practical reality, preparing quantitative estimates of the needs of the homeless population in a given city or county or region is more useful for political advocacy than for programme planning or management, because governments' responsiveness to the needs of homeless people is generally such that resources allocated for services for them are inadequate. It is rarely possible to contemplate addressing all of their needs. The usual problem to be addressed is which interventions will be most cost-effective in addressing the needs of homeless people in the context of inadequate resources. Thus, understanding the range of the needs of homeless people and the effectiveness of methods for meeting those needs is most important.

Characteristics of homeless people that affect service provision

The particular characteristics of homeless people, already alluded to, affect the way services must be provided if their needs are to be met.

These include the distrust that many homeless mentally ill people have of the mental health service system, their relative lack of the supports upon which patients and therapists in other situations can usually rely, the co-occurrence of medical and substance use disorders, and poverty.

Distrust

Those whose needs seem greatest may be the most reluctant to accept help. Their distrust of helpers and helping agencies has several likely roots. Paranoia may reflect paranoid personality disorders or major mental illnesses such as schizophrenia, mania or dementia. In some cases, suspicion of others may be an understandable response to past experiences. Service programmes for homeless people must be prepared to encounter this mistrust and adjust their expectations and approaches accordingly.

Many outreach workers employ strategies first developed in New York City (Cohen, 1990; Barrow *et al*, 1991) to gain the trust of homeless street people. Workers at first may be able to do nothing more than to give a person a sandwich; months may be required to establish even a minimally trusting relationship. Susser has described the reluctance of women in a shelter to trust a psychiatrist. One of the strategies he used to gain their confidence was to conduct a weekly Bingo game in the shelter (Susser, 1992). The Simon Community in England has adopted a philosophy of unconditional acceptance, 'no questions asked' and a minimum of rules in their shelters, as a way of minimising the barriers to the acceptance of help (Leach, 1979), a principle underlying the concept of Safe Havens in the USA (Federal Task Force on Homelessness and Severe Mental Illness, 1992).

Lack of supports

Research has demonstrated the relative isolation of homeless people (Roth *et al*, 1985), including those who are severely mentally ill: they are rarely in an active marital relationship; more often than expected, they have never been married; they report few friends and few confiding relationships; and they tend to describe themselves as loners. They do not have the relationships found in a normal workplace or neighbourhood. More often than expected, they have childhood histories of disruptive family relationships, for instance they have been placed in foster care (Susser *et al*, 1991*b*). Providing services for such a population is very different from providing services for a typical domiciled population, where one can assume that a person is supported by a certain array of relationships. What is more, for homeless people, other supportive factors are lacking, such as a permanent place to sleep and live, personal safety, a reasonable diet and a degree of financial security. Their extremely precarious circumstances should be reflected in treatment and rehabilitation approaches.

Physical illness

The frequency of physical disease in homeless populations poses additional challenges for mental health service providers. Conventional primary care providers are in many cases unwilling or unequipped to respond to their needs for general health care. In addressing the needs of their patients, therefore, mental health programmes for homeless people must be prepared to deal with complex health problems in several domains. Either they should be part of a health care organisation that can address the interrelated health care needs or they should have close and smoothly working linkages with primary health care practitioners or clinics in the area.

The care of chronic diseases that are not necessarily associated with homelessness, but for which homeless mentally ill individuals may have difficulty in obtaining adequate care, represents another important domain of service needs. Diabetes is an example of a condition that is extremely difficult to control, either by diet or medication, under conditions of homelessness (Brickner *et al*, 1985; Wright & Weber, 1987). For mentally ill homeless people, the difficulty in managing a chronic illness such as this is compounded by the psychiatric impairment.

Substance misuse

Dependence on alcohol or other drugs is very prevalent in homeless people, as has already been described. Whatever the treatment issue, it is likely to be complicated by addiction. Any treatment programme that fails to attend to addictions will be limited in its capacity to assist homeless people. Psychotropic medicines, general medical care, rehabilitation efforts, placement in housing and psychotherapeutic interventions are all complicated by a concurrent substance use disorder.

Poverty

Homeless people are among the poorest of the poor. Even where relatively good social security systems are in place, their resources are clearly inadequate to meet their basic needs. Mentally ill persons in general often have difficulty in obtaining entitlements (Allen, 1989).

This is certainly the case for mentally ill homeless people, in part because of their inability to tolerate the cumbersome procedures for obtaining these resources. The amount of public assistance is generally based upon poverty indices and provides minimally adequate resources for survival. An intelligent, healthy and well-organised person may be able to sustain a minimal standard of living with supports of this sort, but for a mentally ill person, the challenge may be too great. Mental health services must be prepared to provide the necessary supports for their clients to meet their basic needs, purchasing medicines, etc.

Principles of service provision

Although each homeless subgroup has its own characteristics and special needs, McMurray-Avila *et al* (1999) point out that several principles of service provision apply to them all:

(a) the importance of outreach to engage clients in treatment;
(b) respect for the individuality of each person;
(c) cultivation of trust and rapport between service provider and client;
(d) flexibility in service provision, including location and hours of service, as well as flexibility in treatment approaches;
(e) the need to attend to the basic survival needs of homeless people and to recognise that until those needs are met health care may not be an individual's priority;
(f) the importance of integrated service provision and case management to coordinate the services needed;
(g) clinical expertise to address complex clinical problems, including access to specialised care;
(h) the need for a range of housing options, including programmes combining housing with services; and
(i) a longitudinal perspective that ensures continuing care until the person's life situation has been stabilised.

The mental health service needs of homeless people are thus complex, requiring the involvement of a variety of clinicians, social service workers and others, focusing on the needs of several subgroups. Services must also be ongoing; returning a homeless person to health and residential stability may require professional support over a period of years.

Target populations for services

In considering service needs, it is important to recognise the several subgroups within the homeless population. Greatest attention has been paid to five categories – the severely mentally ill, addicts, women and children, unattached youths, and the elderly – recognising that an individual may fall into more than one category.

People with severe mental illnesses

It has become accepted that services for homeless people are an essential part of a comprehensive treatment system for the seriously mentally ill (APA, 1997). Clinical experience over two decades has enabled service providers to gain an appreciation for their special needs (Thomison & Cook, 1987; Blackwell *et al*, 1990; Brent-Smith & Dean, 1990; Susser *et al*, 1990; Roderick *et al*, 1991; Breakey, 1992; McMurray-Avila *et al*, 1999). In many respects, these needs are similar to those of other homeless people. Above all, they need a place to live that will offer safety, privacy and a degree of permanence. They need dignity, acceptance and friendship. They need financial support and access to primary health care.

Over and above these needs shared with homeless people in general, the homeless mentally ill have particular needs for treatment, rehabilitation and support. While many have had little contact with the mental health service system, many others have been in treatment (Marshall, 1989). Thus, a problem for many is lack of access to services, while the problem for others is that whatever services have been rendered have clearly not enabled them to be resettled in permanent and adequate housing. Their needs are not recognised, or are not adequately met, or they have not been able or willing to accept services in the manner in which they were offered.

Meeting the mental health service needs of homeless mentally ill persons may be tackled through the establishment of a special programme, or by making existing programmes more responsive to their special needs (Brent-Smith & Dean, 1990). Whichever approach is taken, in view of the complexity of the clinical problems presented, a high level of clinical expertise is required, which generally can only be provided by a team of professionals, rather than a single clinician. This team will develop expertise in several areas: diagnosis of psychiatric disorders may be complicated by aspects of the homeless lifestyle; prescribing practices need to be adapted to the particular circumstances of homeless people and their ability or inability to tolerate certain drugs; special methods may need to be adopted to maximise compliance with treatment plans; and counselling approaches need to be mindful of the special circumstances of life on the street or in a shelter.

Certain elements are required for a comprehensive and responsive service. A US government task force summarised them as follows: assertive outreach; integrated care management; safe havens; housing;

alcohol and/or other drug misuse treatment; health care; income support and benefits; rehabilitation, vocational training and employment assistance; consumer and family involvement; and legal protections (Federal Task Force on Homelessness and Severe Mental Illness, 1992). These service elements are described in the next section.

In addition, close linkages with other parts of the mental health care network are needed, so that people may move on into the mainstream as soon as possible.

Addicts

Major efforts have been expended to explore methods of treating substance use disorders in homeless people. The National Institute on Alcohol Abuse and Alcoholism (NIAAA) supported two rounds of community demonstration projects to identify effective approaches for providing substance misuse treatment for homeless people (Argeriou & McCarthy, 1990; Conrad *et al*, 1993). The following general conclusions were drawn regarding necessary and desirable programme characteristics (Stahler, 1995):

(a) the need to develop treatment programmes that focus not only on the addiction, but also address the tangible needs of people without homes;
(b) the need to develop flexible, low-demand interventions that can accommodate clients who are not initially willing to commit to more extended care;
(c) the need for longer-term, continuous interventions for this population. After-care needs to address not only the maintenance of sobriety, but also the tangible needs and social isolation of clients; and
(d) the need to match clients to appropriate treatment services based on characteristics such as educational attainment, cultural background, severity of substance use, criminal involvement and level of social isolation.

Families

The needs of homeless families with young children have caused great concern in the USA. Studies have documented the high prevalence of anxiety disorders, depression and developmental delay in the children, pointing to the need not only for housing and security of these families but also for mental health services and special educational support for the children. Such families need to be moved out of temporary shelter and into transitional or permanent housing as quickly as possible, so that the family as a whole and the children in particular can experience a greater sense of permanence and security. If they have been victims of abuse, they need to be protected from further abuse and to be provided with whatever counselling or therapy is needed to deal with its emotional consequences. For school children, frequent moves of school can be extremely disruptive. School systems should be persuaded not to move a child to another school if the family is forced to move to a different district to obtain permanent, safe housing.

Youths

Adolescents, unaccompanied by parents, constitute another group with special needs. Craig's 1997 London survey and one-year follow-up of young homeless people compared with a general practice population of young homeless people found that family crises were the most commonly reported cause of the most recent episode of homelessness and that only 25% of the homeless sample came from 'intact' families, compared with 50% of the domiciled sample. Forty per cent of the homeless sample (4% of the domiciled sample) had been taken into statutory care during their childhood. In terms of adverse childhood experiences, parental indifference, lack of care and antipathy were the most significant distinguishing features between the homeless and domiciled groups. Most were still unemployed at one-year follow-up, although most had gained access to their welfare entitlements, mainly owing to the work of voluntary sector agencies.

Adolescents who are homeless and apart from their families are often reluctant to acknowledge their need for services until the situation is extreme. Psychiatric disorders are likely to be ignored, covered up or denied. Their status as minors, issues of consent and confidentiality, and their distrust of adults provide significant barriers to care (Robertson, 1996). Clinicians working with this group should be well versed in the usual health needs of adolescents, but particularly prepared to deal with the physical and emotional effects of violence, sexually transmitted diseases, pregnancy and mental illness. Services should be available in youth shelters, but also on the street, through outreach, because many homeless adolescents do not use shelters (New York State Council on Children and Families, 1984; Robertson, 1996). Health promotion, disease prevention and harm-reduction strategies focused on this group are essential.

The elderly

Most surveys of homeless people find relatively few individuals over the age of 60 years, particularly in street populations. This has been attributed to high death rates, greater access to social security supports, 'mellowing' of persons with personality disorders and less substance dependence in older people. However, there is a distinct group of older homeless people, who have been studied in both the US and the UK. Crane (1993), in London, noted that almost 40% suffered from cognitive impairment and almost 30% were substance-dependent. Cohen *et al* (1988) examined homeless men in New York and identified about one-quarter as suffering from psychosis, one-third as suffering from depression and only 9% as evidencing mild to severe dementia. Doolin (1986), in Boston, commented on the vulnerability of older people to robbery and violence on the streets.

Service models

In response to the varied needs of homeless people, a number of models of providing care have been developed. These differ in terms of settings, target populations and strategies. In general, they have a primary objective of increasing access for people who have difficulty obtaining services through traditional channels.

Street outreach programmes

To address more vigorously the problem of prospective patients' reluctance to seek treatment, most programmes have found it essential to have outreach workers, whose job it is to seek out people who need treatment. Some individuals accept offers of help relatively easily, but others may be extremely resistant, so that repeated contacts may be needed before the person can be persuaded to accept help (Cohen *et al*, 1984; Cohen, 1990; Wobido *et al*, 1990; Lam & Rosenheck, 1998). The outreach team may conclude that a person is in clear danger through self-neglect or failure to protect him- or herself. In this situation, workers may have to use involuntary admission procedures to persudae a person to accept treatment, a process that may bring the team into conflict with advocacy or libertarian groups (Cournos, 1989).

Special clinical services for homeless people

Because of the reluctance of many homeless people to make use of regular health care facilities, and the reluctance of some health care providers to accept homeless people for treatment, special clinics have been set up in many places, where access for homeless people will be easier. Often, such clinics are designed to provide primary health care, but also serve the needs of the mentally ill (Thomison & Cook, 1987; Wright & Weber, 1987; Brickner *et al*, 1990; Joseph, 1990; McMurray-Avila, 1997).

Shelter-based interventions

An alternative approach has been to move the mental health (or primary care) service providers into shelters or other places where homeless people are served. This approach has been employed, for example, in the very large shelters in New York City (Caton *et al*, 1990; Gounis & Susser, 1990).

A range of housing options

Housing is a *sine qua non* of services for homeless people. Resettling mentally ill homeless people requires a range of housing options with a range of levels of supervision (Pollio *et al*, 1997). No single model suits every patient; some will need 24-hour supervision, particularly at first, and others will need, or tolerate, very little supervision. Some will prefer a group setting, while others will want to be alone.

Case management programmes

Case management has emerged in recent years as a vital component of mental health programmes (Morse, 1999). The variety of services that are needed to meet individuals' needs, and the complexity of the processes required to obtain services and entitlements, require both expertise and a level of organisation beyond the capacities of many mentally ill people. Case management for homeless people requires special knowledge of the situations they face and of the various systems to bring together services for income maintenance, housing, treatment and rehabilitation. There is some evidence that case management may have a specific effect in assisting a person to develop networks of supportive relationships (Wasylenki *et al*, 1993; Thornicroft *et al*, 1995) and may thus have a particularly valuable role with homeless people.

Services integration

In most places, service provision for homeless people is hampered by the fractionation of the human services system into different agencies and offices that may even compete with one another. Services can be provided most effectively if there is an organising structure to promote integration of service delivery. A recent multi-site test of this concept in the USA concluded that services integration could be promoted where an inter-agency coordinating body was established, a strategic plan was developed and a specific paid member of staff was assigned the responsibility of promoting integration (Rosenheck *et al*, 1998; Fosburg & Dennis, 1999).

Mobile assertive treatment programmes

An extension of the outreach and case management principles is the development of mobile treatment teams. The treatment model may be based on the Program for Assertive Community Treatment (PACT; Stein & Test, 1985), adapted for a homeless population. In this model, rather than the outreach worker bringing the patient in to the centre, the treatment team goes out to the patient wherever their intervention is needed. What is more, instead of this being thought of as a temporary expedient to improve access to treatment, it is a long-term commitment to the patient, for as long as the treatment programme is needed. This model has been carefully tested as an approach to serving severely mentally ill homeless people, with very positive outcomes (Dixon *et al*, 1995; Lehman *et al*, 1997, 1999).

Linked housing and case management

Many of the most successful initiatives for resettling homeless people who have mental illnesses have involved linking the provision of housing to the provision of case management, or equivalent support services. A good example in the USA is the Shelter Plus Care programme, jointly funded by the Department of Health and Social Services and the Department of Housing and Urban Development. This programme provides subsidies for rented accommodation, contingent upon the tenant accepting support services provided by a mental health organisation. The Thamesreach project in South London provides another example of linking psychiatric services to housing. Hough and his colleagues (Hough *et al*, 1997) examined the effectiveness of arrangements of this sort, concluding that the nature of the case management provided was less critical than the provision of a housing subsidy.

Critical time intervention

Susser and colleagues (Susser *et al*, 1997*b*), working with mentally ill men in a large shelter, and helping them to make the transition to conventional housing arrangements, concluded that the greatest risk of the person falling back into homelessness occurred at the time of transition. They therefore developed a strategy to follow people very closely with social and psychiatric services through the transition, and were able to demonstrate that the likelihood of relapse was reduced.

Safe havens

This term has come to be applied in the USA to an approach that has been employed in a number of places in the USA and UK, to provide a 'low-demand' setting for homeless mentally ill people to obtain shelter, food and protection. They may be encouraged to seek psychiatric services, but it is not a requirement for residence there. The hope is that this may be a stepping stone to reintegration into the community and participation in mental health services in due course (Federal Task Force on Homelessness and Severe Mental Illness, 1992).

Rehabilitation

Rehabilitation is important for people whose skills in everyday living have been affected by disease or by the effects of years lived in conditions of deprivation. By and large, traditional rehabilitation programmes serving domiciled clients are not well equipped to address the particular problems of homeless people. A rehabilitation focus needs to be a strong emphasis in the overall treatment and case management planning for homeless people.

Consumer involvement

The role of consumers, people who have experienced mental illness, homelessness, or both, is becoming widely accepted. Whether as professionally trained colleagues, or as non-professional helpers, such individuals can speak with authority and authenticity in a way that most professionals can not. They can provide valuable insights for the development of the programme and can establish its credibility with prospective patients (Breakey *et al*, 1996; Dixon *et al*, 1997).

Legal protection

Homeless people are, in a conventional sense, powerless and disenfranchised. Mentally ill people are generally at a disadvantage in demanding their rights. Legal advocacy organisations can play a very important part in assisting homeless persons to obtain their rights and helping service providers to cope with bureaucratic obstructions.

Defining need at the local level

In developing a needs assessment for mental health services for homeless people in a specific geographic area, the following approach can be used to define needs with a sufficient level of accuracy for programme planning:

(a) Make use of all sources of information about the nature of the homeless population: welfare agencies, health services, police, homeless shelter programmes (staff and clients), housing authorities, etc.

(b) Define which are the subgroups of homeless people most in need: single adults, families and children, substance misusers, dually diagnosed persons, etc.

(c) Catalogue existing services based on knowledge of the special needs of homeless people and demonstrated programme effectiveness in other places, as discussed above.

(d) Identify gaps in the array of services for the specific populations of concern.

(e) With input from all the stakeholders identified in step 1, develop a list of priorities for new programme development.

Prevention

Mental health service programmes for homeless people are essential, but in essence are merely palliative and do not address the basic causes of the problem. The greater need is for prevention: it should be accepted that part of the role of the generic mental health service system in the era of community care is to provide a system of services that prevent mentally ill people from becoming homeless. Effective mental health service strategies are needed to prevent individuals from falling through the cracks, and mental health services should be evaluated in terms of the extent to which they actively implement preventive strategies.

It should be emphasised once again that, in many respects, the problems of homeless people with psychiatric disorders are little different from those of homeless people in general. The prevention of homelessness for them, as for other homeless people, begins with a consideration of the causes of poverty, the shortage of low-income housing, changes in the employment market, deficiencies in the educational systems and other broad societal issues that are beyond the scope of mental health agencies to address.

Considering the particular problems of the seriously mentally ill, however, it is still not clearly established what the critical factors are that cause a particular person to become homeless. A first stage in developing rational preventive strategies is the identification of risk factors. Childhood placement in foster care, for example, is a risk factor for homelessness later in life (Susser *et al*, 1987, 1993*a*), as is substance misuse co-occurring with mental illness (Belcher, 1989; Drake *et al*, 1989). For women, lack of social supports and pregnancy are also risk factors (Bassuk *et al*, 1997; Weitzman, 1989). If risk profiles can be established, a basis for identifying people at risk can be established and special preventive interventions can be developed in mental health programmes.

Critical Time Intervention (CTI) provides a means of 'secondary prevention', in that people who have been homeless and are now moving from shelters to more stable residences are prevented from 'relapsing' into homelessness once again (Susser *et al*, 1993*b*).

Computerised case registers, care plans and crisis cards appear to be useful in some settings (Sutherby *et al*, 1999) to facilitate continuity and consistency of care for severely disabled mentally ill patients. Their use should be further investigated to assist service systems in reducing the risk of homelessness.

Most importantly, however, a range of housing options, with varying degrees of supervision to meet the varied needs of disabled persons, is essential to a well-developed mental health service system, and basic to preventing homelessness. Mentally ill people, like the general population, have preferences about the setting in which they live. If their preferences are ignored, one response is to leave, even to become homeless, rather than to stay in an unsatisfactory situation. The provision of a variety of good housing options would be calculated to decrease the likelihood of a mentally ill person becoming homeless. District or catchment area service systems can be evaluated on the extent to which they provide appropriate housing for mentally ill people in the service area, and the frequency with which individuals drop out of the system or become homeless.

Summary and conclusion

People with psychiatric disorders constitute a substantial subgroup of the homeless populations of North America and Europe. Their needs for mental health services can be judged from the high prevalence of major mental illnesses, the extent of comorbidity with substance use disorders, their high levels of functional impairment, their lack of social supports and their poverty. Individual assessments indicate that only a small number would be considered, by contemporary criteria, to require long-term hospital care, but many need a complex and well-coordinated system of community-based care. Experience with mental health services for homeless people indicates that special clinics oriented to their needs may be more effective than trying to integrate homeless people straight away into the mainstream mental health service system. Outreach to shelters and street locations is essential and close integration with primary care is advantageous, in view of the high prevalence of somatic illness in the homeless population. Case management has a particularly valuable role in advocacy, coordinating needed services and assisting homeless clients to develop supportive relationships. Above all, access to a range of housing options is important for rehabilitation of homeless people, and to reduce the risk of homelessness for people with psychiatric vulnerabilities.

References

ALLEN, D. S. (1989) The uptake of social security benefits among psychiatric day hospital patients. *Psychiatric Bulletin*, **13**, 626–627.

AMERICAN PSYCHIATRIC ASSOCIATION (1980) *Diagnostic and Statistical Manual of Mental Disorders. Third revision (DSM–III)*. Washington, DC: APA.

—— (1997) Practice guidelines for the treatment of patients with schizophrenia. *American Journal of Psychiatry*, **154** (Suppl., April).

ARCE, A. A., TADLOCK, M., VERGARE, M. H., ET AL (1983) A psychiatric profile of street people admitted to an emergency shelter. *Hospital and Community Psychiatry*, **34**, 812–817.

ARGERIOU, M. & McCARTHY, D. (EDS) (1990) Treating alcoholism and drug abuse among men and women: nine community demonstration grants. *Alcoholism Treatment Quarterly*, **7**(1).

BACHRACH, L. L. (1984) Interpreting research on the homeless mentally ill: some caveats. *Hospital and Community Psychiatry*, **35**, 914–916.

BAKER, R. & HALL, J. N. (1988) REHAB: a new assessment instrument for chronic psychiatric patients. *Schizophrenia Bulletin*, **14**, 97–111.

BALL, F. L. J. & HAVASSY, B. E. (1984) A survey of the problems and needs of homeless consumers of acute psychiatric services. *Hospital and Community Psychiatry*, **35**, 917–921.

BARROW, S. M., HELLMAN, F., LOVELL, A. M., ET AL (1989) *Effectiveness of Programs for the Mentally Ill Homeless. Final Report: Community Support Systems Evaluation Program*. New York: New York Psychiatric Institute.

——, ——, ——, ET AL (1991) Evaluating outreach services: Lessons from a study of five programs. *New Directions in Mental Health Services*, **52**, 29–45.

——, HERMAN, D. B., CORDOVA, P., ET AL (1999) Mortality among homeless shelter residents in New York City. *American Journal of Public Health*, **89**, 529–534.

BASSUK, E. L., RUBIN, L. & LAURIAT, A. S. (1984) Is homelessness a mental health problem? *American Journal of Psychiatry*, **141**, 1546–1550.

——, —— & —— (1986) Characteristics of sheltered homeless families. *American Journal of Public Health*, **76**, 1097–1101.

—— & ROSENBERG, L. (1988) Why does family homelessness occur? A case control study. *American Journal of Public Health*, **78**, 783–788.

——, BUCKNER, J., WEINREB, L., BROWNE, A., ET AL (1997) Homelessness in female-headed families: childhood and adult risk and protective factors. *American Journal of Public Health*, **87**, 241–248.

BELCHER, J. R. (1989) On becoming homeless: a study of chronically mentally ill persons. *Journal of Community Psychology*, **17**, 173–185.

BENTO, A. & MARMELEIRO, C. (1989) Doentes mentais sem casa ('Homeless') em Lisboa. *Hosp. Julio de Matos*, **20**, 11–21.

BLACKWELL, B., BREAKEY, W. R., HAMMERSLEY, D., *ET AL* (1990) Psychiatric and mental health services. In: *Under the Safety Net: The Health and Social Welfare of the Homeless in the United States* (eds P. W.Brickner, L. K. Scharer, B. A. Conanan, *et al*), 184–203. New York: Norton.

BOGUE, D. J. (1963) *Skid Row in American Cities*. Chicago: University of Chicago Press.

BOOTH J. C. (1998) Chronic hepatitis C: the virus, its discovery and the natural history of the disease. *Journal of Viral Hepatitis*, **5**, 213–222.

BREAKEY, W. R. (1992) Mental health services for homeless people. In: *Homeless People: A National Perspective* (eds M. Robertson & M. Greenblatt), pp. 101–108. New York: Plenum.

—— (2001) Service needs of individuals and populations. In: *New Oxford Textbook of Psychiatry* (eds M. G. Gelder, N. C. Andreasen & J. Lopez-Ibor), vol. 24, pp. 1523–1532. Oxford: Oxford University Press.

——, FISCHER, P. J. & KRAMER, M. (1989) Health and mental health problems of homeless men and women living in Baltimore. *Journal of the American Medical Association*, **262**, 1352–1357.

—— & FISCHER, P. J. (1995) Mental illness and the continuum of residential stability. *Social Psychiatry and Psychiatric Epidemiology*, **30**, 147–151.

——, FLYNN, L. & VAN TOSH, L. (1996) Citizen and consumer participation. In: *Integrated Mental Health Services: Modern Community Psychiatry* (ed. W. R. Breakey), 160–174. New York: Oxford University Press.

BRENT-SMITH, H. & DEAN R. (1990) *Plugging the Gaps: Providing a Service for Mentally Ill People*. London: Lewisham and North Southwark Health Authority.

BRESNAHAN, M. (1999) *The Health Sequelae of Homelessness*. PhD Dissertation. New York: Columbia University.

BREWIN, C., WING, J., MANGEN, S., *ET AL* (1987) Principles and practice of measuring needs in the long-term mentally ill: the MRC Needs for Care Assessment. *Psychological Medicine*, **17**, 971–981.

BRICKNER, P. W., SCHARER, L. K., CONANAN, B., *ET AL* (eds) (1985) *Health Care of Homeless People*. New York: Springer Publishing Company.

——, ——, ——, *ET AL* (EDS) (1990) *Under the Safety Net: The Health and Social Welfare of the Homeless in the United States*. New York: Norton.

BROOKE, D., TAYLOR, P., GUNN, J., *ET AL* (1996) Point prevalence of mental disorder in un-convicted male prisoners in England and Wales. *British Medical Journal*, **313**, 1497–1498.

BUCKNER, J. C. & BASSUK, E. L. (1997) Mental disorders and service utilisation among youths from homeless and low-income housed families. *Journal of the American Academy of Child and Adolescent Psychiatry*, **46**, 890–900.

BURROUGHS, J., BOUMA, P., O'CONNOR, E., *ET AL* (1990) Health concerns of homeless women. In: *Under the Safety Net: The Health and Social Welfare of the Homeless in the United States* (eds P. W.Brickner, L. K. Scharer, B. A. Conanan, *et al*), pp. 139–150. New York: Norton.

CAPLOW, T., BAHR, H. M. & STEINBERG, D. (1968) Homelessness. *International Encyclopedia of the Social Sciences*, **6**, 494–499.

CATON, C., WYATT, J. W., GRUNBERG, J., *ET AL* (1990) An evaluation of a mental health program for homeless men. *American Journal of Psychiatry*, **147**, 286–289.

COHEN, C. I. & SOKOLOWSKY, J. (1983) Toward a concept of homelessness among aged men. *Journal of Gerontology*, **38**, 81–89.

COHEN, N. L. (1990) *Psychiatry takes to the Streets*. New York: Guilford.

——, PUTNAM, J. F. & SULLIVAN, A. (1984) The mentally ill homeless: Isolation and adaptation. *Hospital and Community Psychiatry*, **35**, 922–924.

——, TERESI, J. & HOLMES, D. (1988) The mental health of old homeless men. *Journal of the American Geriatrics Society*, **36**, 492–501.

—— & THOMPSON, K. S. (1992) Homeless mentally ill or mentally ill homeless? *American Journal of Psychiatry*, **149**, 816–823.

CONRAD, K. J., HULTMAN, C. I. & LYONS, J. S. (eds) (1993) Treatment of chemically dependent homeless: Theory and implementation in fourteen American projects. *Alcoholism Treatment Quarterly*, **10**.

COMMANDER, M., ODELL, S. & SASHIDHARAN, S. (1997) Birmingham community mental health team for the homeless. *Psychiatric Bulletin*, **21**, 74–76

COURNOS, F. (1989) Involuntary medication and the case of Joyce Brown. *Hospital and Community Psychiatry*, **40**, 736–740.

COWAN, C. W., BREAKEY, W. R. & FISCHER, P. J. (1988) The methodology of counting the homeless. In: *Homelessness Mental and Human Needs*. Institute of Medicine publication. Washington DC: National Academies Press.

CRAIG, T. K. & HODSON, S. (1998) Homeless youth in London: I. Childhood antecedents and psychiatric disorder. *Psychological Medicine*, **28**, 1379–1388.

—— & TIMMS, P. (1992) Out of the wards and onto the streets? Deinstitutionalization and homelessness in Britain. *Journal of Mental Health*, **1**, 265–275.

——, HODSON, S., WOODWARD, S., *ET AL* (1996) *Off to a Bad Start – A Longitudinal Study of Homeless Young People in London*. London: Mental Health Foundation.

CRANE, M. (1993) *Elderly Homeless People Sleeping on the Streets in Inner London: An Exploratory Study*. London: Age Concern Institute of Gerontology.

D'ERCOLE, A. & STRUENING, E. (1990) Victimization among homeless women: implications for service delivery. *Journal of Community Psychology*, **18**, 141–152.

DAYSON, D. (1993) The TAPS Project. 12: Crime, vagrancy, death and readmission of the long-term mentally ill during their first year of local reprovision. *British Journal of Psychiatry*, **162** (Suppl. 19), 40–44.

DIXON, L., KRAUS, N., KERNAN, E., *ET AL* (1995) Modifying the PACT model to serve homeless persons with severe mental illness. *Psychiatric Services*, **46**, 684–688.

——, HACKMAN, A. & LEHMAN, A. (1997) Consumers as staff in assertive community treatment programs. *Administration and Policy in Menta Health*, **25**, 199–208.

DONNELLY, M., McGILLOWAY, S., MAYS, N., *ET AL* (1997) A 3- to 6-year follow-up of former long-stay psychiatric patients in Northern Ireland. *Social Psychiatry and Psychiatric Epidemiology*, **32**, 451–458.

DOOLIN, J. (1986) Planning for the special needs of the homeless elderly. *The Gerontologist*, **26**, 229–231.

DRAKE, R. E. & WALLACH, M. A. (1989) Substance abuse among the chronic mentally ill. *Hospital and Community Psychiatry*, **40**, 1041–1046.

——, OSHER, F. C. & WALLACH, M. A. (1991) Homelessness and dual diagnosis. *American Psychologist*, **46**, 1149–1160.

——, WALLACH, M. A., HOFFMAN, J. S. (1989) Housing instability and homelessness among aftercare patients of an urban state hospital. *Hospital Community Psychiatry*, **40**, 46–51.

EDDINS, E. (1993) Characteristics, health status and service needs of sheltered homeless families. *Association of Black Nursing Faculty Journal*, **4**, 40–44.

EDWARDS, G., WILLIAMSON, V., HAWKER, A., *ET AL* (1968) Census of a reception centre. *British Journal of Psychiatry*, **114**, 1031–1039.

FEDERAL TASK FORCE ON HOMELESSNESS AND SEVERE MENTAL ILLNESS (1992) *Outcasts on Main Street*. Washington, DC: Center for Mental Health Services.

FERNANDEZ, J. (1984) "In Dublin's Fair City": the mentally ill of no fixed abode. *Psychiatric Bulletin*, **8**, 187–190.

FIERMAN, A. H., DREYER, B. P., QUINN, L., *ET AL* (1991) Growth delay in homeless children. *Pediatrics*, **88**, 918–925.

FISCHER, P. J. (1991) *Alcohol, drug abuse and mental health problems among homeless persons: a review of the literature, 1980–1990*. Washington, DC: US Department of Health and Human Services, ADAMHA.

—— & BREAKEY, W. R. (1986) Homelessness and mental health: An overview. *International Journal of Mental Health*, **14**, 6–41.

——, SHAPIRO, S., BREAKEY, W. R., *ET AL* (1986) Mental health and social characteristics of the homeless: A survey of Baltimore shelter users. *American Journal of Public Health*, **76**, 519–524.

FOSBURG, L. & DENNIS, D. (eds) (1999) *Practical Lessons: The 1998 National Symposium on Homelessness Research*. Washington, DC: US Departments of Housing and Urban Development and Health and Social Services.

GELBERG, L., LINN, L. S., USATINE, R. P., *ET AL* (1988) Health, homelessness and poverty: A study of clinic users. *Archives of Internal Medicine*, **145**, 191–196.

——, LINN, L. S. & MAYER-OAKES, S. A. (1990) Differences in health status between older and younger homeless adults. *Journal of American Geriatrics Society*, **38**, 1220–1229.

——, GALLAGHER, T. C., ANDERSEN, R. M., *ET AL* (1997) Competing priorities as a barrier to medical care among homeless adults in Los Angeles. *American Journal of Public Health*, **87**, 217–220.

GILL, B., MELTZER, H., HINDS, K., *ET AL* (1996) *Psychiatric Morbidity among Homeless People. OPCS Surveys of Psychiatric Morbidity in Great Britain, Report 7*. London: HMSO.

GOODMAN, L. A., DUTTON, M. A. & HARRIS, M. (1995) Episodically homeless women with serious mental illness: prevalence of physical and sexual assault. *American Journal of Orthopsychiatry*, **65**, 468–478.

GOUNIS, K. & SUSSER, E. (1990) Shelterization and its implications for mental health services. In: *Psychiatry takes to the Streets* (ed. N. Cohen), pp. 231–255. New York: Guilford Press.

GUNN, J. (1974) Prisons, shelters and homeless men. *Psychiatric Quarterly*, **48**, 505–512.

HAMID, W. A., WYKES, T. & STANSFELD, S. (1995*a*) The social disablement of men in hostels for homeless people. I. Reliability and prevalence, *British Journal of Psychiatry*, **166**, 806–808.

——, —— & —— (1995*b*) The social disablement of men in hostels for homeless people. II. A comparison with patients from long-stay wards, *British Journal of Psychiatry*, **166**, 809–812.

HANZLICK, R. & PARRISH, R. (1993) Death among the homeless in Fulton County, Georgia, 1988–1990. *Public Health Reports*, **108**, 488–491.

HERMAN, D. & SUSSER, E. (eds) (1998) *Homeless in America*. Washington, DC: American Public Health Association.

HERZBERG, J. L. (1987) No fixed abode: a comparison of men and women admitted to an East London psychiatric hospital. *British Journal of Psychiatry*, **150**, 621–627.

HIBBS, J. R., BENNER, L., KLUGMAN, L., *ET AL* (1994) Mortality in a cohort of homeless adults in Philadelphia. *New England Journal of Medicine*, **331**, 304–309.

HOGG, L. I. & MARSHALL, M. (1992) Can we measure need in the homeless mentally ill? Using the MRC Needs for Care Assessment in hostels for the homeless. *Psychological Medicine*, **22**, 1027–1034.

HOUGH, R. L., HARMON, S., TARKE, H., *ET AL* (1997) Supported independent housing: Implementation issues and solutions in the San Diego Project. In: *Mentally Ill and Homeless: Special Programs for Special Needs* (eds W. R. Breakey & J. W. Thompson), pp. 95–118. Amsterdam: Harwood Academic Publishers.

HWANG, S. W., GRAY, J., O'CONNELL, J. J., *ET AL* (1997) Causes of death in homeless adults in Boston. *Annals of Internal Medicine*, **126**, 625–628.

JARMAN, B. & HIRSCH, S. (1992) Statistical models to predict district psychiatric morbidity. In: *Measuring Mental Health Needs* (eds G. Thornicroft, C. R. Brewin & J. Wing), pp. 62–80. London: Gaskell.

JOSEPH, P. L. A. (1990) A psychiatric clinic for the single homeless in a primary care setting in Inner London. *Psychiatric Bulletin*, **14**, 270–271.

KENNEDY, J. T., PETRONE, J., DEISHER, R. W., *ET AL* (1990) Health care for familyless, runaway street kids. In: *Under the Safety Net: The Health and Social Welfare of the Homeless in the United States* (eds P. W.Brickner, L. K. Scharer, B. A. Conanan, *et al*), pp. 82–117. New York: Norton.

Koegel, P., Burnam, A., & Farr, R. K. (1988). The prevalence of specific psychiatric disorders among homeless individuals in the inner city of Los Angeles. *Archives of General Psychiatry*, **45**,1085–1092.

Lam, J. A. & Rosenheck, R. (1998) *Street Outreach for Homeless Persons with Serious Mental Illness: Is it Effective?* Rockville Maryland: Center for Mental Health Services.

Lamb, H. R. (1992) Deinstitutionalization in the Nineties. In: *Treating the Homeless Mentally Ill* (eds H. H. Lamb, L. L. Bachrach & F. I. Kass), pp. 41–54. Washington, DC: American Psychiatric Association.

— & Weinberger, L. E. (1998) Persons with severe mental illness in jails and prisons: a review. *Psychiatric Services*, **49**, 483–492.

Leach, J. (1979). Providing for the destitute. In: *Community Care for the Mentally Disabled* (eds J. K. Wing & R. Olson), pp. 90–105. Oxford: Oxford University Press.

Lehman, A. F., Dixon, L. B., Kernan, E., *et al* (1997) A randomized trial of assertive community treatment for homeless persons with severe mental illness. *Archives of General Psychiatry*, **54**, 1038–1043.

—, —, Hoch, J. S., *et al* (1999) Cost-effectiveness of assertive community treatment for homeless persons with severe mental illness. *British Journal of Psychiatry*, **174**, 346–352.

Link, B., Susser, E., Stueve, A., *et al* (1994) Lifetime and five-year prevalence of homelessness in the United States. *American Journal of Public Health*, **84**, 1907–1912.

—, Phelanm J., Bresnahanm M., *et al* (1995) Lifetime and five-year prevalence of homelessness in the United States: new evidence on an old debate. *American Journal of Orthopsychiatry*, **65**, 347–354.

Lodge-Patch, I. (1970) Homeless men in a London survey. *Proceedings of the Royal Society of Medicine*, **63**, 437–441.

Marshall, E. J. & Reed, J. L. (1992) Psychiatric morbidity in homeless women. *British Journal of Psychiatry*, **160**, 761–769.

Marshall, M. (1989) Collected and neglected: Are Oxford hostels for the homeless filling up with disabled psychiatric patients? *British Medical Journal*, **299**, 706–709.

Maslow, A. H. (1954) *Motivation and Personality*. New York: Harper and Row.

McHugh, P. R. (1992) Psychiatric Misadventures. *American Scholar*, **61**, 497–510.

McMurray-Avila, M. (1997) *Organizing Health Services for Homeless People*. Nashville, TN: National Health Care for the Homeless Council.

—, Gelberg, L. & Breakey, W. R. (1999) Balancing act: clinical practices that respond to the needs of homeless people. In: *Practical Lessons: The 1998 National Symposium on Homelessness Research* (eds L. Fosburg, & D. Dennis), pp. 8.1–8.44. Washington, DC: US Departments of Housing and Urban Development and Health and Social Services.

Miller, D. & Lin, E. (1988) Children in sheltered homeless families: Reported health status and use of health services. *Pediatrics*, **81**, 668–673.

Morbidity and Mortality Weekly Report (1991) Deaths among homeless persons – San Francisco, 1985–1990. *Morbidity and Mortality Weekly Report*, **40**, 877–880.

Morse, G. (1999) A review of case management for people who are homeless: implications for practice, policy and research. In: *Practical Lessons: The 1998 National Symposium on Homelessness Research* (eds L. Fosburg & D. Dennis), pp. 7.1–7.34. Washington, DC: US Departments of Housing and Urban Development and Health and Social Services.

Morse, G. & Calsyn, R. (1986) Mentally disturbed homeless people in St. Louis: Needy, willing, but underserved. *International Journal of Mental Health*, **14**, 74–94.

Munoz, M., Vazquez, C., Koegel, P., *et al* (1998) Differential patterns of mental disorders among the homeless in Madrid (Spain) and Los Angeles (USA). *Social Psychiatry and Psychiatric Epidemiology*, **33**, 514–520.

Nestadt, G., Breakey, W. R., Fischer, P. J., *et al* (1989) Personality disorders in Baltimore's homeless. Paper presented at the annual meeting of the American Public Health Association, Chicago, October.

New York State Council on Children and Families (1984) *Meeting the Needs of Holesless Youth*. Albany, NY: New York State Council on Children and Families.

NORDENTOFT, M., KNUDSEN, H. C. & SCHULSINGER, F. (1992) Housing conditions and residential needs of psychiatric patients in Copenhagen. *Acta Psychiatrica Scandinavica*, **85**, 385–389.

NORTH, C. S. & SMITH, E. M. (1993) A comparison of homeless men and women: different populations, different needs. *Community Mental Health Journal*, **29**, 423–431.

——, —— & SPITZNAGEL, E. L. (1993) Is antisocial personality a valid diagnosis among the homeless? *American Journal of Psychiatry*, **150**, 578–583.

——, —— & SPITZNAGEL, E. L. (1994) Violence and the homeless: an epidemiologic study of victimization and aggression. *Journal of Traumatic Stress*, **7**, 95–110.

PADGETT, D. K. & STRUENING, E. L. (1992) Victimization and traumatic injuries among the homeless: associations with alcohol, drug, and mental problems. *Journal of the American Orthopsychiatric Association*, **62**, 525–534.

PHELAN, J. C. & LINK, B. G. (1999) Who are "the homeless"? Reconsidering the composition and stability of the homeless population. *American Journal of Public Health*, **98**, 1334–1338.

POLLIO, D. E., NORTH, C. S., THOMPSON, S., *ET AL* (1997) Predictors of achieving stable housing in a mentally ill homeless population. *Psychiatric Services*, **48**, 528–530.

PRIEST, R. G. (1976) The homeless person and the psychiatric services: an Edinburgh survey. *British Journal of Psychiatry*, **128**, 128–136.

REGIER, D. A., BOYD, J. H., BURKE, J. D., *ET AL* (1988) One month prevalence of mental disorders in the United States. *Archives of General Psychiatry*, **45**, 977–986.

REULER, J., BAX, M. & SAMPSON, J. (1986) Physician house call services for medically needy, inner-city residents. *American Journal of Public Health*, **76**, 1131–1134.

RIDGELY, M. S., GOLDMAN, H. H. & TALBOTT, J. A. (1986) *Chronically Mentally Ill Young Adults with Substance Abuse Problems: A Review of Relevant Literature and Creation of a Research Agenda.* Baltimore, MD: University of Maryland School of Medicine.

RINGWALT, C. L., GREENE, J. M., ROBERTSON, M., *ET AL* (1998) The prevalence of homelessness among adolescents in the United States. *American Journal of Public Health*, **88**, 1325–1329.

ROBERTSON, M. J. (1996) *Homeless Youth on their Own.* Berkeley, CA: Alcohol Research Group.

——, ZLOTNICK, C. & WESTERFELT, A. (1997) Drug use disorders and treatment contact among homeless adults in Alameda County, California. *American Journal of Public Health*, **87**, 221–228.

ROBINS, L. N., HELZER, J. E., CROUGHAN, J., *ET AL* (1981) National Institute of Mental Health Diagnostic Interview Schedule. *Archives of General Psychiatry*, **38**, 381–389.

RODERICK, P., VICTOR, C. & CONNELLY, J. (1991) Is housing a public health issue? A survey of directors of public health. *British Medical Journal*, **302**, 157–160.

ROSENHECK, R., GALLUP, P. & LEDA, C. A. (1991) Vietnam era and Vietnam combat veterans among the homeless. *American Journal of Public Health*, **81**, 643–646.

—— & KOEGEL, P. (1993) Characteristics of veterans and nonveterans in three samples of homeless men. *Hospital and Community Psychiatry*, **44**, 858–863.

——, MORRISSEY, J., LAM, J., *ET AL* (1998) Service system integration, access to services, and housing outcomes in a program for homeless persons with severe mental illness. *American Journal of Public Health*, **88**, 1610–1615.

ROTH, D., BEAN, J., LUST, N., *ET AL* (1985) *Homelessness in Ohio: A Study of People in Need.* Colombus, OH: Ohio Department of Mental Health.

—— & ——(1986) The Ohio study: A comprehensive look at homelessness. *Psychosocial Rehabilitation Journal*, **9**, 31–38.

ROY, L. & READ S. (1992) The psychiatric careers of male shelter users in Nottingham. *Psychiatric Bulletin*, **16**, 685–687.

SAKAI, J., KIM. M., SHORE, J., *ET AL* (1998) The risk of Purified Protein Derivative positivity in homeless men with psychotic symptoms. *Southern Medical Journal*, **91**, 345–348.

SCOTT, J. (1991) *A Survey of Female Users of Resettlement Units.* Newcastle-upon-Tyne: Department of Psychiatry, University of Newcastle-upon-Tyne.

SHERMAN, D. J. (1992) The neglected health care needs of street youth. *Public Health Report*, **107**, 433–440.

SHINN, M., KNICKMAN, J. R. & WEIZMAN, B. C. (1991) Social relationships and vulnerability to becoming homeless among poor families. *American Psychologist*, **46**, 1180–1187.

SMITH, E. M., NORTH, C. S. & SPITZNAGEL, E. L. (1991) Are hard-to-interview street dwellers needed in assessing psychiatric disorders in homeless men? *International Journal of Methods in Psychiatric Research*, **1**, 69–78.

——, —— & —— (1992) A systematic study of mental illness, substance abuse, and treatment in 600 homeless men. *Annals of Clinical Psychiatry*, **4**, 111–120.

——, —— & —— (1993) Alcohol, drugs, and psychiatric comorbidity among homeless women: an epidemiologic study. *Journal of Clinical Psychiatry*, **54**, 82–87.

SNOW, D. A. & BAKER, S. G., ANDERSON, L., *ET AL* (1986) The myth of pervasive mental illness among the homeless. *Social Problems*, **33**, 407–423.

SOCIAL EXCLUSION UNIT (1998) *Rough Sleeping*. London: The Stationery Office.

SPITZER, R. L., COHEN, G., MILLER J. D., *ET AL* (1969) The psychiatric status of 100 men on skid row. *International Journal of Social Psychiatry*, **15**, 230–234.

STAHLER, C. J. (1995) Social interventions for homeless substance abusers. Evaluating treatment outcomes (editorial). *Journal of Addictive Diseases*, **14** (4).

STARK, C., SCOTT, J., HILL, M., *ET AL* (1989) *A Survey of the 'Long-stay' Users of DSS Resettlement Units*. Newcastle-upon-Tyne: Department of Social Policy, University of Newcastle-upon-Tyne.

STEIN, L. & TEST, M. A. (1985) *The Training in Community Living Model: A Decade of Experience*. San Francisco: Jossey Bass.

SUSSER, E. (1992) Working with people who are mentally ill and homeless: the role of the psychiatrist. In: *Homelessness and its prevention* (ed. R. Jahiel), pp. 207–217. Baltimore, MD.: Johns Hopkins University Press.

——, STRUENING, E. L. & CONOVER, S. (1987) Childhood experiences of homeless men. *American Journal of Psychiatry*, **144**,1599–1601.

——, —— & —— (1989) Psychiatric problems in homeless men. *Archives of General Psychiatry*, **46**, 845–850.

——, GOLDFINGER, S. M. & WHITE, A. (1990) *Community Mental Health Journal*, **26**, 463–480.

——, LIN, S., CONOVER, S., *ET AL* (1991*a*) Childhood antecedents of homelessness in psychiatric patients. *American Journal of Psychiatry*, **148**, 1026–1030.

——, —— & —— (1991*b*) Risk factors for homelessness in patients admitted to a state mental hospital. *American Journal of Psychiatry*, **148**, 1659–1664.

——, VALENCIA, E., GOLDFINGERM, S. M., *ET AL* (1993*a*) Injection drug use among homeless adults with severe mental illness. *American Journal of Public Health*, **87**, 854–856.

——, MOORE, R. & LINK, B. (1993*b*) Risk factors for homelessness. *Epidemiology Reviews*, **15**, 546–556.

——, BETNE, P., VALENCIA, E., *ET AL* (1997*a*) Injection drug use among homeless adults with severe mental illness. *American Journal of Public Health*, **87**, 854–856.

——, VALENCIA, E., CONOVER, S., *ET AL* (1997*b*) Preventing recurrent homelessness among mentally ill men: a critical time intervention after discharge from a shelter. *American Journal of Public Health*, **87**, 256–262.

SUTHERBY, K., SZMUKLER, G. I., HALPERN, A., *ET AL* (1999) A study of "crisis cards" in a community psychiatric service. *Acta Psychiatrica Scandinavica*, **97**, 1–6.

THOMISON, A. R. & COOK, D. A. G. (1987) Rootlessness and mental disorder. *British Journal of Clinical and Social Psychiatry*, **5**, 5–8.

THORNICROFT, G., BREAKEY, W. R. & PRIMM, A. B. (1995) Case management and network enhancement of the long-term mentally ill. In: *Social Support and Psychiatric Disorder* (ed. T. S. Brugha), pp. 239–256. Cambridge: Cambridge University Press.

TIDMARSH, D. & WOOD, S. (1972) Psychiatric aspects of destitution. In: *Evaluating a Community Psychiatry Service: The Camberwell Register 1964–71* (eds J. K. Wing & A. M. Hailey), pp. 327–340. London: Oxford University Press.

TIMMS, P. (1996) Homelessness and mental illness: a brief history. In: *Homelessness & Mental Health* (ed. D. Bughra), pp. 11–25. Cambridge University Press: Cambridge.

—— & FRY, A. H. (1989) Homelessness and mental illness. *Health Trends*, **21**,70–71.

US CONFERENCE OF MAYORS (1989) *A Status Report on Hunger and Homelessness in America's Cities.* Washington, DC: The US Conference of Mayors.

VASQUEZ, C., MUNOZ, M. & SANZ, J. (1997) Lifetime and 12-month prevalence of DSM–III–R mental disorders among the homeless in Madrid: a European study using the CIDI. *Acta Psychiatrica Scandinavica*, **94**, 1–8.

VERNEZ, G., BURNAM, M A., MCGLYNN, E. A., *ET AL* (1988) *Review of California's Program for the Homeless Mentally Disabled.* Santa Monica, CA: RAND Corporation.

VICTOR, C. R. (1992) Health status of the temporarily homeless population and residents of North West Thames Region. *British Medical Journal*, **305**, 387–391.

VOSTANIS, P., GRATTAN, E., CUMELLA, S., *ET AL* (1998) Mental health problems of homeless children and families: longitudinal study. *British Medical Journal*, **316**, 899–902.

WASYLENKI, D. A., GOERING, P. N., LEMIRE, D., *ET AL* (1993) The hostel outreach program: assertive case management for homeless mentally ill persons. *Hospital and Community Psychiatry*, **44**, 848–853.

WEITZMAN, B. C. (1989) Pregnancy and childbirth: risk factors for homelessness? *Family Planning Perspectives*, **21**, 175-178.

——, KNICKMAN, J. & SHINN, M. (1992) Predictors of shelter use among low-income families: Psychiatric history, substance abuse, and victimization. *American Journal of Public Health*, **82**, 1547–1550.

WESTLAKE, L. & GEORGE, S. L. (1994) Subjective health status of single homeless people in Bradford. *Public Health*, **108**, 111–119.

WHITBECK, L. B. & SIMONS, R. L. (1990) Life on the streets: the victimisation of runaway and homeless adolescents. *Youth and Society*, **22**, 108–125.

WHITELEY, J. S. (1955) Down and out in London: Mental illness in the lower social groups. *Lancet*, **2**, 608–610.

WHYNES, D. K., MLITT, B. A. & GIGGS, J. A. (1992) The health of the Nottingham homeless. *Public Health*, **106**, 307–314.

WINKLEBY, M. A. (1990) Comparison of risk factors for ill health in a sample of homeless and nonhomeless poor. *Public Health Reports*, **105**, 404–410.

WOBIDO, S. L., FRANK, T., MERRITT, B., *ET AL* (1990) Outreach. In: *Under the Safety Net: The Health and Social Welfare of the Homeless in the United States* (eds P. W.Brickner, L. K. Scharer, B. A. Conanan, *et al*), pp. 328–339. New York: Norton.

WOOD, D., VALDEZ, B., HAYASHI, T., *ET AL* (1990) Homeless and housed families in Los Angeles: A study comparing demographic, economic, and family function characteristics. *American Journal of Public Health*, **80**, 1049–1052.

WORLD HEALTH ORGANIZATION (1989) *Composite International Diagnostic Interview. Core Version 1.0.* Geneva: WHO.

WRIGHT, J. D. & WEBER, E. (1987) *Homelessness and Health.* Washington, DC: McGraw-Hill.

WYATT, R. J. & DE RENZO, E. G. (1986) Scienceless to Homelessness. *Science*, **234**, 1309.

WYKES, T. & STURT, E. (1986) The measurement of social behaviour in psychiatric patients: and assessment of the reliability and validity of the SBS Schedule. *British Journal of Psychiatry*, **148**, 1–11.

ZIMA, B., BUSSING, R. & FORNESS, S. (1997) Sheltered homeless children: their eligibility and unmet need for special education evaluations. *American Journal of Public Health*, **87**, 236–240.

——, WELLS, K. B. & FREEMAN, H. E. (1994) Emotional and behavioral problems and severe academic delays among sheltered homeless children in Los Angeles county. *American Journal of Public Health*, **84**, 260–264.

ZOLOPA, A., HAHN, J., GORTER, R., *ET AL* (1994) HIV and tuberculosis infection in San Francisco's homeless adults. *Journal of the American Medical Journal*, **272**, 455–461.

19 Needs of carers

ELIZABETH KUIPERS

Carers of those with psychiatric problems are not given a choice in the matter. It happens that someone with whom they have contact and a relationship has mental health difficulties. Thus, for this group – the carers of those with schizophrenia or depression – the needs are not so much about their own functioning, or lack of it, as about the demands placed on them by their acceptance of the caring role. In the literature, the needs of relatives are not even considered unless they are also carers. Thus, the impact of a severe mental illness on those who relinquish a caring role or who do not take it up is not taken into account. 'Peripheral' relatives such as grandparents or siblings, who do not take on caring as a primary role, also tend to be ignored. Up until now, relatives' needs have been documented almost exclusively for the main carers of the psychiatrically ill – often elderly mothers (Scazufca & Kuipers, 1997). Carers of the psychiatrically ill are likely to be female, but unlike other groups a proportion of other carers, such as spouses, siblings (Lively *et al*, 1995) or adult children, will be male.

Needs for care, as defined elsewhere in this volume, do not apply to relatives: they do not initially have an 'illness' or disability for which there is an acceptable and effective treatment or cure. However, in the process of remaining involved with someone who becomes mentally ill, they do develop problems associated with this caring role. These problems can be defined as relatives' needs. Unfortunately, these problems have often not been recognised; the idea that relatives have needs for care on their own behalf has taken a remarkably long time to be accepted, let alone acted upon. In the past, relatives have been blamed, ignored or just left to cope by professionals concerned only with the 'patient'.

This situation has now begun to change. Self-help groups such as the National Schizophrenia Fellowship (NSF) and the Manic-Depressive Fellowship were effective in pushing such changes through and remain influential; relatives' views are beginning to be taken seriously. However, the proportion of relatives who belong to self-help groups is still small and, as a group, carers remain poor advocates on their own behalf. The Community Care Act (1992) incorporated the idea that carers must be consulted, must be included in discharge and care planning, and can ask for help, a 'needs assessment', in their own right. The impact of this legislation is now beginning to be felt, as it is no longer unusual for clinical teams to ask for relatives' views and for carers to attend planning meetings. However, whether this has yet changed practice and led to carers feeling more supported is not so clear.

The existence of carers is now becoming even more essential. Mental health beds continue to be reduced and admission time in remaining ones tends to be short. Alternative provision such as hostel accommodation or group homes remains unevenly distributed around the country and increasingly dependent on local and charitable initiatives. Figures on those with major mental illnesses who return home to live with relatives vary, but are about 60% for first admission (McMillan *et al*, 1986) and 50% if first and subsequent admissions are included (Gibbons *et al*, 1984). Even in the case of long-term patients, between 40% and 50% either live with or are in close contact with relatives or have other patients in their network who take on this caring role (Creer *et al*, 1982). The central role of families in providing long-term care is not in dispute (Gibbons *et al*, 1984). Without relatives, it seems likely that professional services would be overwhelmed by the needs of patients trying to live in the community. However, in order both to maximise the care that such patients receive and to ensure it is not delivered at the cost of another vulnerable group in society – unpaid carers (Lefley, 1987) – it is necessary to consider in detail the impact of caregiving for those with long-term severe mental illness.

The measurement of family burden, or the impact of care

Since the 1950s, when patients first began to return to live in the community after the introduction of the phenothiazines, there has been interest in, and studies of, the effect that this had on relatives. However, the sobering fact emerges that a great deal of what was documented then is still being documented 50 years later. This seems to reflect a basic difficulty that professionals have in accepting that relatives have needs and require services on their own behalf. There remains a tendency for professionals to think that relatives are still 'someone else's job', particularly now that the pressures in community teams focus on averting crises and maintaining contact with difficult-to-engage clients. In the past 15 years, opportunities for working in partnership with relatives have developed, and there are some signs that carers are seen as a resource with needs of their own (Kuipers & Bebbington, 1985, 1990; Mintz *et al*, 1987; Department of Health, 1999: National Service Framework Standard 6). However, being offered appropriate support and help (so that those who want to can continue in a caring role without being exploited or made to feel guilty if they refuse) still seems to be problematic.

To explore the problems that families may experience as a consequence of their caring role, the concept of family burden was developed, reviewed by Schene *et al* (1994). Platt (1985) discussed the issues involved in measuring burden, and defined it as "the presence of problems, difficulties or adverse events which affect the life (lives) of the psychiatric patients' significant others (e.g. members of the household and/or the family)" (p. 385). There are other definitions, but in Platt's view they share a common underlying frame of reference: "the effect of the patient upon the family" (Goldberg & Huxley, 1980, p. 127); "the impact of living with a [psychiatric] patient on the way of life, or health of family members" (Brown, 1967, p. 53); and "the difficulties felt by the family of a psychiatric patient" (Pai & Kapur, 1981, p. 334).

Hoenig & Hamilton (1966) were the first to make a clear attempt to distinguish between two dimensions of burden; the 'objective' and 'subjective' burden of caring. Objective burden is any disruption of family life that is potentially verifiable and observable, such as financial problems, social isolation or having to cope with violent behaviour. Subjective burden refers to the personal feelings that relatives attribute to the caring role, such as distress or upset. In the better studies, these are assessed independently (e.g. Fadden *et al*, 1987*b*).

There have also been attempts to distinguish between an event and its perceived cause – what has been called 'patient relatedness' (e.g. Platt *et al*, 1983). This enables independent analysis of an event and its specificity to the problems of living with a psychiatric patient. Families may have financial problems that may or may not be attributable to a patient living in the household.

Measures of burden vary in what they ask about, how well they separate objective and subjective burden, and which informants they use. However, what they attempt to examine is the basic loss of reciprocity in relationships that can be caused by severe mental illness, which breaks down the usual mechanisms that maintain an equable and supportive relationship. It seems to be this imbalance that may prevent the relationship from being intrinsically self-perpetuating and lead carers to feel that they need external support in order to maintain the caring role. The degree of burden that relatives of patients with severe psychiatric disorders report has been reviewed in the past (e.g. Fadden *et al*, 1987*a*; MacCarthy, 1988). As MacCarthy (1988) discussed, the evidence of burden has varied depending on the criteria used and on the fact that relatives, as a group, are remarkably uncomplaining. Nevertheless, it is clear that burden exists and is usually extensive. Recent research in developing countries confirms that even with extended families, the burden of care is similar and leads to increased stress in relatives (Martyns-Yellowe, 1992; Salleh, 1994).

Mandelbrote & Folkard (1961*a,b*) estimated the degree to which families were restricted or disturbed by the presence of someone with schizophrenia in the home. Despite a rather crude method of assessment, they found that over half of the families were disturbed in some way, although only 2% reported severe stress. Mills (1962) studied psychiatric patients without selecting for diagnosis and found that most were a source of some anxiety to their relatives. More than half were described as difficult at home, and only a small minority caused no practical problems. In Grad & Sainsbury's study (1963*a,b*), almost two-thirds of the families had been experiencing hardship because the patient was living at home and in one-fifth the burden was severe. Two years later, 20% of their initial sample remained heavily burdened.

Wing *et al* (1964) followed 113 patients with schizophrenia for a year after discharge. When patients returned to live with their families, social relations were strained in nearly two-thirds of cases. Waters & Northover (1965) similarly reported that many men with schizophrenia occasioned moderate to severe hardship to their relatives in terms of social embarrassment, inconvenience and behaviour that frightened them or caused tension in the family. Hoenig & Hamilton (1966, 1969) found that three-quarters of their patients had some kind of adverse effect on the household.

Creer *et al* (1982) interviewed 52 relatives of long-term patients and found that up to 60% of households had to contend with at least moderate levels of disturbed behaviour. Gibbons *et al* (1984), in a sample of 141 patients, found a similar proportion suffered hardship, often severe. In their study, only 10% of the sample gave no evidence of family hardship. Carers were coping with high levels of disability; 65% of patients showed disturbed behaviour and 78% had restricted social performance. In these last two studies, as MacCarthy (1988) pointed out, supportive relatives were included even if they did not always live with the patient; as even a short break from continuous care ('respite') seems to reduce subjective burden, these high levels of hardship may still underestimate the problems faced by full-time carers.

The problems that severe mental illness can cause to relationships are reflected in high rates of divorce and separation in marriages where one member is mentally ill. As early as 1966, Brown *et al* noted that in many cases the patient's illness had been instrumental in bringing about divorce and separation, and in their study the rates for patients were three times the national average for women and four times for men. Clinically, it appears that if a carer is a spouse, they will have considered separation or divorce. However, the guilt engendered by a decision to leave, when a partner is in obvious difficulties, will mitigate against it; several studies note this. An early study of spouses (Yarrow *et al*, 1955*a*) found that even those contemplating separation or divorce had elected to give the relationship another try. Fadden *et al* (1987*b*), in a study of the spouses of long-term depressive patients, found a similar adherence to the marriage despite considerable difficulties. Whereas marital status was not associated with burden by Biegel *et al* (1994), Carpentier *et al* (1992) found that women single parents reported more burden than women living with partners. This was also found by Scazufca & Kuipers (1997).

Effects on social and leisure activities

An obvious consequence of living with a relative with persistent mental illness is the damaging effect on social and leisure activities. This is often considerably worse for women, who are more likely to be the main carers (Fadden *et al*, 1987*b*). Yarrow *et al* (1955*b*) noted that wives (carers) consistently believed that mental illness was stigmatised by others and expressed fears of social discrimination. As a consequence, one-third of them adopted a pattern of 'aggressive concealment', making drastic changes in order to avoid former friends; some even moved house. Another third had told only members of the family, or close friends who either understood the problem or had been in a similar situation themselves.

A number of other studies have documented the restriction of social activities experienced by those who live with and care for patients with schizophrenia (e.g. Mandelbrote & Folkard, 1961*a,b*; Wing *et al*, 1964; Waters & Northover, 1965). This can be especially marked when the relative is elderly (Leff *et al*, 1982). Similar observations have also been made for spouses of patients with severe depression (Fadden *et al*, 1987*b*). These relatives spent over 60 hours per week in face-to-face contact with the patient and were correspondingly socially isolated. In MacCarthy *et al*'s study (1989*b*), relatives averaged 49 hours per week contact with long-term patients. Anderson *et al* (1984) found a decrease in the social networks of some relatives who lived with a person with schizophrenia. MacCarthy (1988) noted that relatives of those attending long-term day care had very few social contacts other than the patient, few were employed and many remained isolated in their own homes. She also pointed out that social isolation is a "pervasive problem, which impairs the relationship between patient and supporter and reduces coping resources more fundamentally than material hardship". A recent first-onset study found that carers were socially isolated and worried about stigma even at this initial stage (Kuipers & Raune, 2000). It is clear that isolation and stigma are not new problems, and may not diminish (Kuipers *et al*, 1989; Kuipers, 1993).

Financial and employment difficulties

These have been emphasised in a number of studies (Yarrow *et al*, 1955*b*; Mandelbrote & Folkard, 1961*a,b*; Mills, 1962; Hoenig & Hamilton, 1966, 1969; Stevens, 1972; Fadden *et al*, 1987*b*). They are likely to be greatest when the carer is a spouse, as caring may interfere quite substantially with the opportunity to stay in work and the spouse may not be able to take on the role of financial provider. Because severe psychiatric disorders may interfere with long-term earning capacity, higher levels of burden may occur when patients who were formerly earning are affected than when the problems begin early in life. In the latter case, expectations and financial commitments may not yet have developed. Many clients in long-term care never become financially independent, and relatives, such as parents, who have always supported them, may find this a less difficult transition. Nevertheless, the loss of potential earnings, whether of a previous main earner or of a person who might have been expected to be economically viable, is likely to have effects on carers and to lead to, at the very least, a more impoverished family setting than otherwise. Because these psychiatric problems are often long-term, these effects are likely to be underestimated. A recent attempt to do so suggested that such costs are very high (Knapp, 1997).

How do relatives adjust to these illnesses?

Viewing disturbed or unusual behaviour as symptomatic of illness or relapse is what professionals are trained to do. Carers are not, however, and they may make various attributions in an attempt to understand and deal with day-to-day difficulties. They may decide an individual is being 'difficult' or 'lazy' and blame them for their behaviour. This is typical of relatives rated as critical or hostile according to the expressed emotion measure (Leff & Vaughn, 1985;

Brewin *et al*, 1991). Alternatively, they may deny, or fail to see, any behaviour as problematic (Jackson *et al*, 1990).

Relatives are likely to feel high levels of anxiety, exacerbated by the fact that often there is a crisis before any professional help can be obtained. It is also likely that guilt, anger and feelings of rejection will surface. These reactions were noted by Clausen *et al* (1955) and Yarrow *et al* (1955*a*). Most of the relatives described by Creer & Wing (1974) had at times expressed anger at the way their lives had been spoiled, and grief when they recalled what the patient had been like before the illness. Fadden *et al* (1987*b*) found that many of the spouses of patients with depression expressed not only anger and guilt but a sense of loss, as if they had been physically bereft of the person they married. This grief has been likened to a bereavement process, in terms of both impact and the length of time it can take to accept the patient as they are now (Lefley, 1987; Kuipers *et al*, 1989).

Things may not become easier over time. Objective hardships are likely to increase (Grad & Sainsbury, 1968; Hoenig & Hamilton, 1969; Lefley, 1987). However, resignation, which is associated with less objective stress, is also more common (Gibbons *et al*, 1984; MacCarthy *et al*, 1989*b*).

Relatives' own mental health

It is only relatively recently that it has become routine to investigate the psychological impact of caring while assessing the severity of burden. Effects were documented initially for those living with partners with depression or neuroses (Kreitman, 1964; Kreitman *et al*, 1970; Ovenstone, 1973*a*) and for those living with people with schizophrenia (Brown *et al*, 1966; Hoenig & Hamilton, 1966, 1969; Stevens, 1972; Creer & Wing, 1974). More recently, relatives have been assessed using standardised measures such as the General Health Questionnaire (GHQ; Goldberg & Hillier, 1979) and the Present State Examination (PSE; Wing *et al*, 1974). The consistent finding then emerged that around one-third of relatives are likely to have raised levels of anxiety and depression connected to the caring role (Creer *et al*, 1982; Fadden *et al*, 1987*b*). MacCarthy *et al* (1989*b*) found that 77% of a sample of 45 carers of long-term patients described at least one symptom of distress and 14 (33%) reported experiencing three or more such symptoms – considerably higher levels of disorder than would be expected in the general population. This is confirmed by more recent studies (Scazufca & Kuipers, 1996; Kuipers & Raune, 2000). As MacCarthy (1988) has pointed out, "calculating the costs of maintaining a patient in need of continual care in the community should include that of providing psychiatric treatment for up to one third of the main dispensers of this care" (p. 216).

Burdensome symptoms

Behavioural problems in patients are the best predictors of complaints from carers and are major correlates of burden (Lefley, 1987). In practice, these seem to fall into two categories – socially disruptive behaviour and social withdrawal.

In Mills' study (1962), carers were commonly concerned that patients might be a danger to themselves or to others. Problems frequently arose with neighbours as a result of patients' behaviour. Many relatives complained of disturbed nights. In Grad & Sainsbury's study (1963*a,b*), people with psychosis were more problematic than those with neurotic problems. Severe burden was related to aggression, delusions, hallucinations, confusion and poor self-care. However, problems that were complained of most often were the frustrating, depressive and hyponchondriacal preoccupations of patients. Brown *et al* (1966) found that the number of problems and the distress experienced by relatives were related to the degree of disturbed behaviour shown by patients with schizophrenia who lived with them. Hoenig & Hamilton (1966, 1969) confirmed that most frequently relatives reported both aggressive behaviour and extreme seclusion and withdrawal as problematic.

Creer & Wing (1974), in a study of 80 long-term carers, 50 of whom were members of the NSF, found that negative symptoms of social withdrawal, lack of conversation, under-activity, slowness and having few leisure interests were rated most often as problems. Socially embarrassing behaviour and obviously disturbed behaviour were also difficult. Gibbons *et al* (1984) reported that disruptive behaviour caused the most distress to relatives. Even though they were minority behaviours, offensive behaviour, rudeness and violence were found by almost all carers to be upsetting if they had to cope with them. According to another study (Fadden *et al*, 1987*b*), sleeplessness was the main problem for carers of patients with depression, followed by misery, worry, guilt and the inactivity of patients.

MacCarthy *et al* (1989*b*) found patients' lack of independent self-help skills and disruptive antisocial behaviour, followed by negative symptoms and difficulties in relating to the patient, to be the main problems named by carers. Tessler & Gamache (1994), in a large study in three American cities, found that 45% of the 305 relatives they interviewed tried to control troublesome behaviour.

The burden of depressive symptoms

The specific burdens of depressive illnesses of carers are not often separated in the literature, and the relatively limited information available is mainly concerned with the effects on spouses – the main carers (Fadden *et al*, 1987*a*; Kuipers, 1987). In these marriages, there is frequently conflict (Hinchcliffe *et al*, 1978), particularly over role functions (Ovenstone, 1973*b*), and a high level of dependence (Birtchnell & Kennard, 1983). With increasing pathology on the part of the husband, fewer joint decisions are made (Collins *et al*, 1971), and the wives of patients with depression may have significantly less independent social activity than controls (Nelson *et al*, 1970). Partners may find it difficult to take over roles in the marriage; spouses not only find that they have increased responsibilities but that they have lost their own support and intimate confidante in the marriage (Fadden *et al*, 1987*b*). Adolescent children living with parents with chronic depression have increased levels of psychiatric morbidity (Hammen *et al*, 1987). These disturbances may be more marked when they have to cope with life events (Hirsch *et al*, 1985). A recent survey comparing the carers of elderly people with dementia or with chronic depression found that both groups met the criteria for caseness on the GHQ, and felt stressed and burdened by the caring role (Rosenvinge *et al*, 1998). Another study of 47 carers of people with schizophrenia or schizo-affective disorder found that the carers were more distressed by depressed behaviour than by any other symptoms (Tucker *et al*, 1998). This suggests that depressive behaviour, either in those with a main diagnosis of depression or in those with psychosis, is often burdensome.

Behaviour of professionals towards relatives

Not many studies have looked at this specifically. The Clausen study (Clausen *et al*, 1955) investigated how attitudes held by both patients' wives and their psychiatrists affected the services provided (Deasy & Quinn, 1955). Wives mainly made requests for information regarding aetiology, diagnosis and prognosis, and advice on how to deal with the patient when he returned home. In nearly two-thirds of cases, however, wives expressed dissatisfaction because they did not receive this information or the professionals were inaccessible. Deasy & Quinn reported that psychiatrists frequently felt that they had to protect patients from their wives, as they believed that factors in the relation-ship had caused the illness.

General dissatisfaction with services, mental health professionals and service delivery systems continues to be expressed by carers (Lefley,

1987). In the past, carers were rarely involved in decision-making, and wished for services that were available continuously, not just in a crisis. Carers of the long-term mentally ill may also have to deal with the complexities not only of the mental health services but also of legal and criminal systems. An NSF survey suggested that carers found the police to be the most useful professional group (Hogman & Pearson, 1995).

MacCarthy *et al* (1989*b*) looked specifically at how adequately a service provides for the needs of relatives of those attending long-term day care. This study was one of a series of surveys of high-contact users of psychiatric services, in which the MRC Needs for Care Assessment (Brewin *et al*, 1987, 1988) was used to measure both functioning and whether interventions had been attempted; this led to judgements of whether needs had been met or not. MacCarthy *et al*'s study (1989*b*) was one of the earliest to adapt these standard-ised measures of need to look at the problems relatives might experience. Subjects were 145 patients attending day care locally. Of these, 61 (42%) were living with at least one other relative. Patient functioning was assessed by interviewing the relatives with a modified version of the MRC Social Behaviour Schedule (Wykes & Sturt, 1986). Questions were asked about difficulties with finances, employment, children and their own physical and mental health in order to assess objective burden. Relatives were also asked the extent to which any particular problem could be attributed to the patient. Finally, they were asked about contact with services and their satisfaction with these.

MacCarthy *et al* found that relatives had problems most frequently in the areas of information and advice, emotional support and respite care. These three areas were also the ones with most unmet need. They found that practical needs such as for housing, child care and help with benefits were most often met. However, information and advice had only been offered successfully to about half of the relatives. Support for emotional burdens had the highest rate of under-provision. Some relatives were being offered help, but one-fifth of the sample needed help that had not yet been offered. Respite care had been rarely identified as a problem and had only been met for one family out of 61. This study confirmed again that relatives tolerated their demanding role, had difficulty articulating what other help they would like and were not likely to complain. Since then, other authors have looked at carers' own needs for care (Biegel *et al*, 1994; Loukissa, 1995; Szmukler *et al*, 1996*a*) and have developed specific programmes for helping carers themselves (Szmukler *et al*, 1996*b*). These studies (Cuijpers & Stam, 2000) suggest that inter-viewing in this way can improve outcome.

Implications for service provision

It is clear from the literature reviewed that carers of those with long-term mental health problems have a demanding role, and may be extensively burdened by it, both objectively and in terms of the emotional impact of these disorders. The degree of burden may be severe and can affect carers' own mental well-being, particularly as caring is likely to last for a lifetime (Lefley, 1987; Prudo & Blum, 1987) without respite (MacCarthy *et al*, 1989*b*). Services seem more likely and able to respond to crises than to the continuous, changing requirements of families as they go through the life cycle. Patients' stability may vary and interact with these changes. Services do provide practical help, but even now, nearly 50 years after the problems were first documented, they have difficulty in providing information and advice, and particularly in providing effective emotional support, even though research evidence shows that this can be done.

Carers have changing needs both for their own mental health and quality of life and to enable them to provide an environment that can be sustained and can also promote recovery. Many relatives do manage this extremely well, but it cannot be assumed. There is also some evidence that the resignation that can characterise long-term caring relationships may be detrimental to clients' functioning and well-being (MacCarthy *et al*, 1989*a*).

There is hardly any mention in the literature of benefits that might occur in the caring role. Lefley (1987) notes that positive aspects have not been adequately assessed. Szmukler *et al* (1996*b*) looked at this specifically and did find some positives. Kuipers & Raune (2000), in a first-episode study found that "feeling useful", "discovering strengths in myself" and "becoming more understanding of others" were some of the more positive aspects mentioned by first-onset carers.

However, the role is often accepted because of a lack of community alternatives and not because it is chosen. This lack runs right through the literature; there may be limited support offered, and carers are not able to choose whether to take up the caring role. Caring appears at present to involve total care, with all the social and personal costs involved; often, the alternative is to reject the role altogether. This may be a position that women have been prepared to accept, but given societal changes, and women's multiple roles, it may not be one that will always continue (Scazufca & Kuipers, 1997).

Specific needs for services

The needs outlined above seem to suggest a rather pessimistic view of whether anything will ever change. There is a danger of professionals and the services available becoming as overwhelmed and even as burdened by families' problems as carers themselves. There is sometimes a sense that whatever is offered it will not be enough. However, consideration of specific services that can be provided, together with evidence on efficacy and effectiveness, make clear how this could be improved.

The need for collaborative rather than adversarial relationships between professionals and carers

Over the past three decades, there is evidence of some changes from professionals 'blaming' families for problems to being willing instead to work with them in partnership, and to use the resources both parties have available to help improve and maintain individuals' recovery. The change has been most noticeable in the literature on successful family interventions in schizophrenia. This was initially based on the earlier work on expressed emotion (Leff & Vaughn, 1985), which suggested that family attitudes have an effect on the course and recovery in psychosis. Despite some contrary views (Hatfield *et al*, 1987), this idea has led to the development of techniques whereby the family can be helped to reappraise and re-attribute difficult symptoms and problem-solve more effectively (Falloon *et al*, 1985; Leff *et al*, 1985; Tarrier *et al*, 1988). There is also evidence that expressed emotion and burden are linked (Jackson *et al*, 1990; Smith *et al*, 1993; Scazufca & Kuipers, 1996; Kuipers & Raune, 2000), and that both are more dependent on appraisal of problems than on actual deficits.

Another requirement of a collaborative stance by professionals is that they are prepared to take the carers' viewpoint seriously, to act if asked rather than wait for a crisis, and to work on prevention of relapse rather than just treating symptoms once a relapse has occurred. Even a 24-hour crisis team can fail to provide adequate long-term support and rehabilitation (Reynolds *et al*, 1990). Carers are well able to assess early signs of relapse in patients who live with them and to decide whether this information can be used with clinicians to prevent more serious symptoms from developing (Birchwood *et al*, 1989). The Community Care Act of 1992, and the requirement of the NSF (1999) to involve carers in care planning and in their own needs assessment, should help to improve this.

Another strand of research that may reduce the distance between professional staff and carers is the recently replicated finding that not only do staff and carers have to cope with many of the same behavioural problems in patients (Creer *et al*, 1982), but they also share a range of expressed emotion ratings (Watts, 1988). Typically, around 40% of staff in long-term care will be rated as 'high expressed' emotion (critical) towards one or more key patients (Moore & Kuipers, 1992; Moore *et al*, 1992; Kuipers & Moore, 1995; Oliver & Kuipers, 1996). This finding has implications for the importance of staff training and for allowing carers access to specialised help for patients' behaviour that staff also have problems in coping with.

Need for understanding

It must now be obvious that informing carers is a necessary first step in any interaction between carers and professionals. Information helps carers to understand the condition they are dealing with and its implications, in terms of both long-term care and emotional impact. Telling carers the name of a condition, such as schizophrenia, psychosis or depression, helps alleviate some of the confusion and misattribution that is otherwise likely to arise. Those most likely to be distressed have both high expressed emotion and long-term problems, and appraise symptoms more negatively (Barrowclough & Parle, 1997). However, giving information to carers is by no means straightforward. Because of the high levels of anxiety that carers might have when first in contact with professionals, there may be considerable difficulties in under-standing and accepting what is said. At best, education provides some clarity and optimism and is the basis for engaging relatives in further intervention (Smith & Birchwood, 1987; Berkowitz *et al*, 1990). Staff must be prepared to continually answer questions, to admit when answers are uncertain or unknown, and to discuss implications for the individual family over many months. Changes in the situation, a cyclical illness or other unpredictability will often mean the whole process starting again.

Help in problem-solving

Difficult behaviour is a correlate of burden in carers. Poor social functioning seems a particular issue (Kuipers & Raune, 2000). Thus, helping carers to cope with it successfully is important, and it can be very frustrating for carers if avoided or handled superficially. Giving advice does not mean that staff tell carers what to do – this is perceived as arrogant, and lacks credibility because staff are seen as not having to cope continuously with these problems. Family members need to be encouraged to try out new and more constructive problem-solving, one problem at a time, broken into manageable steps, with possible solutions negotiated rather than imposed on all involved, including the client. There is now considerable literature available on the techniques that can be successfully applied (Falloon *et al*, 1984; Anderson *et al*, 1986; Kuipers & Bebbington, 1990; Kuipers *et al*, 1992; Barrowclough & Tarrier, 1992).

Need for emotional support

The emotional impact of illness, particularly severe mental illness, continues to be underestimated. Families are likely to have a wide range of emotional responses. Shock and denial can characterise first contacts with professional services. Later, guilt, loss, anger and rejection are likely, as is worry about the future and the person's vulnerability, given perceived and actual deficits in role performance. Isolation, stigma, and poor understanding from friends and family are common. Clients may themselves feel depressed and lose confidence and hope (Birchwood *et al*, 1993; Rooke & Birchwood, 1998). Hopelessness and final resignation – "nothing ever changes" – may set in. It is not surprising that professionals may feel daunted and not attempt to get involved. However, there is good evidence that help can be given successfully (Penn & Mueser, 1996; Pharoah *et al*, 2000; Bustillo *et al*, 2001). Most of the intervention studies with a positive outcome offered at least nine months of treatment, saw whole families together and offered information, problem-solving and support.

Need for care to continue

One of the worst aspects of professional services that carers discuss is high staff turnover. Busy community teams are not ideal places for staff to form long-term relationships as advocates for families because as staff move on, carers have to start again with new professionals. However, in the same way that continuity of care is a reasonable aim for long-term patients (Watts & Bennet, 1983), so it can be for long-term carers. The self-help groups have taken on this role over the past 25 years, offering support groups and help-lines. Professional services can, via a keyworker system, ensure that even if staff change, information is handed on effectively and monitoring and intervention strategies are not lost, and this is one of the functions of the Enhanced Care Programme Approach and the new Standard 6 of the NSF (1999).

Need to look after themselves

The damage to a carer's own health from the caring role, including the personal and social costs (Noh & Turner, 1987), is now well documented. Carers risk increased psychological problems, such as depression and anxiety (Salleh, 1994; Tessler & Gamache, 1994), isolation, family impoverishment and a likelihood that the family will become enmeshed and over-dependent (Lefley, 1987). Nevertheless, carers often want to offer help and see what they do as a positive contribution – one that can enhance client recovery and social functioning. The issue seems to be the lack of choice. Feeling forced into a difficult and often unrewarding role will not make it work to either carers' or patients' advantage. Carers can offer a valuable resource, a possible lifetime commitment to a patient and a 'normal' setting in the community. They provide contact with a social network for patients whose own networks are likely to be restricted (Hamilton *et al*, 1989). If carers feel exploited and left to cope unaided, this resource will not necessarily continue to be available.

In order to look after themselves, carers are likely to need time off (respite) and to develop their own independent interests, or a sense of perspective. A recent study found that carers with jobs were more likely to be less distressed (Scazufca & Kuipers, 1996). This may not be causal, but it is likely that being able to maintain other roles and not have caring as the only focus is helpful. It is difficult to accept that it can be caring to leave a patient to cope alone some of the time. However, such interventions have been shown to be effective, both in changing overprotective relationships and in allowing relatives to enjoy themselves without experiencing guilt (Leff *et al*, 1982, 1989).

If there were more alternatives available in the community, in the range of accommodation and in the flexibility of support, and greater importance attributed to the caring role and some choice in it, it is possible that the burden would diminish. However, this has yet to be demonstrated in ordinary service contexts.

Need for respite care

The specific use of respite care for long-term mental health problems is not established. It is accepted that elderly patients can be admitted to relieve carers, but it is not now seen as justified for clients to be given a hospital bed *just* for social reasons, given current bed shortages. Another model is not to rely on hospital beds – an increasingly scarce and expensive resource – but to offer other accommodation in the community specifically for this use. The NSF have pioneered the use of houses in local areas for this purpose.

The needs of 'peripheral' relatives

Relatives who are not the main carer, but who are often still involved with the patients' concerns, are hardly ever considered by services. In recent years, there have been some local attempts to form support groups that will consider these needs; so far, these are groups for siblings of patients and for children of patients.

Siblings have particular problems that include feelings of anger and resentment at the attention the patient is receiving in the family and fear that they themselves will have mental illness problems as well. Later on, siblings report feeling guilt at the anger and fear, and also guilt at their own achievements that may highlight the continuing difficulties and lack of progress of a brother or sister. There is often also misunderstanding of the problems, followed by avoidance and leaving home early to make sure the burden of care is not passed on to them. Ambivalent feelings may remain in the relationship between an ill and a well sibling (Lively *et al*, 1995).

Children share some of these feelings, and often also have a very confused relationship with the ill parent, who may not be able to offer consistent care. Gibbons *et al* (1984) reported that children were adversely affected in 63% of the households with children. Children will often blame themselves, and later feel anger and resentment if care is lacking or sporadic. It seems likely that at least one capable parent or carer is necessary to a child's development, and children from settings where this has not been possible because of mental illness may have specific problems.

Services need to be aware that 'peripheral' relatives exist, but may be neither as vocal nor as easy to contact as the main carer. They are likely to have similar needs to the main carer: for basic information, for advice, for help to cope with specific problems, for reassurance and for emotional support.

Conclusions

At present, the needs of relatives of the long-term mentally ill living in the community are extensive and unlikely to be met in full. We have known about these needs for 50 years, and they have not changed substantially. There is now awareness of the problems, but still a 'scatter shot' approach (Kreisman & Joy, 1974) to the implementation of solutions. There is evidence suggesting that the existing needs do not have to be overwhelming for services and that outcome can improve. Provision of support for carers will enable them to make informed decisions about their commitment, level of involvement and how they take up the role. Meeting needs is also likely to be cost-effective as it can prevent aspects of future morbidity in both carers and people who live with them.

Carers may have little choice over the position they find themselves in and its impact. Their needs are intrinsic to the role and are likely to develop over time, as they attempt a valuable and difficult job. At the start of this new millennium, it is time to stop simply cataloguing the problems and to provide services routinely that meet these needs effectively.

References

ANDERSON, C. M., HOGARTY, B., BAYER, T., *ET AL* (1984) EE and social networks in parents of schizophrenic patients. *British Journal of Psychiatry*, **144**, 247–255.

——, REISS, D. J. & HOGARTY, C. E. (1986) *Schizophrenia in the Family: A Practitioner's Guide to Psychoeducation and Management.* New York: Guilford Press.

BARROWCLOUGH, C. & PARLE, M. (1997) Appraisal, psychological adjustment and expressed emotion in relatives of patients suffering from schizophrenia. *British Journal of Psychiatry*, **171**, 26–30.

—— & TARRIER, N. (1992) *Families of Schizophrenic Patients: Cognitive Behavioural Interventions.* London: Chapman & Hall.

BERKOWITZ, R., SHAVIT, N. & LEFF, J. P. (1990) Educating relatives of schizophrenic patients. *Social Psychiatry and Psychiatric Epidemiology*, **25**, 216–220.

BIEGEL, D. E., MILLIGAN, S. E., PUTNAM, P. L., *ET AL* (1994) Predictors of burden among lower socioeconomic status caregivers of persons with chronic mental illness. *Community Mental Health Journal*, **30**, 473–494.

BIRCHWOOD, M., SMITH, J., MACMILLAN, F., *ET AL* (1989) Predicting relapse in schizophrenia: the development and implementation of an early signs monitoring system using patients and families as observers, a preliminary investigation. *Psychological Medicine*, **19**, 649–656.

——, MASON, R., MACMILLAN, F., *ET AL* (1993) Depression, demoralization and control over psychotic illness: a comparison of depressed and non-depressed patients with a chronic psychosis. *Psychological Medicine*, **23**, 387–395.

BIRTCHNELL, J. & KENNARD, J. (1983) Does marital maladjustment lead to mental illness? *Social Psychiatry*, **18**, 79–88.

BREWIN, C. R., MACCARTHY, B., DUDA, K., *ET AL* (1991) Attribution and expressed emotion in the relatives of patients with schizophrenia. *Journal of Abnormal Psychology*, **100**, 546–554.

——, WING, J. K., MANGEN, S. P., *ET AL* (1987) Principles and practice of measuring needs in the long-term mentally ill: the MRC Needs for Care Assessment. *Psychological Medicine*, **17**, 971–981.

——, ——, ——, *ET AL* (1988) Needs for care among the long-term mentally ill: a report from the Camberwell High Contact Survey. *Psychological Medicine*, **18**, 457–468.

BROWN, G. W. (1967) The family of the schizophrenic patient. In: *Recent Developments in Schizophrenia* (eds A. J. Coppen & A. Walk), pp. 43–59. London: Royal Medico-Psychological Association.

——, BONE, M., DALISON, B., *ET AL* (1966) *Schizophrenia and Social Care.* Oxford: Oxford University Press.

BUSTILLO, J. R., LAURIELLO, J., HORAN, W. P., *ET AL* (2001) The psychosocial treatment of schizophrenia: an update. *American Journal of Psychiatry*, **158**, 163–175.

CARPENTIER, N., LESAGE, A., GOULET, J., ET AL (1992) Burden of care of families not living with young schizophrenic relatives. *Hospital and Community Psychiatry*, **43**, 38–43.

CLAUSEN, J. A. & YARROW, M. R. (1955) The impact of mental illness on the family. *Journal of Social Issues*, **11**, 3–64.

——, ——, DEASY, L. C., ET AL (1955) The impact of mental illness: research formulation. *Journal of Social Issues*, **11**, 6–11.

COLLINS, J., KREITMAN, N., NELSON, B., ET AL (1971) Neurosis and marital interaction: III. Family roles and function. *British Journal of Psychiatry*, **119**, 233–242.

CREER, C. & WING, J. K. (1974) *Schizophrenia at Home*. Surbiton: National Schizophrenia Fellowship.

——, STURT, E. & WYKES, T. (1982) The role of relatives. In: *Long-Term Community Care: Experience in a London Borough* (ed. J. K. Wing), pp. 29–39. Psychological Medicine Monograph Supplement No. 2.

CUIJPERS, P. & STAM, H. (2000) Burnout among relatives of psychiatric patients attending psychoeducational support groups. *Psychiatric Services*, **51**, 357–359.

DEASY, L. C. & QUINN, O. W. (1955) The wife of the mental patient and the hospital psychiatrist. *Journal of Social Issues*, **11**, 49–60.

DEPARTMENT OF HEALTH (1999) *National Service Framework for Mental Health: Modern Standards and Service Models*. London: Department of Health.

FADDEN, G. B., BEBBINGTON, P. E. & KUIPERS, L. (1987*a*) The burden of care: the impact of functional psychiatric illness on the patient's family. *British Journal of Psychiatry*, **150**, 285–292.

——, KUIPERS, L. & BEBBINGTON, P. E. (1987*b*) Caring and its burdens: a study of the relatives of depressed patients. *British Journal of Psychiatry*, **151**, 660–667.

FALLOON, I. R. H., BOYD, J. L., MCGILL, C. W., ET AL (1984) *Family Care of Schizophrenia*. New York: Guilford Press.

——, ——, ——, ET AL (1985) Family management in the prevention of morbidity of schizophrenia. Clinical outcome of a two year longitudinal study. *Archives of General Psychiatry*, **42**, 887–896.

GIBBONS, J. S., HORN, S. H., POWELL, J. M., ET AL (1984) Schizophrenic patients and their families. A survey in a psychiatric service based on a district general hospital. *British Journal of Psychiatry*, **144**, 70–77.

GOLDBERG, D. P. & HILLIER, V. G. (1979) A scaled version of the GHQ. *Psychological Medicine*, **9**, 139–146.

—— & HUXLEY, P. (1980) *Mental Illness in the Community*. London: Tavistock.

GRAD, J. & SAINSBURY, P. (1963*a*) Evaluating a community care service. In: *Trends in Mental Health Services* (eds J. Farndale & H. Freeman), pp. 303–317. New York: Macmillan.

—— & —— (1963*b*) Mental illness and the family. *Lancet*, *i*, 544–547.

—— & —— (1968) The effects that patients have on their families in a community care and a control psychiatric service: a two-year follow-up. *British Journal of Psychiatry*, **114**, 265–278.

HAMILTON, N. G., PONZOHA, C. A., CUTLER, P. L., ET AL (1989) Social networks and negative versus positive symptoms of schizophrenia. *Schizophrenia Bulletin*, **15**, 625–633.

HAMMEN, C., ADRIAN, C., GORDON, D., ET AL (1987) Children of depressed mothers: maternal strain and symptoms as predictors of dysfunction. *Journal of Abnormal Psychology*, **96**, 190–198.

HATFIELD, A., SPANIOL, L. & ZIPPLE, A. M. (1987) Expressed emotion: a family perspective. *Schizophrenia Bulletin*, **13**, 221–226.

HINCHCLIFFE, M. K., HOOPER, D. & ROBERTS, F. J. (1978) *The Melancholy Marriage*. Chichester: Wiley.

HIRSCH, B. J., MOOR, R. H. & REISCHL, T. L. (1985) Psychological adjustment of adolescent children of a depressed, arthritic or normal parent. *Journal of Abnormal Psychology*, **94**, 154–164.

HOENIG, J. & HAMILTON, M. W. (1966) The schizophrenic patient in the community and his effect on the household. *International Journal of Social Psychiatry*, **12**, 165–176.

—— & —— (1969) *The Desegregation of the Mentally Ill*. London: Routledge and Kegan Paul.

HOGMAN, G. & PEARSON, G. (1995) *The Silent Partners: The Needs and Experiences of People who care for People with a Severe Mental Illness*. London: National Schizophrenia Fellowship.

JACKSON, H. T., SMITH, N. & MCGORRY, P. (1990) Relationship between EE and family burden in psychotic disorders: an exploratory study. *Acta Psychiatrica Scandinavia*, **82**, 243–249.

KNAPP, M. (1997) Costs of schizophrenia. *British Journal of Psychiatry*, **171**, 509–518.

KREISMAN, D. E. & JOY, V. D. (1974) Family response to the mental illness of a relative: a review of the literature. *Schizophrenia Bulletin*, **10**, 34–57.

KREITMAN, N. (1964) The patient's spouse. *British Journal of Psychiatry*, **110**, 159–173.

——, COLLINS, J., NELSON, B., *ET AL* (1970) Neurosis and marital interaction: I. Personality and symptoms. *British Journal of Psychiatry*, **117**, 33–46.

KUIPERS, E. (1987) Depression and the family. In: *Coping with Disorder in the Family* (ed. J. Orford), pp. 194–216. London: Croom Helm.

—— (1993) Family burden in schizophrenia: implications for services. *Social Psychiatry and Psychiatric Epidemiology*, **28**, 207–210.

—— & BEBBINGTON, P. (1985) Relatives as a resource in the management of functional illness. *British Journal of Psychiatry*, **147**, 465–470.

—— & —— (1990) *Working in Partnership: Clinicians and Carers in Management of Longstanding Mental Illness*. Oxford: Heinemann Press.

—— & MOORE, E. (1995) Expressed emotion and staff–client relationships: implications for community care of the severely mentally ill. *International Journal of Mental Health*, **24**, 13–26.

—— & RAUNE, D. (2000) The early development of expressed emotion and burden in the families of first onset psychosis. In: *Early Intervention in Psychosis* (eds M. Birchwood, D. Fowler & C. Jackson), pp. 128–140. Chichester: Wiley.

——, MACCARTHY, B., HURRY, J., *ET AL* (1989) Counselling the relatives of the long-term adult mentally ill: II. A low cost supportive model. *British Journal of Psychiatry*, **154**, 775–782.

——, LEFF, J. & LAM, D. (1992) *Family Work for Schizophrenia: A Practical Guide*. London: Gaskell.

LEFF, J., & VAUGHN, C. (1985) *Expressed Emotion in Families*. London: Guilford Press.

——, KUIPERS, L., BERKOWITZ, R., *ET AL* (1982) A controlled trial of social intervention in the families of schizophrenic patients. *British Journal of Psychiatry*, **141**, 121–134.

——, ——, ——, *ET AL* (1985) A controlled trial of social intervention in the families of schizophrenic patients. Two year follow up. *British Journal of Psychiatry*, **146**, 594–600.

——, BERKOWITZ, R., SHAVIT, N., *ET AL* (1989) A trial of family therapy versus a relatives' group for schizophrenics. *British Journal of Psychiatry*, **154**, 58–66.

LEFLEY, H. P. (1987) Ageing parents as care givers of mentally ill children: an emerging social problem. *Hospital and Community Psychiatry*, **38**, 1063–1070.

LIVELY, E., FRIEDRICH, R. M. & BUCKWALTER, K. C. (1995) Sibling perception of schizophrenia: impact on relationships, roles, and health issues. *Mental Health Nursing*, **16**, 225–238.

LOUKISSA, D. A. (1995) Family burden in chronic mental illness: a review of research studies. *Journal of Advanced Nursing*, **21**, 248–255.

MACCARTHY, B. (1988) The roles of relatives. In: *Community Care in Practice* (eds A. Lavender & F. Holloway), pp. 207–227. Chichester: Wiley.

——, KUIPERS, L., HURRY, J., *ET AL* (1989*a*) Counselling the relatives of the long-term adult mentally ill: evaluation of the impact on relatives and patients. *British Journal of Psychiatry*, **154**, 768–775.

——, LESAGE, A., BREWIN, C. R., *ET AL* (1989*b*) Needs for care among the relatives of long-term users of day-care. *Psychological Medicine*, **19**, 725–736.

MANDELBROTE, B. M. & FOLKARD, S. (1961*a*) Some problems and needs of schizophrenics in relation to a developing psychiatric community service. *Comprehensive Psychiatry*, **2**, 317–328.

—— & —— (1961*b*) Some factors related to outcome and social adjustment in schizophrenia. *Acta Psychiatrica Scandinavica*, **37**, 223–235.

MARI, J. J. & STRIENER, D. L. (1994) An overview of family interventions and relapse on schizophrenia: meta-analysis of research findings. *Psychological Medicine*, **24**, 565–578.

MARTYNS-YELLOWE, I. S. (1992) The burden of schizophrenia on the family. A study from Nigeria. *British Journal of Psychiatry*, **161**, 779–782.

McMILLAN, J. F., GOLD, A., CROW, T. J., ET AL (1986) The Northwick Park Study of first episodes of schizophrenia: IV. Expressed emotion and relapse. *British Journal of Psychiatry*, **148**, 133–143.

MILLS, E. (1962) *Living with Mental Illness: A Study in East London*. London: Routledge and Kegan Paul.

MINTZ, L. I., LIBERMAN, R. P., MIKLOWITZ, D. J., ET AL (1987) Expressed emotion: a call for partnership among relatives, patients and professionals. *Schizophrenia Bulletin*, **13**, 227–235.

MOORE, E., & KUIPERS, L. (1992) Behavioural correlates of EE in staff patient interactions. *Social Psychiatry and Psychiatric Epidemiology*, **27**, 298–303.

——, BALL, R. A. & KUIPERS, L. (1992) Expressed emotion in staff working with the long-term adult mentally ill. *British Journal of Psychiatry*, **161**, 802–808.

NELSON, B., COLLINS, J., KREITMAN, N., ET AL (1970) Neurosis and marital interaction: II. Time-sharing and social activity. *British Journal of Psychiatry*, **117**, 47–58.

NOH, S. & TURNER, R. J. (1987) Living with psychiatric patients: implications for the mental health of family members. *Social Science and Medicine*, **25**, 263–272.

OLIVER, N. & KUIPERS, E. (1996) Stress and its relationship to EE in community mental health workers. *International Journal of Social Psychiatry*, **42**, 150–159.

OVENSTONE, I. M. K. (1973*a*) The development of neurosis in the wives of neurotic men. Part I: Symptomatology and personality. *British Journal of Psychiatry*, **122**, 33–43.

—— (1973*b*) The development of neurosis in the wives of neurotic men. Part 2: Marital role functions and marital tension. *British Journal of Psychiatry*, **122**, 711–717.

PAI, S. & KAPUR, R. L. (1981) The burden on the family of a psychiatric patient: development of an interview schedule. *British Journal of Psychiatry*, **138**, 332–335.

PENN, D. L. & MUESER, K. T. (1996) Research update of the psychosocial treatment of schizophrenia. *American Journal of Psychiatry*, **153**, 607–617.

PHAROAH, F. M., MARI, J. J. & STREINER, D. (2000) Family intervention for schizophrenia. Cochrane Review. *Cochrane Library*, Issue 2. Oxford: Update Software.

PLATT, S. (1985) Measuring the burden of psychiatric illness in the family: an evaluation of some rating scales. *Psychological Medicine*, **15**, 383–393.

——, WEYMAN, A. & HIRSCH, S. (1983) *Social Behaviour Assessment Schedule (SBA)* (3rd edn). Windsor, Berks: NFER, Nelson.

PRUDO, R. & BLUM, H. M. (1987) Five-year outcome and prognosis in schizophrenia: a report from the London Field Research Centre of the International Pilot Study of Schizophrenia. *British Journal of Psychiatry*, **150**, 345–354.

REYNOLDS, I., JONES, J. E., BERRY, D. W., ET AL (1990) A crisis team for the mentally ill: the effect on patients, relatives and admissions. *Medical Journal of Australia*, **152**, 646–652.

ROOKE, O. & BIRCHWOOD, M. (1998) Loss, humiliation and entrapment as appraisals of schizophrenic illness: A prospective study of depressed and non-depressed patients. *British Journal of Clinical Psychology*, **37**, 259–268.

ROSENVINGE, H., JONES, D., JUDGE, E., ET AL (1998) Demented and chronic depressed patients attending a day hospital: stress experienced by carers. *International Journal of Geriatric Psychiatry*, **13**, 8–11.

SALLEH, M. R. (1994) The burden of care of schizophrenia in Malay families. *Acta Psychiatrica Scandinavica*, **89**, 180–185.

SCAZUFCA, M. & KUIPERS, E. (1996) Links between expressed emotion and burden of care in relatives of patients with schizophrenia. *British Journal of Psychiatry*, **168**, 580–587.

—— & —— (1997) Impact on women who care for those with schizophrenia. *Psychiatric Bulletin*, **21**, 469–471.

SCHENE, A. H., TESSLER, R. C. & GAMACHE, G. M. (1994) Instruments measuring family or caregiver burden in severe mental illness. *Social Psychiatry and Psychiatric Epidemiology*, **29**, 228–240.

SMITH, J. & BIRCHWOOD, M. J. (1987) Specific and non-specific effects of educational intervention with families living with a schizophrenic relative. *British Journal of Psychiatry*, **150**, 645–652.

——, ——, COCHRANE, R., ET AL (1993) The needs of high and low expressed emotion families: a normative approach. *Social Psychiatry and Psychaitric Medicine*, **28**, 11–16.

STEVENS, B. (1972) Dependence of schizophrenic patients on elderly relatives. *Psychological Medicine*, **2**, 17–32.

SZMUKLER, G. I., HERRMAN, L., COLUSA, S., ET AL (1996*a*) Caring for relatives with serious mental illness: The development of Experience of Caregiving Inventory. *Social Psychiatry and Psychiatric Epidemiology*, **31**, 137–148.

——, ——, ——, ET AL (1996*b*) A controlled trial of a counselling intervention for caregivers of relatives with schizophrenia. *Social Psychiatry and Psychiatric Epidemiology*, **31**, 149–155.

TARRIER, N., BARROWCLOUGH, C., BAMRAH, J. S., ET AL (1988) The community management of schizophrenia: a controlled trial of behavioural intervention with families to reduce relapse. *British Journal of Psychiatry*, **153**, 532–542.

TESSLER, R. & GAMACHE, G. (1994) Continuity of care, residence, and family burden in Ohio. *Milbank Quarterly*, **72**, 149–169.

TOOK, M. & EVANS, T. (1990) *Provision of Community Services for Mentally Ill People and their Carers: A Survey for the Department of Health, the View of the Members of the NSF on Community Services*. London: NSF.

TUCKER, C., BARKER, A. & GREGOIRE, A. (1998) Living with schizophrenia: caring for a person with a severe mental illness. *Social Psychiatry and Psychiatric Epidemiology*, **33**, 305–309.

WATERS, M. A. & NORTHOVER, J. (1965) Rehabilitated long-stay schizophrenics in the community. *British Journal of Psychiatry*, **111**, 258–267.

WATTS, F. N. & BENNETT, D. H. (1983) *Theory and Practice of Psychiatric Rehabilitation*. Chichester: Wiley.

WATTS, S. (1988) *A Descriptive Investigation of the Incidence of High EE in Staff Working with Schizophrenic Patients in a Hospital Setting*. Unpublished dissertation for Diploma in Clinical Psychology. Leicester: British Psychological Society.

WING, J. K., MONCK, E., BROWN, G. W., ET AL (1964) Morbidity in the community of schizophrenic patients discharged from London mental hospitals in 1959. *British Journal of Psychiatry*, **110**, 10–21.

——, COOPER, J. E. & SARTORIUS, N. (1974) *The Measurement and Classification of Psychiatric Symptoms*. Cambridge: Cambridge University Press.

WYKES, T. & STURT, E. (1986) The measurement of social behaviour in psychiatric patients: an assessment of the reliability and validity of the SBS schedule. *British Journal of Psychiatry*, **148**, 1–11.

YARROW, M., CLAUSEN, J. & ROBBINS, P. (1955A) The social meaning of mental illness. *Journal of Social Issues*, **11**, 33–48.

——, SCHWARTZ, C. G., MURPHY, H. S., ET AL (1955*b*) The psychological meaning of mental illness in the family. *Journal of Social Issues*, **11**, 12–24.

20 Mental health needs of children and young people

ROBERT JEZZARD

Mental health needs assessment for children and young people is, as yet, an imprecise and complex science. In this chapter, I shall address definitions of need in this group, conceptual issues, measurement limitations, policy questions and epidemiological approaches to needs assessment. Subsequently, I shall examine the evidence base in this field, and shall use the example of assessing the mental health needs of young people at particular risk of developing problems to illustrate the relevant challenges.

I will argue that mental health needs assessment for children and young people should be a continuing and iterative process that is constantly revised as new information emerges. It is also a multi-agency activity that, to be effective, requires the participation of a range of commissioning authorities and service providers. It should incorporate a comprehensive range of needs from those related to mental health promotion and primary prevention affecting large groups of children to highly specialised needs of much smaller groups, such as those with complex neuropsychiatric problems. The apparently daunting nature of this task is probably sufficient to explain the current inadequacies in many authorities' needs assessments.

It is a task, therefore, that requires a pragmatic approach in the first instance, but it needs to be placed in an evolutionary framework that allows for constant refinement. Many important questions cannot yet be answered with precision, but gaps in knowledge and understanding both at national and local level are gradually being filled. Too often, needs assessment is seen as a one-off exercise that for reasons of incompleteness seems hard to utilise for service development.

The complexity and variable quality of the information that informs any needs assessment demands an approach that can provide structure to the process. Such a structure was specified by the National Health Service Management Executive (1991) as incorporating epidemiology, the evidence base and stakeholder views. However, it is arguable that an audit of resources and an assessment of service provision are also necessary components to feed into what is essentially a circular process.

It can be viewed as a jigsaw puzzle that can not be completed because there are pieces missing. Parts of the picture are more developed than others and some pieces do not seem to fit well together. To complicate matters further, the picture is changing over time and some pieces will need to be removed and new ones added. While this jigsaw may never be fully completed, there are enough pieces to work with. The first step is to lay out the pieces that are available to us.

Definition of need

"Need is at best a relative concept and the definition of need depends primarily upon those who undertake the identification and assessment effort" (Siegel *et al*, 1978). Within child and adolescent mental services (CAMHS), this statement is particularly pertinent in the light of the various views about the breadth of the concept of children's mental health and also the services that are needed to prevent, identify and treat child mental health problems.

The Handbook on Child and Adolescent Mental Health (Department of Health and Department of Education, 1995) set the policy context for CAMHS in England:

> "All people, agencies and services in contact with children have a part to play even though the promotion, maintenance and restoration of mental health may not be their prime purpose."

It is evident, therefore, that a mental health needs assessment for children and young people must take into account a wide range of opinions and multiple sources of information. Siegel *et al* (1978) described the exercise as a "co-operative venture within a human service network – a venture designed to enhance and monitor program integration, relevance, adequacy and planned change".

Concepts of mental health and ill health

Although the components of good mental health, as outlined in the NHS Health Advisory Service (HAS) thematic review, *Together We Stand* (1995), have acquired broad acceptance, there is not the same level of agreement about the concept of mental ill health in children and young people. The language used to describe and categorise children's problems varies, particularly between agencies, where it is the specific and different functions of each agency that often determine the way children's needs are grouped together (Kurtz, 1996). Even within specialist CAMHS, there are differences of view largely focused on the relative merits of the diagnostic *versus* the symptomatic or problem-oriented approach to categorisation. To some, the imposition of certain 'labels' to describe children's difficulties serves to medicalise what others would see as social or otherwise understandable phenomena and leads to the negative consequence of stigmatisation of the child. The issue of language can therefore present a significant challenge to a cooperative approach to mental health needs assessment. It needs to be understood that there is no perfect system of categorising children's mental health needs and that each has strengths and weaknesses and is better suited for some functions more than others.

Purpose

Given the complexity of assessing the mental health needs of a population, it is perhaps not so surprising that most services have not been established on the basis of need (Kurtz *et al*, 1994). Where a needs assessment has been undertaken, it has often not been used strategically for the development and improvement of services. An appreciation of its purpose is essential if it is to be both carried out well and used to maximum benefit.

Increased emphasis is now placed on improving the clinical and cost-effectiveness, efficiency and overall quality of public services. A strategic approach to the planning and development of services is now an essential requirement if these objectives are to be realised and, for CAMHS, if the mental health of children and young people is to improve. As Kurtz *et al* highlighted in the 1994 national survey, there are considerable variations in CAMHS around the country. These differences are ones of size, scope, composition and delivery; differences that are historical and rarely entirely logical. Now that CAMHS have been given a place on the NHS agenda, expectations are high and increased expenditure on services will be expected to deliver better outcomes for children and young people. This can only occur if service development is based upon sound information. No service currently meets all needs and need is usually estimated to be much in excess of potential sources of help (Subotsky, 1992). Coupled with this is increasing concern that for identified need, interventions are not always based upon the best evidence. While a needs assessment will not give all the answers, it is an essential starting point for rational decisions about service change, resource allocation and economic evaluation of services (Knapp, 1997). Priorities will still have to be determined, but preferably on a logical and considered basis.

Present situation

Since the 1994 survey, a number of other inquiries into CAMHS have been undertaken. The House of Commons Health Select Committee report (1997) recognised the efforts being made to improve services, but also voiced a number of concerns, particularly the relative paucity of nationally available information upon which to undertake strategic planning. Most recently, the Audit Commission published a report (1999) that does indicate that improvements have taken place, but that there is still more work to be done. Fifty per cent of the participating health authorities in this study considered their needs assessments to be just adequate or worse. Forty-four per cent of NHS trusts said that they had not been involved with their health authority in any assessment of needs. The degree to which other relevant stakeholders were involved also varied greatly. While the basis upon which services are now commissioned may be better than that outlined by Vanstraelen & Cottrell (1994), it is evident that there are still many shortcomings in the conduct of needs assessments. Whether this is related to the complexity of the task, the resources allocated to the process or a lack of appreciation of its importance is not clear. What is clear, however, is that there is an expectation that all relevant authorities should base their strategy for improving CAMHS on a mental health needs assessment.

The overall approach

As indicated in the introduction, the structure outlined by the NHS Management Executive (1991) has been the starting point for all the most comprehensive guides to mental health needs assessment for children and young people (HAS, 1995; Kurtz, 1996; Wallace *et al*, 1997). None has limited its attention to the three components alone, as to do so artificially detaches it from the process of utilising information for strategic planning, service improvement and priority setting.

Wallace *et al* (1997) highlight the multiple sources of information that should be incorporated and Kurtz (1996) emphasises the need for an iterative process or 'argument' to take place in order to integrate the information obtained. If services are provided within an inter-agency context, then a needs assessment must be an inter-agency exercise too (Epstein *et al*, 1996). The need for inter-agency collaboration has been readily illustrated by Zahner *et al* (1992). In their study of 6–11-year-old children, the information from both parents and teachers among others was needed to define the at-risk population.

Cohen & Eastman (1997), when describing needs assessments for mentally disordered offenders, also a complex group, recommended the use of a number of separate approaches in order to provide a range of perspectives that shed light on different aspects of need. The fact that perspectives of need vary depending on who is consulted further emphasises the importance of multiple informants.

Most of the available literature has given relatively little attention to two additional elements. First, an appreciation of the policy context in which CAMHS operates can provide information about the priorities of the day and therefore also some focus on important areas of need. This is relevant not only to individuals or groups of children and young people but also to the utilisation of the evidence base and the organisation and resource profile of services. Second, little attention has been given to needs assessment as a continuing exercise entailing a process akin to the audit cycle. Priorities change, the needs profile of a population can change and the evidence base continues to develop. As the methodologies for evaluating services also develop and the monitoring of outcomes becomes more of a component of day-to-day clinical activity, so too will this information need to feed back into the process of needs assessment. Likewise, resource availability must also be taken into account and provides a useful means of helping to identify unmet need (Kurtz, 1996).

The policy context

While national priorities for our public services are subject to change according to the political imperatives of the day, there are some themes that are likely to stand the test of time, for example:

(a) partnership and collaboration between agencies;
(b) the need for high-quality, clinically effective and cost-efficient services; and
(c) the importance of health gain.

Mental health promotion, prevention and early intervention have more recently gained additional prominence within the health and social agenda, and if increased investment in these aspects of mental health service provision is rewarded by a reduction in the prevalence of mental health problems, then these too are likely to remain. The evidence that this will be so is promising, but not conclusive, and gains in the short term will need to be sustained over longer periods than exist within most of the current evidence of effectiveness. Whether the social and environmental factors that appear to have played a part in the increase in psychosocial disorders in young people in the Western world over the past 50 years or so (Rutter & Smith, 1995) can be stemmed or even reversed by a re-orientation of services and changes in social policy remains to be seen. Whatever the success of preventive approaches, those children and young people with established problems will continue to require services, and as the evidence base for intervention improves so the requirement for specific service availability will increase.

Apart from the overarching policy determinants, there may be specific population groups that are given priority status, either at national or at local level. At the time of writing, concern about the mental health needs of both looked after children and young offenders has placed them high on the agenda for national action. At a local level, policy priorities may be targeted on other particular areas of need, for example refugee children from war-torn countries.

Finally, the policy framework set out for CAMHS needs to be taken into account. Currently, this is set out in a Department of Health handbook (1995) and further elaborated within the HAS thematic review (1995). Services are conceptualised as being provided in four tiers of provision. These tiers reflect the level of need, expertise required and organisational context in which services are provided. This concept is of value in helping to understand the process of needs assessment and the need to consider all levels of need from primary care through to highly specialist in-patient care. However, these tiers are not firm structures and neither children and young people nor those professionals providing services can be rigidly contained within a tier. Ideal services will allow a degree of movement and flexibility.

A full appreciation of the policy context will help to determine the manner in which a needs assessment is carried out, but becomes particularly important during the process of utilising the information in service planning.

Epidemiology

Jenkins (1998) has outlined the essential relevance of epidemiology and disability measurement in ensuring that development of policy and service planning is responsive to local needs. The relevance is at all levels of service provision and in all the contexts in which need may become apparent. However, prevalence figures from epidemiological surveys may vary. This is despite many studies both in the UK and from other countries in the world. Although a prevalence figure of up to 20% of children having moderate to severe mental health problems severe enough to require intervention is frequently quoted, figures both for overall prevalence and for each individual condition can vary widely. Sampling methods, types of measure employed and case definition profoundly affect these estimates (Brandenburg *et al*, 1990). Consideration also needs to be given to severity, perceived need for treatment and concordance of symptom reports by multiple informants. Prevalence figures for individual conditions are also not consistent across the age range, between genders and between communities with different demographic characteristics. Care must also be taken when information based upon identified patients is translated into the needs of a population (Summerfelt *et al*, 1997). In the survey of the Mental Health of Children and Adolescents in Great Britain (Meltzer *et al*, 2000), 10% of 5–15-year-olds were found to have a common mental disorder. This survey also provides information on a range of socio-demographic variables, the impact of the disorder on the child and family, and the use of services. It is the most comprehensive national epidemiological information available. Epidemiological data, while extremely important, does not provide certain answers, and figures based upon national estimates have to be adjusted according to local circumstances.

Rutter & Graham (1968) provided a useful definition of child psychiatric disorder:

> "An abnormality of emotion, behaviour or relationships which is developmentally inappropriate and of sufficient duration and severity to cause persistent suffering or handicap to the child and/ or distress or disturbance to the family or community."

This definition, however, relates to established conditions and does not necessarily address all problems that may be of concern to professionals and service users nor problems that may benefit from intervention early in their development. Severity and impairment are of course important issues to consider, but 'sub-threshold' disorders that do not fulfil diagnostic criteria in childhood may predict psychopathology in adolescence (Costello *et al*, 1999) and hence be a focus for prevention. This is particularly relevant for conduct disorders, but less so for emotional disorders, except to some degree in girls. Both diagnostic categories and elevated symptom scores have their place (Jensen & Watanabe, 1999), but there is a danger in reifying either.

Wallace *et al* (1997) addressed some of these difficulties by highlighting the importance of a number of dimensions that can be used to assess severity and by dividing the 'patterns of behaviour, emotions or relationships' that may be of concern to children, young people and others into problems and disorders, each of which in turn can be affected by the association of particular risk factors.

In each individual case, the characteristics, complexity and presence of risk factors in addition to diagnostic classification define the severity and likely need for service provision. An outline of the proposed core data as published by the Association for Child Psychology and Psychiatry (Berger *et al,* 1993) was developed in order to make it more possible for services to collect information that incorporates all these necessary elements. Also, being less dependent upon formal diagnosis, it has the advantage of being acceptable to a broader range of professional viewpoints. Despite this development, the most reliable epidemiological research data in the UK are still largely based upon the ICD–10 (World Health Organization (WHO), 1992), although there is also information about the prevalence of some of the more minor problems. A detailed account of the available epidemiological research is beyond the scope of this chapter but is comprehensively reviewed by Wallace *et al* (1997).

The quoted ranges for many problems and disorders are often quite large and reasons for this have already been outlined. While detailed and in-depth surveys from locality to locality are clearly unrealistic, there needs to be a mechanism for translating the available knowledge of prevalence within the research literature into locally relevant information. Some problems and disorders are more prevalent in populations with higher levels of psychosocial adversity, for example, conduct disorders and depression. Others are less linked to local demography. Hence, knowledge of both the prevalence of risk factors in any population and their relevance to specific conditions is required. Kurtz (1996) suggests that more use needs to be made of data about risk factors and provides a helpful summary of information sources. Morbidity indices such as those derived from Jarman (1983) are helpful, but do not necessarily sufficiently reflect the mental health needs of children and young people in a community.

Information about the numbers of children 'looked after', with statements of special educational need or who are in trouble with the law, for instance, enhances the local specificity of the needs assessment. By directly addressing the needs of such groups of children, not only is the overall assessment of needs likely to be more accurate, but also the opportunity arises to highlight a potential focus for service provision. Some mental health needs may be more effectively or easily met by shifting the emphasis from a focus on the individual or on specific disorders to groups of children at risk. A focus on children with special educational needs or those looked after by social services for instance is consonant with the manner in which education or social services are provided, hence creating greater opportunities for collaboration in the needs assessment. It also encourages some flexibility in the consideration of the needs, not only of individual children and young people, but also of the staff working with them and the institution as a whole. Specialist CAMHS are never likely to be able to meet all the mental health needs of children and young people, but they can assist other professionals in meeting those needs by offering consultation and training.

Relatively few studies exist on the prevalence of mental health problems for young people looked after by local authorities, although they have been long recognised as a vulnerable and needy group. There is, however, a much higher prevalence of mental health problems in this group than in those who are living at home. In one study (McCann *et al*, 1996), a number of young people with severe and potentially treatable disorders such as psychoses were identified in addition to a significant number with major depression and even more with conduct disorder. Comorbidity levels were high, which may account for some of the difficulties in helping these young people (Arcelus *et al*, 1999).

Young people who are at risk

A group of young people who tend not to access conventional mental health care but who also find difficulties in accessing it is the young homeless. Craig and colleagues (1996) undertook a longitudinal study of homeless young people in London and found that almost two-thirds of the homeless respondents were suffering from psychiatric disorder in the month prior to the first interview. Only 27% of those with psychiatric disorder in the past year had had any contact with mental health services.

Young offenders, also, as a group, are at higher risk of having a mental health problem and tend to have a low level of contact with primary health care, with many unregistered with a general practitioner (GP) (Dolan *et al*, 1999). Their mental health needs are neither well recognised and widely understood nor adequately met (Kurtz *et al*, 1998). It is only by looking at their needs as a group that the level of unmet need and the degree to which specialist and innovative service provision is required become appreciated. The development of youth offending teams will no doubt enhance the urgency for developments in ways of working with these young people.

The mental health needs of some children will demand very specific skills that are not likely to be readily available in most localities. Hearing-impaired children in schools for the deaf, for instance, have been found to have a prevalence of psychiatric disorder of up to 42% (Hindley, 1997). Hence, the presence of a special school for children with a sensory impairment may require specific attention in any needs assessment.

Whether it be about groups as defined above or about others such as the children of mentally ill parents, children with chronic illness or children excluded from school, such information can offer a number of advantages:

(a) it adds to the accuracy of the overall profile of need;
(b) it helps identify unmet need;
(c) it helps make epidemiological data more locally relevant; and
(d) it helps define types of service need.

The evidence base

In the face of finite resources and considerable unmet need, it is self-evident that resources must be used to the best effect and interventions be based upon the best evidence of effectiveness. The research base for CAMHS has improved considerably, but there are still many gaps, as there are in most areas of mental health and social care practice. Were services only to deliver interventions of proven effectiveness, then many children would be left without help and support.

The status of evidence-based medicine is itself under some scrutiny (Naylor, 1995; Black, 1998). Sackett & Rosenberg (1995) suggested that "the problem determines the nature and source of evidence to be sought" and that there needs to be an integration of clinical experience with evidence from systematic research. The complexity of some problems and their individual manifestations means that, for the present, the randomised controlled trial will not provide all the answers. Greenhalgh & Hurwitz (1999) maintain that the core clinical skills of listening, questioning and explaining may influence the outcome for the patient as much as the more scientific and technical aspects of treatment. Greenhalgh (1999) also described the dissonance that can occur when attempting to apply research findings in day-to-day clinical encounters if the 'narrative–interpretative paradigm' is ignored.

Where good evidence exists for the efficacy of interventions, it is usually based upon research into individual disorders for a particular age group, delivered by a particular type of therapist in a specific setting, and hence it may be difficult to generalise into day-to-day clinical practice (Kurtz, 1996). So, it is also important to monitor the effectiveness of interventions when applied in ordinary clinical settings, where multiple variables such as individual circumstances, comorbidity, the setting and resource availability have considerable influence.

The overall quality of the evidence base varies, and not simply because of the quality of the research. There are conflicting and uncertain findings to consider as well as the gaps. Target & Fonagy (1996) reviewed the evidence for a number of psychotherapeutic approaches for particular disorders in children and young people and the strength of evidence for particular treatments varies from disorder to disorder.

A number of other comprehensive reviews are available, such as that by Kazdin (1997), who looked at the evidence for psychosocial treatments for children with conduct disorder. As he points out, while problem-solving skills training, parent management training, functional family therapy and multi-systemic therapy are all promising treatments, many important questions remain unanswered. Likewise, a review of treatments for depression in children and adolescents (Harrington *et al*, 1998) pointed to increasing evidence for the value of cognitive–behavioural treatments for mild depressive disorders, promising evidence for interpersonal psychotherapy and encouraging evidence for the use of fluoxetine. However, it is also important to note that there is now little evidence to support the use of tricyclic antidepressants in adolescents, a piece of evidence no less important simply because it is negative.

There remains the question of what to do with young people with serious and complex problems but for whom evidence of effective interventions is entirely lacking. GPs in one survey (Jones & Bhadrinath, 1998) indicated that the issue of treatability did not affect their view of the prioritisation of a case if the problem presented was sufficiently anxiety-provoking. There will always be calls for 'something to be done', and for these children and other vulnerable groups care will be required to be provided by someone. Social services, in particular, care for many children and young people who are difficult to help, and CAMHS must take a share of the responsibility even if they do not have all the answers. In these situations, there are other effective outcomes to be considered. If those caring for severely disturbed children, whether formally or informally, are able to come to a common understanding of the child's difficulties, develop similar expectations and agree on future plans, then that in itself may be of sufficient value, even if major change in the child does not take place (Wiener *et al*, 1999).

In making use of the evidence base, we must place it in an ethical framework, learn from the science, integrate it with individual clinical expertise, adapt it to the circumstances and wishes of individual patients and the setting in which they are seen, and acknowledge not only what we know but what we do not know about a topic.

Stakeholder views

While epidemiological research aims to achieve objective evidence of prevalence and an evidence-based scientific validity for interventions, neither may count for much if they are out of tune with other perceptions of need and the demands of the stakeholders, whether they be referrers to CAMHS or the service users themselves. Appropriate weight should be given to epidemiology and the evidence base, but in addition the views of other relevant parties should be taken into account.

A needs assessment that, from the outset, is truly participatory is less likely to run into difficulties. None the less, most evidence points to perceptions of need showing considerable variation, even within single professional groups or between members within the same family. Experience of service usage too will have an impact upon expressed need, both positively and negatively, and will affect the demands made for particular types of service (HAS, 1995). For instance, a study of the perceptions of admission and outcome in a child psychiatric unit (Chessman *et al*, 1997) showed that there was a lack of congruence between parents and children's views, especially at the final interview. Hence, the incorporation of service users' perspectives is no straightforward matter. Where there appears to be little overlap between an objective assessment of need and the articulated demand for service provision, constructive dialogue and debate is required.

When such consultations do take place, important and enlightening information usually emerges and there are often common themes, for example concern about length of waiting lists, too many exclusion criteria for referrals and the inflexibility of service provision. A survey of primary case-workers in the USA indicated that many children needed school- and home-based services, and they further differentiated the service needs of female and male children. A survey conducted by the Health Education Authority (Aggleton *et al*, 1995) found that few young men expressed any confidence in the belief that talking about problems helped. The report concluded that creative and innovative approaches are required to reach young men. Low-cost opportunities for physical activity and creativity may be more appropriate to them than counselling. Fisher *et al* (1999) have formalised this approach and recommend the use of trained community development workers to contribute to locally focused needs assessments.

While local circumstances will vary, a certain amount is known already. GPs tend to be concerned that waiting times for assessment by specialist CAMHS are too long and that services often seem inaccessible to those for whom they have the greatest concern (Jones & Bhadrinath, 1998). Problems involving risk are a particular priority. Social services departments have also voiced similar concerns and feel that their particular needs to help discharge their statutory duties are not supported by child mental health professionals.

Service usage

Another way of assessing the views and perceptions of service users is to study the take-up and usage of services. A service that considers that it has been developed according to the best scientific evidence available, but that does not reach those who most need it is clearly not doing its job properly. Armbruster & Schwab-Stone (1994) studied the drop-outs from a child guidance clinic. They were higher among those of minority status and from single-parent families, and, being a US study, Medicaid status also had its impact. Severe disorder, maternal stress and high levels of socio-economic disadvantage were important predictors for treatment drop-outs in another study (Kazdin, 1991). It is important, however, not to generalise reasons for non-attendance and drop-out from treatment. Ubeysekara & Cox (1998) highlighted a number of reasons for non-attendance at a child psychiatric clinic, including improvement during the waiting period, financial and transportation problems, parental anxiety and poor preparation by referrers. Coulter (1998) emphasises the importance both of patients needing to be better informed and the need for ensuring that referrals are appropriate.

A study of overall use of health services by children and young people (Cooper *et al*, 1998) highlighted the importance of ethnicity. While there was no significant variation of service usage according to social class, Black Caribbean, Indian, Pakistani and Bangladeshi children and young people were less likely to use hospital in-patient and out-patient services than their White counterparts.

Information utilisation

As has been indicated earlier, the needs assessment process should be a circular process. The information about need must then be matched against the services, which may or may not be meeting that need, and the effectiveness of service delivery assessed. The more specific and defined the service, the easier this task is to perform. Hence, a specialist in-patient service for young people with psychoses can be described in some detail, costed and evaluated more readily than early intervention programmes for pre-school children with behavioural difficulties. The latter may be seen by a range of professionals in a range of agency settings offering a variety of different approaches, and the measurement of effectiveness is not only challenging but also a long-term task.

Mapping available resources within a specified area is clearly a multi-agency activity and needs to encompass generic agency services as well as specialist services. This will involve not only health, social services and education, but also the voluntary sector and other public services, such as those in the youth justice arena. A narrow and restricted viewpoint may lead to duplication of provision, and an unwarranted assumption about the activities of another agency may lead to the perpetuation of unmet need. For example, a defined need to provide treatment services for young people who have been convicted of sexually abusive behaviour may be being met within a voluntary sector project and may therefore not be a priority for service development. Likewise, an erroneous assumption that such a service is already being provided by the youth justice sector might mean that the needs of these young people are simply forgotten.

A degree of critical appraisal of current service provision will of course be required. The mere existence of a service does not mean that it is undertaking effective work or that it is using the best available evidence to guide its activity. Even the reassurance that a service evaluation is being undertaken may be insufficient reassurance if the methodologies are inappropriate or unsatisfactory.

References

AGGLETON, P., MCCLEAN, C., TAYLOR-LABOURN, A. T., ET AL (1995) *Young Men Speak Out: A Report to the Health Education Authority*. London: Health Education Authority.

ARCELUS, J., BELLERBY, T. & VOSTANIS, P. (1999) A mental health service for young people in the care of the local authority. *Clinical Child Psychology and Psychiatry*, **4**, 233–245.

ARMBRUSTER, P. & SCHWAB-STONE, M. E. (1994) Sociodemographic characteristics of drop-outs from a child guidance clinic. *Hospital and Community Psychiatry*, **45**, 804–808.

AUDIT COMMISSION (1999) *Children in Mind. Child and Adolescent Mental Health Services*. London: Audit Commission.

BERGER, M., HILL, P., SEIN, E., ET AL (1993) *A Proposed Core Date Set for Child and Adolescent Psychology and Psychiatric Services*. London: Association for Child Psychology and Psychiatry.

BLACK, D. (1998) The limiation of evidence. *Journal of the Royal College of Physicians*, **32**, 23–26.

BRANDENBURG, N. A., FRIEDMAN, R. M. & SILVER. S. E. (1990) The epidemiology of child psychiatric disorders: Prevalence findings from recent studies. *Journal of the American Academy of Child and Adolescent Psychiatry*, **29**, 76–83.

CHESSMAN, R., HARDING, L., HART, C., *ET AL* (1997) Do parents and children have common perceptions of admission, treatment and outcome in a child psychiatric unit? *Clinical Child Psychology and Psychiatry*, **2**, 251–270.

COHEN, A. & EASTMAN, N. (1997) Needs assessment for mentally disordered offenders and others requiring similar services. Theoretical issues and a methodological framework. *British Journal of Psychiatry*, **171**, 412–416.

COOPER, H., SMAJE, C. & ABER, S. (1998) Use of health services by children and young people according to ethnicity and social class: secondary analysis of a national survey. *British Medical Journal*, **317**, 1047–1051.

COSTELLO, E. J., ANGOLD, A. & KEELER, G. P. (1999) Adolescent outcomes of childhood disorders: the consequences of severity and impairment. *Journal of the American Academy of Child and Adolescent Psychiatry*, **38**, 121–128.

COULTER, A. (1998) Managing demand at the interface between primary and secondary care. *British Medical Journal*, **316**, 1974–1976.

CRAIG, T. K. J., HODSON, S., WOODWARD, S., *ET AL* (1996) *Off to a Bad Start. A Longitudinal Study of Homeless Young People in London.* London: Mental Health Foundation.

DEPARTMENT OF HEALTH AND DEPARTMENT FOR EDUCATION (1995) *A Handbook on Child and Adolescent Mental Health.* London: Department of Health.

DOLAN, M., HOLLOWAY, J., BAILEY, S., *ET AL* (1999) Health status of juvenile offenders. A survey of young offenders appearing before the juvenile courts. *Journal of Adolescence*, **22**, 137–144.

EPSTEIN, M. H., QUINN, K., CUMBLAD, C., *ET AL* (1996) Needs assessment of community-based services for children and youth with emotional or behavioral disorders and their families: Part 1. A conceptual model. *Journal of Mental Health Administration*, **23**, 418–431.

FISHER, B., NEVE, H. & HERITAGE, Z. (1999) Community development, user involvement and primary health care. *British Medical Journal*, **318**, 749–750.

GREENHALGH, T. (1999) Narrative based medicine in an evidence based world. *British Medical Journal*, **318**, 323–325.

—— & HURWITZ, B. (1999) Why study narrative? *British Medical Journal*, **318**, 48–50.

HARRINGTON, R., WHITTAKER, J. & SHOEBRIDGE, P. (1998) Psychological treatment of depression in children and adolescents. A review of treatment research. *British Journal of Psychiatry*, **173**, 291–298.

HAWTON, K., FAGG, J., SIMKIN, S., *ET AL* (1997) Trends in deliberate self-harm in Oxford, 1985–1995. Implications for clinical services and the prevention of suicide. *British Journal of Psychiatry*, **171**, 556–560.

HEALTH ADVISORY SERVICE (1995) *Together We Stand: The Commissioning, Role and Management of Child and Adolescent Mental Health Services.* London: HMSO.

HINDLEY, P. (1997) Psychiatric aspects of hearing impairment. *Journal of Child Psychology and Psychiatry*, **38**, 101–117.

HOUSE OF COMMONS HEALTH SELECT COMMITTEE (1997) *Child and Adolescent Mental Health Services: Report from the Health Select Committee. Session 1996–1997.* HC 26-1. London: The Stationery Office.

JARMAN, B. (1983) Identification of underprivileged areas. *British Medical Journal*, **286**, 1705–1709.

JENKINS, R. (1998) Linking epidemiology and disability measurement with mental health service policy and planning. *Epidemiologia e Psichiatria Sociale*, **7**, 120–126.

JENSEN, P. S. & WATANABE, H. (1999) Sherlock Holmes and child psychopathology assessment approaches: the case of the false positive. *Journal of the American Academy of Child and Adolescent Psychiatry*, **38**, 138–146.

JONES, S. M. & BHADRINATH, B. R. (1998) GPs' views on prioritisation of child and adolescent mental health problems. *Psychiatric Bulletin*, **22**, 484–486.

KAZDIN, A. E. (1991) The effectiveness of psychotherapy with children and adults. *Journal of Consulting and Clinical Psychology*, **59**, 785–798.

—— (1997) Psychosocial treatments for conduct disorder in children. *Journal of Child Psychology and Psychiatry*, **38**, 161–178.

KNAPP, M. (1997) Economic evaluations and interventions for children and adolescents with mental health problems. *Journal of Child Psychology and Psychiatry*, **38**, 3–25.

KURTZ, Z. (1996) *Treating Children Well: A Guide to Using the Evidence Base in Commissioning and Managing Services for the Health of Children and Young People*. London: Mental Health Foundation.

——, THORNES, R. & WOLKIND, S. (1994) *Services for the Mental Health of Children and Young People in England. A National Review*. London: Maudsley Hospital and South Thames (West) Regional Health Authority.

——, THORNES, R. & BAILEY, S. (1998) Children in the criminal justice and secure care systems: how their mental health needs are met. *Journal of Adolescence*, **21**, 543–553.

MCCANN, J. B., JAMES, A., WILSON, S., *ET AL* (1996) Prevalence of psychiatric disorders in young people in the care system. *British Medical Journal*, **313**, 1529–1530.

MELTZER, H., GATWARD, R., GOODMAN, R., *ET AL* (2000) *Mental Health of Children and Adolescents in Great Britain*. ONS. London: The Stationery Office.

MENTAL HEALTH FOUNDATION (1999) *Bright Futures: Promoting Children and Young Peoples's Mental Health*. London: Mental Health Foundation.

NHS MANAGEMENT EXECUTIVE (1991) *Assessing Health Care Needs: A DHA Project Discussion Paper*. London: Department of Health.

NAYLOR, C. D. (1995) Grey zones of clinical practice; some limits to evidence-based medicine. *The Lancet*, **345**, 840–842.

RUTTER, M. & GRAHAM, P. (1968) The reliability and validity of the psychiatric assessment of the child: I. Interview with the child. *British Journal of Psychiatry*, **114**, 563–579.

—— & SMITH, D. (1995) *Psychosocial Disorders in Young People: Time Trends and their Causes*. Chichester: John Wiley & Sons.

SACKETT, D. L. & ROSENBERG, W. M. (1995) On the need for evidence-based medicine. *Journal of Public Health Medicine*, **17**, 330–334.

SIEGEL, L. M., ATTKISSON, C. & CARSON, L. G. (1978) Need identification and program planning in the community context. In *Evaluation of Human Service Programs* (eds C. Atkisson, W. A. Hargreaves, M. J. Horowitz, *et al*), pp. 215–252. New York: Academic Press.

SUBOTSKY, F. (1992) Psychiatric treatment for children – the organisation of services. *Archives of Diseases in Childhood*, **67**, 971–975.

SUMMERFELT, W. M. T., SALZER, M. S. & BICKMAN, L. (1997) Interpreting differential rates of service use: Avoiding myopia. *Clinical Child Psychology and Psychiatry*, **2**, 591–595.

TARGET, M. & FONAGY, P. (1996) The psychological treatment of child and adolescent psychiatric disorders. In: *What Works for Whom? A Critical Review of Psychotherapy Research* (eds A. Roth & P. Fonagy), pp. 263–320. New York: Guilford Press.

UBEYSEKARA, A. & COX, N. (1998) Attendance at child psychiatric clinics. *Psychiatric Bulletin*, **22**, 435–437.

VANSTRAELEN, M. & COTTRELL, D. (1994) Child and adolescent mental health services: purchaser's knowledge and plans. *British Medical Journal*, **309**, 259–261.

WALLACE, S. A., CROWN, J. M., BERGER, M., *ET AL* (1997) Child and adolescent mental health. In: *Health Care Needs Assessment: Second Series* (eds A. Stevens & J. Raftery), pp. 55–128. Oxford: Radcliffe Medical Press

WIENER, A., WITHERS, K., PATRICK, M., *ET AL* (1999) What changes are of value in severely disturbed children? *Clinical Child Psychology and Psychiatry*, **4**, 201–213.

WORLD HEALTH ORGANIZATION (1992) *International Statistical Classification of Diseases and Related Health Problems. Tenth revision (ICD–10)*. Geneva: WHO.

ZAHNER, G. E. P., PAWELKIEWICZ, W., DE FRANCESCO, J. J., *ET AL* (1992) Children's mental health service needs and utilization patterns in urban community: An epidemiological assessment. *Journal of the American Academy of Child and Adolescent Psychiatry*, **31**, 951–960.

21 Measurement of needs in people with learning disabilities and mental health problems

KIRIAKOS XENITIDIS and NICK BOURAS

The increased risk of people with learning disabilities to develop mental health problems compared with the general population has only in recent years become the focus of interest among mental health professionals. The reasons are mainly historical. Many professionals believed that people with learning disabilities were not capable of developing mental illness like the rest of the population. The behavioural disorders frequently exhibited by people with learning disabilities were attributed entirely to their impaired cognitive development (Schroeder *et al*, 1979). However, in recent years, consensus has emerged that learning disabilities and mental illness can coexist and that people with learning disabilities can develop a wide range of mental health problems (Eaton & Menolascino, 1982; Sovner & Hurley, 1983; Reiss, 1988*a*, 1994).

Reports on the prevalence of mental health problems in people with learning disabilities vary from less than 10% to more than 80% (Borthwick-Duffy, 1994). The main reasons for this wide discrepancy are the different criteria applied in defining 'learning disabilities' and 'mental health problems', and the diversity of study samples used (Crews *et al*, 1994).

It is important to note that 'learning disabilities' is the term currently used in the UK to describe the group of people exhibiting a combination of low intelligence quotient (IQ) and substantially impaired adaptive behaviour. 'Mental handicap', 'intellectual disability', 'developmental disabilities' and 'mental impairment' are other terms currently in use. 'Mental retardation' is the term used in both major psychiatric classification systems, ICD–10 (World Health Organization (WHO), 1992) and DSM–IV (American Psychiatric Association (APA), 1994).

Service provision

The extensive de-institutionalisation programmes for people with learning disabilities, which have been implemented in the USA, the UK and other parts of the world during the past two decades, have raised important issues relating to the delivery of services (Bouras & Holt, 2001). Jacobson (1999), in the USA, reported a fall of 46% in the institutional population of people with learning disabilities, while Emerson & Hatton (1998) predicted that in the UK over 40 000 people with learning disabilities would have been resettled in the community by the year 2000. Two fairly recent national surveys in the UK revealed widespread deficits in local service planning and a variety of unmet mental health needs for people with learning disabilities (Gravestock & Bouras, 1997; Bailey & Cooper, 1998). The resettlement of adults with learning disabilities from large institutions to smaller residences in the community was accelerated in the UK with the implementation of the National Health Service (NHS) and Community Care Act (House of Commons, 1990), which also distinguished between 'social care' and 'health care'. The intention was that social services departments would provide social care, and health care would be provided by health services. However, the distinction between social care and health care is not clear cut for people with learning disabilities and the majority of service providers are currently operating a mixed care system. Furthermore, more recently there has been an increasing tendency for services for people with learning disabilities to be commissioned jointly by social and health services (Department of Health, 2001).

Needs assessment

Policy changes under the new legal framework highlighted the concept of needs assessment. It became a statutory duty for social services to assess the needs of people, including those with learning disabilities, who may require community care. One of the main aims of the needs assessment approach is to shift care provision from being service-led or demand-led to being needs-led, and thus to enhance the link between individual clinical practice and health gain at a population level (Stevens & Raftery, 1994). Financial cost is an important dimension of population-based needs assessment and it is estimated that in relation to adults with learning disabilities, the NHS has spent over £1.4 billion on services; in addition, local authorities have spent approximately £1.6 billion (Department of Health, 2001).

Although there seems to be agreement about the importance of providing services according to need, there is a lack of consensus about the definition of need, and this issue is dealt with in detail in other parts of this book. Among the most relevant definitions of need for people with learning disabilities are "the requirement of individuals to enable them to achieve acceptable quality of life" (Department of Health Social Services Inspectorate, 1991) and "a problem which can benefit from an existing intervention" (Stevens & Gabbay, 1991). People with learning disabilities often have a complex constellation of difficulties commonly referred to as 'special needs'. It has not, however, been established whether either the 'quality of life' or 'ability to benefit' (or indeed any other) approach contains the necessary and sufficient information for defining need in this population. In addition, there is a lack of agreement as to who should assess need. Mooney (1986) suggests, from a health economics point of view, that need can only be assessed by professionals, whereas others (Bradshaw, 1972) use a sociological perspective to argue that individuals' assessments of their own needs are valid as 'felt' and 'expressed' needs. Slade (1994) highlighted, in the context of mental health services, the importance of taking users' views into account, especially if they differ significantly from those of their carers or the professionals. The concept of mental health needs in people with learning disabilities was reviewed by Gravestock (1999).

A number of instruments have been developed to measure mental health problems and/or needs in people with learning disabilities. These instruments can be divided into the following broad categories.

Assessment and diagnostic instruments

The most commonly used instruments include:

(a) The Psychopathology Instrument for Mentally Retarded Adults (PIMRA; Kazdin *et al*, 1983), which focuses on psychiatric symptoms and is available in self-report and informant versions.
(b) The Aberrant Behaviour Checklist (ABC; Aman *et al*, 1985), which is a research-oriented checklist of behavioural problems, originally developed for measurement of treatment outcome.
(c) The Reiss Screen for Maladaptive Behaviour (Reiss, 1988*b*), which is a screening instrument for behavioural problems.
(d) The Psychiatric Assessment Schedule for Adults with Developmental Disabilities (PAS–ADD; Moss *et al*, 1998), which is a psychopathology measure based on the Present State Examination tradition (Wing *et al*, 1974).

Service needs instruments

The following are examples of commonly used instruments:

(a) The Hampshire Assessment for Living with Others (HALO; Shackleton-Bailey & Pidcock, 1983), which was developed for the purpose of planning for residential placement and training needs of children and adults with learning disabilities.

(b) The Vineland Social Maturity Scale (Doll, 1965), which was designed to assist the development of individual care programmes for children and adults with learning disabilities.

(c) The Disability Assessment Schedule (DAS; Holmes *et al*, 1982), which is a rating scale completed through interview with an informant and assesses the level of impairment in 12 life domains for the purpose of planning of placement and management.

(d) The Adaptive Behaviour Scale (ABS; Nihira *et al*, 1974), which was developed for individual programme planning and evaluation of services. It is divided in two parts: Part I (adaptive behaviour) assesses the individual's functioning in 10 life domains and Part II assesses maladaptive behaviour and examines 14 specific types of behaviour.

The instruments mentioned above either measure mental health or behavioural problems or indirectly assess service needs of people with learning disabilities. However, several of them are lengthy and require special training for their administration. Also, most of them are completed by professionals only and do not take into consideration the views of service users or their carers.

The Camberwell Assessment of Need for Adults with Developmental and Intellectual Disabilities (CANDID; Xenitidis *et al*, 2000) was developed in order to fill the existing gap in measuring needs for people with learning disabilities and mental health problems.

Development of the CANDID

The CANDID was developed by modifying the Camberwell Assessment of Need (CAN; Phelan *et al*, 1995) to address specifically the needs of adults with learning disabilities and mental health problems. As with the CAN, the following pre-development criteria were set, that it should:

(a) have known and acceptable validity and reliability;

(b) be brief and suitable for use by a range of professionals;

(c) require no formal training;

(d) record the points of view of service users, informal carers and staff;

(e) measure met and unmet need;

(f) measure the help provided by informal carers and services separately; and

(g) be suitable for use in research and clinical practice.

The questions in each need area of the CANDID are divided into four sections:

(a) Section I assesses the absence or presence of need and, if need is present, whether it is met or not met.

(b) Section II rates the help received from informal carers.

(c) Section IIIa asks about how much help local services are *providing* and IIIb about how much help the respondent believes that the person *needs* from local services.

(d) Section IV enquires about the respondent's satisfaction with the *type* (IVa) and *amount* (IVb) of help received from local services.

Development process

Focus groups of service users, informal carers and staff were conducted that identified broad areas of needs relevant to people with learning disabilities and mental health problems. Health and social services professionals with expertise in working with adults with learning disabilities and mental health problems were consulted and invited to make comments on the first draft. On the basis of these consultations, the second draft was developed, comprising 25 areas of needs. This was then subjected to reliability testing. The term 'developmental and intellectual disabilities' was preferred over the ambiguous official UK term 'learning disabilities' to make clear the target population of the instrument when used outside the UK, where a range of designations are used for this group of people.

Validity studies

Content validity

A questionnaire was designed to enquire about the views of service users (*n*=45) and their informal carers on the list of need areas identified through the process described above. They were asked to score on a scale of 1–3 each need area according to its relevance and importance, and also to suggest any additional items that should have been included. Adults with a range of learning disabilities and additional mental health problems were included in this sample. For those with a level of learning disabilities severe enough to interfere significantly with the comprehension of the questionnaire, this was completed by the carers alone. All 45 users and carers approached responded to the questionnaire. Following the survey, a total score, the sum of the individual respondents' score for each need item, was calculated. No additional items were consistently suggested by more than two respondents.

Consensual validity

Fifty-five experts in the field of mental health in learning disabilities were targeted on a national level in the UK. They were selected from a range of professional backgrounds including nursing, psychiatry, clinical psychology, public health, speech and language therapy, social work, physiotherapy and occupational therapy. Their opinions were sought on the content, language and structure of the draft instrument. Forty-five out of the 55 experts who were approached responded by completing and returning a postal questionnaire. As far as the content of the instrument was concerned, no item was rated as irrelevant or redundant by more than one respondent. Apart from 'Communication', no other need item was consistently suggested for inclusion in the scale by more than two respondents.

Criterion validity

No 'gold standard' instrument exists currently for the assessment of needs of people with learning disabilities and mental health problems. In order to establish the *concurrent validity* of the CANDID in relation to external criteria, two standardised tools were used: the DAS (Holmes *et al*, 1982), and the Global Assessment of Functioning (GAF; APA, 1994). For the estimation of concurrent validity, the CANDID summary scores (total number of needs) were compared with the total DAS and GAF scores. In both DAS and GAF, the higher the score the higher the level of functioning, whereas a high score on the CANDID indicates a high level of high need. Both correlations were statistically significant and the Spearman's P correlation coefficients were −33 ($P<0.05$) and −47 ($P<0.01$) respectively.

Reliability

In total, 40 service users were enrolled in the reliability study from two separate learning disabilities mental health services, one community-based and one in-patient service, from two NHS trusts. Their characteristics are shown in Table 21.1. The total number of needs (mean ±s.d.) per service user identified by the member of staff ($n=40$) during the first interview was 13.98±2.97 (95% CI 13.03–14.92). This was almost identical with that identified by the informal carer ($n=27$) (14.10±2.34; 95% CI 13.11–14.96) and both were higher

TABLE 21.1
Characteristics of patients enrolled in the reliability study (n=40)

Age in years, mean (range)	37.5	(20.0–67.0)
Gender, *n* (%)		
Male	27	(67.5)
Female	13	(32.5)
Ethnic origin, *n* (%)		
Caucasian	38	(95.0)
Afro-Caribbean	1	(2.5)
Asian	1	(2.5)
Patient status, *n* (%)		
Out-patient	15	(37.5)
In-patient	9	(22.5)
Residential	6	(40.0)
Level of learning disability, *n* (%)		
Mild	26	(65.0)
Moderate	19	(22.5)
Severe/profound	5	(12.5)
Living situation, *n* (%)		
Alone	2	(5.0)
With partner	2	(5.0)
With parents	9	(22.5)
With others	27	(67.5)
Marital status, *n* (%)		
Single	37	(92.5)
Married	3	(7.5)
Clinical conditions, *n* (%)		
Psychotic illness	20	(50.0)
Autism	10	(25.0)
Epilepsy	11	(27.5)

than the user's ($n=31$) assessment of their own needs (11.55 ± 2.51; 95% CI 10.63–12.47). The ratings of carers and staff did not differ significantly, whereas the difference between the ratings of users and carers as well as between users and staff were significant ($P<0.01$). Table 21.2 shows the needs assessment results of the reliability study sample.

Five interviewers/raters were used: a psychiatrist, an occupational therapist, a social worker and two nurses (one with general psychiatric and one with learning disabilities training). The second raters rated the interviews either live or from audiotape. Interviewing the service user, his or her informal carer and the member of staff took on average approximately 1.5 hours.

TABLE 21.2
Assessment of need for the 25 areas of the CANDID

		No serious need		Met need		Unmet need		Not known	
Area of need		n	%	n	%	n	%	n	%
1	Accommodation	0.0	0.0	36.0	90.0	4.0	10.0	0.0	0.0
2	Food	1.0	2.5	38.0	95.0	0.0	0.0	1.0	2.5
3	Looking after the home	6.0	15.0	30.0	75.0	2.0	5.0	2.0	5.0
4	Self-care	6.0	15.0	33.0	82.5	0.0	0.0	1.0	2.5
5	Daytime activities	3.0	7.5	33.0	82.5	4.0	10.0	0.0	0.0
6	General physical health	22.0	55.0	18.0	45.0	0.0	0.0	0.0	0.0
7	Eyesight and hearing	24.0	60.0	16.0	40.0	0.0	0.0	0.0	0.0
8	Mobility	35.0	87.5	5.0	12.5	0.0	0.0	0.0	0.0
9	Seizures	32.0	80.0	7.0	17.5	1.0	2.5	0.0	0.0
10	Major mental health problems	21.0	52.5	16.0	40.0	3.0	7.5	0.0	0.0
11	Minor mental health problems	6.0	15.0	28.0	70.0	6.0	15.0	0.0	0.0
12	Information	28.0	70.0	8.0	20.0	0.0	0.0	4.0	10.0
13	Safety to self	21.0	52.5	17.0	42.5	2.0	5.0	0.0	0.0
14	Exploitation risk	11.0	27.5	27.0	67.5	2.0	5.0	0.0	0.0
15	Safety to others	18.0	45.0	14.0	35.0	8.0	20.0	0.0	0.0
16	Inappropriate behaviour	20.0	50.0	16.0	40.0	4.0	10.0	0.0	0.0
17	Substance misuse	37.0	92.5	3.0	7.5	0.0	0.0	0.0	0.0
18	Communication	20.0	50.0	18.0	45.0	2.0	5.0	0.0	0.0
19	Social relationships	6.0	15.0	26.0	65.0	7.0	17.5	0.0	0.0
20	Sexual expression	25.0	62.5	10.0	25.0	4.0	10.0	1.0	2.5
21	Caring for someone else	37.0	92.5	1.0	2.5	2.0	5.0	0.0	0.0
22	Basic education	3.0	7.5	27.0	67.5	8.0	20.0	2.0	5.0
23	Transport	6.0	15.0	28.0	70.0	4.0	10.0	2.0	2.0
24	Money budgeting	3.0	7.5	18.0	45.0	18.0	45.0	1.0	2.5
25	Welfare benefits	20.0	50.0	4.0	10.0	1.0	2.5	15.0	37.5

Data from staff interviews were used (*n*=40).

Overall reliability

Intra-class correlations between summary scores of the two raters (for interrater reliability) and at two points in time T_1 and T_2 (for test–retest reliability) were calculated using variance components analysis. For interrater reliability, the overall intra-class correlation coefficient (r) for the total number of needs was 0.93 for user ratings, 0.90 for carer ratings and 0.97 for staff ratings. For test–retest reliability, the coefficient was 0.71, 0.69 and 0.86 respectively. On the basis of paired *t*-tests, there was no evidence of relative bias between the two time points or between live and taped interviews. In addition to total number of needs (Section I), the interrater and test–retest reliability of the summary scores for Sections II, III and IVa of the CANDID were calculated. The correlations were generally higher for interrater than test–retest reliability and the results are shown in Table 21.3.

Item-by-item reliability

Interrater and test–retest reliability were also examined for each need item individually and two measures of agreement calculated: percentage of complete agreement and k coefficients. For interrater reliability, the range of complete agreement on exact rating was 71–100% for users, 85.1–100% for carers and 77.5–100% for staff. For test–retest reliability the range was 58.3–100% for users, 66.6–100% for carers and 71–100% for staff. Table 21.4 shows the percentages of complete agreement and k coefficients for each need item.

TABLE 21.3
Test–retest interrater reliability for the CANDID

CANDID section	Type of reliability	User ratings	Carer ratings	Staff ratings
I (total number of needs)	Test–retest	0.71	0.69	0.86
	Interrater	0.93	0.90	0.97
II (help given by relatives/friends)	Test–retest	0.93	0.95	0.96
	Interrater	0.96	0.91	0.96
IIIa (help given by services	Test–retest	0.75	0.90	0.88
	Interrater	0.98	0.96	0.92
IIIb (help needed by services)	Test–retest	0.72	0.87	0.84
	Interrater	0.94	0.93	0.94
IVa (right kind of help?)	Test–retest	0.65	0.76	0.64
	Interrater	0.84	0.86	0.88

TABLE 21.4

Interrater and test–retest reliability for identification of need in the 25 areas of the CANDID

Item	User Interrater (n=31) %	k	User Test–retest (n=24) %	k	Carer Interrater (n=27) %	k	Carer Test–retest (n=21) %	k	Staff Interrater (n=40) %	k	Staff Test–retest (n=31) %	k
1 Accommodation	90.3	*	87.5	*	96.3	*	95.2	*	97.5	0.84	96.8	0.84
2 Food	93.5	0.77	95.8	0.78	96.3	0.79	100.0	1.0	90.0	0.33	96.8	*
3 Looking after the home	90.4	0.74	83.3	0.50	100.0	1.00	85.7	*	100.0	1.00	90.3	0.63
4 Self-care	93.6	0.87	66.6	0.29	100.0	1.00	100.0	1.00	100.0	1.00	93.5	0.48
5 Daytime activities	90.4	0.76	75.0	*	92.6	0.80	95.2	0.78	92.5	0.77	87.1	0.44
6 General physical health	96.8	0.91	95.8	0.88	96.3	0.91	90.4	0.80	100.0	1.00	90.3	0.81
7 Eyesight and hearing	93.5	0.87	87.5	73.00	96.3	0.93	95.2	0.91	97.5	0.95	96.8	0.92
8 Mobility	96.8	0.96	95.8	0.78	96.3	0.91	90.5	0.77	100.0	1.00	100.0	1.00
9 Seizures	100.0	1.00	95.8	0.88	100.0	1.00	100.0	1.00	100.0	1.00	96.7	91.00
10 Major mental health problems	96.8	0.94	75.0	0.54	92.5	0.86	81.0	0.64	92.5	0.87	77.4	0.61
11 Minor mental health problems	87.1	0.77	70.8	0.46	85.1	0.75	71.4	0.47	92.5	0.82	83.9	0.70

12 Information	83.8	0.75	62.6	0.40	100.0	1.00	66.6	0.50	100.0	1.00	87.0	0.68
13 Safety to self	87.1	0.70	75.0	0.47	96.3	0.93	100.0	1.00	97.5	0.96	93.6	0.88
14 Exploitation risk	90.4	0.89	87.5	0.73	85.2	0.73	71.5	0.46	100.0	1.00	87.1	0.71
15 Safety to others	90.3	0.80	83.3	0.64	93.6	0.86	90.5	0.82	95.0	0.92	83.9	0.75
16 Inappropriate behaviour	96.8	0.96	87.5	0.68	96.3	0.93	71.4	0.48	100.0	1.00	77.5	0.62
17 Substance misuse	96.7	0.96	91.7	0.46	100.0	1.00	95.2	0.50	97.5	0.82	100.0	1.00
18 Communication	96.8	0.94	83.3	0.69	92.6	0.87	81.0	0.66	97.5	0.95	80.6	0.65
19 Social relations	93.6	0.89	70.8	0.48	92.6	0.85	90.4	0.76	95.0	0.90	74.2	0.93
20 Sexual expression	100.0	1.00	75.0	*	92.6	0.86	81.0	0.53	90.0	0.81	87.2	0.82
21 Caring for someone else	100.0	1.00	95.9	0.66	100.0	1.00	100.0	1.00	100.0	1.00	100.0	1.00
22 Basic education	87.1	0.77	79.1	0.77	88.8	0.81	80.9	0.70	77.5	0.60	71.0	0.47
23 Transport	87.1	0.70	79.2	0.52	92.6	0.72	100.0	1.00	95.0	0.90	93.6	0.86
24 Money budgeting	71.0	0.58	79.2	0.62	85.1	0.72	76.2	0.53	90.0	0.83	74.2	0.53
25 Welfare benefits	93.6	0.90	58.3	0.29	88.8	0.78	90.5	0.79	95.0	0.92	90.3	0.84

* Kappa coefficients were not calculated because of one variable being a constant, distribution highly skewed or size too small.

Kappa values in the range of 0.81–1.00 indicate 'almost perfect' agreement, 0.61–0.80 'substantial' agreement and 0.41–0.60 'moderate' agreement (Landis & Koch, 1977). Kappa values in some instances were very low despite high complete agreement. Examination of the raw data in such instances showed that this was owing to a highly skewed distribution of scores. This difficulty with misleading κ values has been recognised before and is discussed in Feinstein & Cicchetti (1990).

Conclusions

The assessment of needs for people with learning disabilities and mental health problems has become increasingly important, especially under the current trends of joint commissioning of social and health services. There is a lack of standardised instruments for the assessment of needs of this group of people. The CANDID is brief and easy to administer by staff from different professional backgrounds and it does not require formal training for its administration. It measures met and unmet needs, and records the contribution of formal services and informal carers in meeting needs. It assesses the views of the service users themselves, their informal carers and members of staff involved in their care.

The CANDID can be used as a tool for planning services for people with learning disabilities at an individual level (shaping individualised care plans) and, with the use of aggregated data, at a population level (designing a service in a geographical area). It can be used to facilitate local authorities' statutory obligation for needs assessment under the NHS and Community Care Act (1990). It can also be used, as an audit or research tool, in conjunction with the Health of the Nation Outcome Scales (HoNOS; Wing *et al*, 1998) to evaluate the effectiveness of specific therapeutic interventions. A modified version of the HoNOS for people with learning disabilities (HoNOS–LD) has been developed (Royal College of Psychiatrists, 2000).

The findings of the CANDID validity and reliability study suggest that this instrument has acceptable validity and reliability when used under research conditions. More data is required on its clinical utility and feasibility that will be established with its longer-term application in routine clinical settings.

References

AMAN, M. G., SIGN, N. N., STEWART, A. W., *ET AL* (1985) The Aberrant Behavior Checklist: A behavior rating scale for the assessment of treatment effects. *American Journal of Mental Deficiency*, **89**, 485–491.

AMERICAN PSYCHIATRIC ASSOCIATION (1994) *Diagnostic and Statistical Manual of Mental Disorders. 4th edition. (DSM–IV).* Washington, DC: APA.

AUDIT COMMISSION (1992) *Community Care: Managing the Cascade of Care.* London: HMSO.

BAILEY, N. M. & COOPER, S.-A. (1998) NHS beds for people with learning disabilities. *Psychiatric Bulletin,* **22**, 69–72.

BORTHWICK-DUFFY, S. A. (1994) Epidemiology and prevalence of psychopathology in people with mental retardation. *Journal of Consulting and Clinical Psychology,* **62**, 17–27.

BOURAS, N. & HOLT, G. (2001) Community mental health services for adults with learning disabilities. In: *Community Psychiatry* (ed. G. Thornicroft & G. Szmukler), pp. 397–408. Oxford: Oxford University Press.

BRADSHAW, J. (1972) A taxonomy of social need. In: *Problems and Progress in Medical Care: Essays on Current Research* (ed. G. McLachlan). Oxford: Oxford University Press.

CREWS, D. W., BONAVENTURA, S. & ROWE, F. (1994) Dual diagnosis: Prevalence of psychiatric disorders in a large state residential facility for individuals with mental retardation. *American Journal on Mental Retardation,* **98**, 688–731.

DEPARTMENT OF HEALTH (2001) *Valuing People: a New Strategy for Learning Disability for the 21st Century.* London: The Stationery Office.

DEPARTMENT OF HEALTH SOCIAL SERVICES INSPECTORATE (1991) *Care Management and Assessment: Summary of Practice Guidance.* London: HMSO.

DOLL, E. A. (1965) *The Vineland Social Maturity Scale.* Minnesota: Circle Pines.

EATON, I. F. & MENOLASCINO, F. J. (1982) Psychiatric disorders in the mentally retarded. Types, problems, and challenges. *American Journal of Psychiatry,* **139**, 1298–1303.

EMERSON, E. & HATTON, C. (1998) Disabilities in England, Wales and Scotland: residential provision for people with intellectual disabilities. *Journal of Applied Research in Intellectual Disabilities,* **1**, 1–14.

FEINSTEIN, A. R & CICCHETTI, D. V. (1990) High agreement but low kappa: 1. The problems of two paradoxes. *Journal of Clinical Epidemiology,* **43**, 543–549.

GRAVESTOCK, S. (1999) Adults with learning disabilities and mental health needs: Conceptual and service issues. *Tizard Learning Disabilities Review,* **4**, 6–13.

—— & BOURAS, N. (1997) Survey of services for adults with learning disabilities. *Psychiatric Bulletin,* **21**, 197–199.

HOLMES, N., SHAH, A. & WING L. (1982) The Disability Assessment Schedule: A brief screening device for use with the mentally retarded. *Psychological Medicine,* **12**, 879–890.

HOUSE OF COMMONS (1990) *The National Health Service and Community Care Act.* London: HMSO.

JACOBSON, J. (1999) Dual diagnosis services: history, progress and perspectives. In: *Psychiatric and Behavioural Disorders in Developmental Disabilities and Mental Retardation* (ed. N. Bouras), pp. 327–358. Cambridge: Cambridge University Press.

KAZDIN, A. E., MATSON, J. L.& SENATOR, V. (1983) Assessment of depression in mentally retarded adults. *American Journal of Psychiatry,* **140**, 1040–1043.

LANDIS, J. R. & KOCH, G. C. (1977) The measurement of observer agreement for categorical data. *Biometrics,* **33**, 159–174.

MOONEY, G. (1986) Need, demand and the agency relationship. In: *Economics, Medicine and Health Care* (ed. G. Mooney), 2nd edition. London: Harvester Wheatsheaf.

MOSS, S., PROSSER, H, COSTELLO, H., *ET AL* (1998) Reliability and validity of the PAS–ADD Checklist for detecting psychiatric disorders in adults with intellectual disability. *Journal of Intellectual Disability Research,* **42**, 173–183.

NIHIRA, K., FOSTER, R., SHELHAAS, M., *ET AL* (1974) *AAMD Adaptive Behavior Scale,* 1974 Revision. Washington, DC: American Association on Mental Deficiency.

PHELAN, M., SLADE, M., THORNICROFT, G., *ET AL* (1995) The Camberwell Assessment of Need: The validity and reliability of an instrument to assess the needs of people with severe mental illness. *British Journal of Psychiatry,* **167**, 589–595.

REISS, S. (1988*a*) Dual diagnosis in the United States. Australia and New Zealand. *Journal of Developmental Disabilities,* **14**, 43–48.

—— (1988*b*) *The Reiss Screen Test Manual.* Orland Park, Ill: International Diagnostic Systems.

—— (1994) Psychopathology in mental retardation. In: *Mental Health in Mental Retardation* (ed. N. Bouras), pp. 67–78. Cambridge: Cambridge University Press.

ROYAL COLLEGE OF PSYCHIATRISTS (2000) *The Health of the Nation Outcome Scales for People with Learning Disabilities (HoNOS–LD)*. London: Royal College of Psychiatrists.

SCHROEDER, S. R., MULLICK, J. A. & SCHROEDER, C. S. (1979) Management of severe behavior problems of the retarded. In: *Handbook of Mental Deficiency, Psychological Theory and Research* (ed. N. R. Ellis), pp. 341–366. Hillsdale, NJ: Erlbaum.

SHACKLETON-BAILEY, M. J. & PIDCOCK B. E. (1983) *Hampshire Assessment of Living with Others* (5th version). Winchester: Hampshire Social Services.

SLADE, M. (1994) Needs assessment: who needs to assess? *British Journal of Psychiatry*, **165**, 287–292.

SOVNER, R. & HURLEY, A. D. (1983) Do the mentally retarded suffer from affective Illness? *Archives of General Psychiatry*, **40**, 61–67.

STEVENS, A. & GABBAY, J. (1991) Needs assessment needs assessment. *Health Trends*, **23**, 20–23.

—— & RAFTERY, J. (1994) *Health Care Needs Assessment*. Oxford: Ratcliffe Medical Press Ltd.

WING, J. K., COOPER, J. E. & SARTORIUS, N. (1974) *The Measurement and Classification of Psychiatric Symptoms*. Cambridge: Cambridge University Press.

——, BEEVOR, A. S, CURTIS, R. H., *ET AL* (1998) Health of the Nation Outcome Scales (HoNOS). Research and development. *British Journal of Psychiatry*, **172**, 11–18.

WORLD HEALTH ORGANIZATION (1992) *International Classification of Diseases and Related Health Problems. Tenth revision (ICD–10)*. Geneva: WHO.

XENITIDIS, K. THORNICROFT, G., LEESE, M., *ET AL* (2000) Reliability and validity of CANDID: A needs assessment instrument for adults with learning disabilities and mental health problems. *British Journal of Psychiatry*, **176**, 473–478.

22 Needs assessment in mental health care for older people

TOM REYNOLDS and MARTIN ORRELL

The increasing size of the older population of the world, and particularly that of the 'oldest old' (those over 85 years), has led to a growing recognition of the potential demands that this will make on health and social care resources worldwide. Although much debate and analysis concentrates on the possible impacts of such demands, there is also a growing awareness of the wider issues involved in such radically changing population demographics. Thus, the United Nations (UN) delegated 1999 as the International Year of Older Persons, and in the UK, acting on the initiative of the charity Age Concern, the 'Debate of the Age' was launched in 1998.

A look at world population figures and projections shows a general trend towards a growing and ageing population over the past 35 years (UN, 1998). The growth in population is expected to continue, with a projected further increase of 45% between 1990 and 2020. Europe is the only continent projected to have a fall in overall population between 1990 and 2020. However, the increasing elderly population in Europe is projected to continue, with the current estimate of 15.8% of Europe's population aged 65 years and over expected to rise to 20.4% by the year 2020.

In the UK, the overall population increased by 12% between 1961 and 1997 to reach a total of 59 million (Office for National Statistics (ONS), 1999). However, over the same period there has been a 34% increase in the population aged 65 years and over. This age group now accounts for 15.7% of the overall population and is expected to rise to account for 20% of the total population by 2020.

Epidemiology of psychiatric morbidity in older people

The prevalence of dementia is about 5% in people aged over 65 years and increases by approximately 5% every five years thereafter (Jorm *et al*, 1987; Cooper, 1991; Skoog *et al*, 1993). Elderly people occupy between 40% and 50% of all hospital beds (Mather, 1997). Studies of elderly people in general hospitals have shown dementia prevalence rates of 30–60% (Ramsay *et al*, 1991; Pitt, 1993). Higher prevalences of 70–90% have been found in nursing homes in the USA (Katzman, 1986; Evans *et al*, 1989; Aronson *et al*, 1990). A survey by Wattis *et al* (1992) in the UK found dementia rates ranging from 59% in private residential homes to 97% in local authority 'elderly mentally infirm' homes. There are currently about 200 000 new cases of dementia identified every year in the UK, with a point prevalence of around 500 000. With the projected increase in the elderly population, this figure will rise by another 100 000 over the next 20 years.

Studies on prevalence rates of depression have yielded remarkable variability in community studies of older people. Beekman *et al* (1999) reviewed 34 studies and found rates from 0.4% to 34%. Although major depression seems to be relatively rare (average prevalence of 1.8%), minor depression is more common (average prevalence of 9.8%) and average prevalence for "all depressive syndromes deemed clinically relevant" is 13.5% (Beekman *et al*, 1999). Higher depression rates of around 20% have been found in general hospital settings (Cooper, 1987; Burn *et al*, 1993).

Neurotic disorders in all age groups have higher prevalence rates in females, but this difference is less marked in the elderly. While the majority of cases in the elderly begin earlier in life, a significant minority first present after the age of 65 years (Bergmann, 1972; Lindesay, 1991).

Needs of older people

Against the background of a rising elderly population, organisations ranging from health and social services to governments and international bodies are eager to be able to survey and measure the demands such changes are likely to have on limited resources. Cassel (1994) highlighted the particular importance of assessing the health care needs of older people in the context of health care rationing. The Medical Research Council's topic review on the health of the elderly people in the UK (Medical Research Council (MRC), 1994) recommended that "research in community care should be focused on areas of particular relevance to the changes in care within the community, notably needs based approaches".

The identification and assessment of mental health needs has been the subject of varied opinions and research approaches in the UK, particularly since the introduction of legislation (National Health

Service (NHS) and Community Care Act; House of Commons, 1990) aimed at generating a more coordinated and comprehensive service provision by Social Services and the NHS. The Community Care Act (1993), which made it a formal requirement to assess the social and health care needs of those with mental illness, highlights a move towards better planning and coordination of care. This is in the context of a culture of ever-increasing awareness of limited resources, the consequent requirement to prioritise efficiently and the import-ance of demonstrating the effectiveness of health and social care interventions.

The frequent coexistence of disability, physical illness and social problems means that older people with mental illness often have complex needs. As problems are often both long-term and multiple, proper evaluation will be more difficult without standardised methods aimed at comprehensive and systematic assessment. Maslow (1954) postulated that certain needs are 'universal' in humans generally. However, different subsections of the population will have additional more specific types of need. Thus, older people with dementia may have specific and unique needs related to their cognitive impairment, but their range of general needs are the same as everyone else (Murphy, 1992).

Needs of special groups of older people

While older adults with mental health problems in general constitute a special group, there are subgroups within this population that warrant more specific attention by virtue of further vulnerability, disability or prejudice. One of the main recommendations of the report of a joint working party of the Royal College of Psychiatrists and Royal College of Physicians (Council Report CR69, 1998) was that "specific attention should be paid to particularly vulnerable groups of older people, including the homeless, those with learning disabilities, ethnic and cultural minorities, and older people in institutions or elsewhere who are exposed to the risk of abuse."

Studies in the USA have shown an increased percentage lifetime prevalence of dementia among homeless populations of around 3.4% (Koegel *et al*, 1988; Breakey *et al*, 1989), compared with 1.3% found in the overall population in the National Institute of Mental Health (NIMH) Epidemiological Catchment Area study in five American cities (Regier *et al*, 1988). In another American study examining the factors that lead to homelessness among elderly people, in addition to factors such as lack of appropriate housing and low income, Keigher & Greenblatt (1992) found that dementia contributed significantly. In a

UK study of homeless people over the age of 60 years, Crane (1994) found that 85% of the men and 100% of the women were suffering from a chronic psychiatric disorder, while 54% of the whole sample had memory problems. Hamid (1997) used the Needs Schedule (Wykes *et al*, 1982, 1985; Brewin *et al*, 1987) to compare the service needs of a sample of London homeless elderly men with those of a younger cohort and found no significant differences except for a higher rate of need for help with self-care and for residential care in the elderly group. Crane (1998) studied homeless older people in four UK cities. She found direct or indirect evidence of mental illness in two-thirds of them and a significantly higher prevalence of mental health problems in homeless women. In addition, mental ill health was a factor in the path to homelessness in many cases, some of the subjects becoming homeless because their needs had been neglected or undetected. The general trend towards overrepresentation of people with mental health problems among a group already severely disadvantaged and traditionally difficult to access and engage poses tough questions as to how their needs can be assessed and managed effectively.

Older people with learning disabilities form a very heterogenous group with an increased risk of other health-related problems, such as sensory impairments, physical disabilities and epilepsy (Holland & Moss, 1997). As such, the requirement for well-coordinated and integrated specialist health and social services is becoming increasingly recognised. Older people with learning disabilities are generally more able than their younger counterparts, owing to the effects of differential mortality rates (Holland & Moss, 1997), and studies have highlighted particular need in areas such as social and recreational activity and community living skills rather than activities of daily living skills (Gow & Chow, 1989; See *et al*, 1990).

The rate of closure of the large psychiatric hospitals means that significant numbers of elderly long-term in-patients will not live out their lives in hospital, as predicted by Arie & Jolley (1982), and their needs for care demand special attention. One indicator of why special attention is required is the reported increased mortality rate after relocation of elderly long-term hospital in-patients (Jackson & Whyte, 1998). Some studies have highlighted that the care needs of some long-stay hospital residents are greater than existing community services can meet (Pryce *et al*, 1991). Other studies have shown different outcomes in transferring long-stay patients from hospital to community settings (Linn *et al*, 1985; Timko *et al*, 1993; Trieman *et al*, 1996). Rodriguez-Ferrera & Vassilas (1998) therefore conclude that it is the quality of the environment, not where it is, that matters in outcomes for older people.

The issue of abuse has been highlighted by the Royal College of Psychiatrists & Royal College of Physicians (1998), particularly with regard to institutional care, and Fisk (1997) points out that the overall prevalence of abuse of around 4% derived from population surveys is a significant underestimation of the extent of the problem, as these surveys exclude the most vulnerable groups, such as those in long-term care settings. Homer & Gilleard (1990) found that 45% of carers admitted to physical or verbal abuse or neglect in one survey.

Cochrane & Bal (1989) reported a number of important findings in a survey of immigrants to England receiving mental health care. They found an excess of diagnosed schizophrenia in people born in the Caribbean and a markedly increased rate of first admissions for schizophrenia compared with English-born subjects. However, for all diagnoses combined, the admission rate of Caribbean-born people was much smaller than for native-born people, particularly for personality disorders, alcohol misuse and neurotic disorders. There is a small number of reports on mental health service use of older people from ethnic minorities that suggest that as a group they are underrepresented (Bahl, 1993; Blakemore & Boneham, 1994; Pharoah, 1994). Abas (1997) concludes that in order to deliver proper care we should be "focusing on needs-based assessment and ensuring that mainstream services can be flexible enough to take in the needs of an ethnically diverse population".

Needs assessment

Until recently, there have been no instruments specifically designed to measure met and unmet need for the range of interventions available from mental health and social care services for older people (Hamid *et al*, 1995). Needs assessment instruments developed in the UK were generally designed to measure the needs of adults with serious mental health problems under the age of 65 years. Examples include the MRC Needs for Care Assessment (MRC NCA; Brewin *et al*, 1987), a modified version – the Cardinal Needs Schedule (CNS; Marshall *et al*, 1995), the Camberwell Assessment of Needs (CAN; Phelan *et al*, 1995) and the Bangor Assessment of Need Profile (BANP; Carter *et al*, 1996).

The MRC NCA (Brewin *et al*, 1987) was designed to measure needs in the long-term mentally ill. A need was deemed to be present if a patient's level of functioning fell below, or threatened to fall below, some minimum specified level and a potentially effective remedy existed. While a number of studies suggest that it has good reliability if used by trained investigators (Brewin & Wing, 1993), some problems were highlighted when it was used in hostels for the homeless (Hogg & Marshall, 1992) and for long-term in-patients (Pryce *et al*, 1993). Hogg & Marshall (1992) concluded that their data was difficult to interpret owing to the failure to take account of patients' and carers' views "in sufficient detail" and therefore went on to develop a modified version, the CNS (Marshall *et al*, 1995).

The BANP (Carter *et al*, 1996) covers 32 items of need and allows patients and their keyworkers to give their opinion. It was specifically intended to assess the needs of those with long-term mental illness and the authors conclude that it is "principally proffered as a research instrument".

The CAN (Phelan *et al*, 1995) was developed to measure the needs of people with severe mental illness in the general adult population. It measures whether a need exists in 22 domains and whether it is met or not. If help is being given, it also allows recording of the level of help being given by different agencies, from friends and relatives to statutory services. It has good reliability and validity. Studies comparing the assessments made by staff and patients showed that both groups tended to rate similar numbers but different types of needs, agreeing moderately on met needs but less often on unmet needs (Slade *et al*, 1996).

Assessing the needs of older people with mental health problems

Assessing the needs of older people with mental health problems has attracted various approaches. Epidemiologically based approaches have been used to look at population needs in older people (Victor, 1991). However, individual approaches have largely concentrated on those with dementia, a group with obvious multiple and enduring needs, whose care, in health and social terms, has probably been more systematically studied than that of other groups of older people with psychiatric disorders (Aronson *et al*, 1992; Wattis *et al*, 1992; McWalter *et al*, 1998). Older people may also have different perceptions of their needs from those of clinicians (McEwan, 1992).

Wattis *et al* (1992) proposed a model for estimating the needs for continuing care of people with dementia, by assessing their level of dependency using the Clifton Assessment Procedures for the Elderly (CAPE; Gilleard & Pattie, 1979) or the Crighton Royal Behaviour Scale (Robinson, 1961). This approach was useful in determining the appropriateness of various continuing care settings. However, the level of dependency did not necessarily equate with level of need generally, in either a qualitative or quantitative sense, and did not define what the needs were. For example, a person with a mild dementia, rated as low dependency and apparently appropriately housed in a residential home, may still have a large number of unmet needs because of poor quality of care or poor understanding of those needs. On the other hand, a person with profound dementia, with very high dependency, may have few if any unmet needs as they receive obvious help or intervention in all aspects of daily living.

Again, with the exception of the Camberwell Assessment of Need for the Elderly (CANE; Reynolds *et al*, 2000), specific needs assessment instruments have tended to be for the older population with dementia. Thus, Gordon *et al* (1997) designed an instrument aimed at gathering data for population needs assessment and service planning for people with dementia. They found that the Tayside Profile for Dementia Planning had satisfactory validity and reliability, but noted that informal carers and professionals perceived needs differently. As it was not clear which group had the more valid opinion, a mix of informal carers and professionals as informants is postulated to offer the best approach when using the profile.

The Care Needs Assessment Pack for Dementia (Care NAP–D; McWalter *et al*, 1998) was designed for use by a multi-disciplinary team to rate met and unmet needs of people with dementia and their carers in the community and related settings such as day hospitals. Although it does not differentiate between information sources (e.g. interviews with the person with dementia, the carer or others involved and information from case notes), it does allow discrepancies or differences of opinion to be recorded at the rater's discretion. Recordings are made on seven sub-scales of need (health and mobility, self-care and toileting, social interaction, thinking and memory, behaviour and mental state, house care and community living). The section specific to the carer allows assessment of need over six domains; health, daily difficulties, support, breaks from caring, feelings and information. Preliminary research suggests that it has validity in a number of domains and demonstrates reasonable reliability (McWalter *et al*, 1998).

The CANE (Reynolds *et al*, 2000) is a relatively new instrument designed for measuring the broad range of needs of older people with mental health problems, including dementia, depression and other disorders. It is intended for use in all settings from the community, out-patients and acute psychiatric wards to day hospitals, dementia assessment wards and continuing care in hospital, nursing homes and residential homes.

The CANE was based on the structural model of the CAN (Phelan *et al*, 1995) and similar criteria were set out before embarking on its development. These were that it should: have adequate psychometric properties; be valid and reliable; be completable within 30 minutes; be usable by a wide range of professionals; be easily learned and used without extensive training; be suitable for routine clinical practice and for research; and be applicable to a wide range of populations and settings. It should also measure both met and unmet needs, incorporate staff, patients' and carers' views of needs and have a section on the needs of carers. Lastly, it should measure level of help received from informal carers as well as from statutory services.

Comprehensive consensus methods resulted in a version containing 24 areas of need for patients and two for their carers (Box 22.1). In each area, there was space for the patient, his or her carer and a key staff member to record their views of need. An example page is shown in Fig. 22.1. The reliability and validity studies showed that the CANE had good content, construct and consensual validity. It also demonstrated appropriate criterion validity with, for example, a

---

Box 22.1
Areas of need covered in CANE (Reynolds et al, 2000)

1 Accommodation
2 Household skills
3 Food
4 Self-care
5 Caring for someone else
6 Daytime activities
7 Memory
8 Eyesight/hearing
9 Mobility/transport
10 Continence
11 Physical health
12 Drugs
13 Psychotic symptoms
14 Psychological distress
15 Information
16 Safety (deliberate self-harm)
17 Safety (inadvertent self-harm)
18 Safety (abuse/neglect)
19 Behaviour
20 Alcohol
21 Company
22 Intimate relationships
23 Money
24 Benefits

Two items for carers:
1 Carer's need for information
2 Carer's psychological distress

14 PSYCHOLOGICAL DISTRESS

ASSESSMENTS
USER   STAFF   CARER

DOES THE PERSON SUFFER FROM CURRENT
PSYCHOLOGICAL DISTRESS?
Have you recently felt very sad or fed up? Have you felt very anxious, frightened or worried?

0 = NO PROBLEM   e.g Occasional or mild distress.
1 = NO/MODERATE PROBLEM
    DUE TO HELP GIVEN   e.g. Needs and gets ongoing support.
2 = SERIOUS PROBLEM   e.g. Distress affects life significantly, e.g. prevents person
                                going out.
9 = NOT KNOWN

IF RATED 0 OR 9 GO TO QUESTION 15

HOW MUCH HELP DOES THE PERSON RECEIVE
FROM FRIENDS OR RELATIVES FOR THIS DISTRESS?

0 = NONE
1 = LOW HELP   e.g. Some sympathy and support.
2 = MODERATE HELP   e.g. Has opportunity at least weekly to talk about distress
                                and get help with coping strategies.
3 = HIGH HELP   e.g. Constant support and supervision.
9 = NOT KNOWN

HOW MUCH HELP DOES THE PERSON *RECEIVE* FROM
LOCAL SERVICES FOR THIS DISTRESS?

HOW MUCH HELP DOES THE PERSON *NEED* FROM
LOCAL SERVICES FOR THIS DISTRESS?

0 = NONE
1 = LOW HELP   e.g. Assessment of mental state or occasional support.
2 = MODERATE HELP   e.g. Specific psychological or social intervention for
                                anxiety. Counselled by staff at least once a week, e.g. at
                                day hospital.
3 = HIGH HELP   e.g. 24 hour hospital care, or crisis care at home.
9 = NOT KNOWN

DOES THE PERSON RECEIVE THE RIGHT TYPE
OF HELP FOR THIS DISTRESS?
(0 = NO   1 = YES   9 = NOT KNOWN)

OVERALL, IS THE PERSON SATISFIED WITH THE
AMOUNT OF HELP THEY ARE RECEIVING FOR THIS
DISTRESS?
(0 = NOT SATISFIED   1 = SATISFIED)

COMMENTS

Fig. 22.1 Example page of the CANE. Section 1 records if need exists. Sections 2 and 3 record level of help given by informal carers and statutory bodies respectively. Section 4 records if right type of help is being given and level of satisfaction with the amount of help.

correlation of 0.66 with the Behaviour Rating Scale from the CAPE (Gilleard & Pattie, 1979). The reliability was generally very high with interrater reliability κ values of >0.85 for all staff ratings (an indication of excellent agreement according to Fleiss (1981)). Correlations of interrater and test–retest reliability of total numbers of needs identified by staff were 0.99 and 0.93 respectively.

Growing interest in the CANE has resulted in its translation into four other European languages (German, Norwegian, Spanish and Swedish). It is in use in a number of studies in various settings in the UK. Current UK studies are using the CANE to evaluate the needs of older people in primary care and to assess needs and social support in sheltered accommodation. Another study is comparing the needs of those in residential care with those in NHS continuing care. The CANE appears to be a reliable and feasible instrument to investigate needs in a wide range of settings.

Conclusions

A 'user-friendly', standardised, comprehensive, reliable and valid schedule for assessing the needs of older adults with mental health problems helps not only in clinical practice but also in research and health and social service planning. Clinicians who helped with the initial trials of the CANE consistently commented on its usefulness in honing assessment skills. An instrument like the CANE not only helps record the level of need of the patient but also allows recording of two important areas of need for their carers (information and psychological distress). A growing body of work points to the importance of taking account of carers' needs (Gwyther & Strulowitz, 1998; Teri, 1999). The recent Royal Commission report (1999) on the funding of long-term care highlights the needs of carers and recommends that "better services should be offered to those who currently have a carer" and "the Government should consider a national carer support package". Systematic, comprehensive, easily comparable data-sets are produced by studies that use the same core instruments. A survey of social service departments in England and Wales by Martin *et al* (1999) showed there were substantial national variations in the ways that needs assessments were carried out for older people with mental health problems. Such differences may lead to significant inequalities in the assessment of those needs and subsequent inequalities in the provision of care for this vulnerable group.

As Richards pointed out in his editorial (1998):

> "At present assessment of 'need' and the response to it is arbitrarily determined by individual local authorities – hence the wide

geographical variations. The case for setting nationally agreed methods of assessment and criteria for eligibility for services is strong."

Martin *et al* (1999) came to similar conclusions in their national survey. The use of standardised, well-validated and reliable instruments to carry out assessments of the needs of older people with mental health problems should not only help at the 'micro' level in the formulation of specific individual care planning but should also, if the instrument is suitable, be very useful at the 'macro' level to help plan health service provision based on the identified needs.

References

ABAS, M. (1997) Functional disorders in ethnic minority elders. In: *Advances in Old Age Psychiatry* (eds C. Holmes & R. Howard), pp. 234–245. Petersfield: Wrightson.

AGE CONCERN (1998) *Debate of the Age*. London: Age Concern.

ARIE, T. & JOLLEY, D. J. (1982) Making services work: organisation and style of psychogeriatric services. In: *The Psychiatry of Late Life* (eds R. Levy & F. Post), pp. 221–251. Oxford: Blackwell.

ARONSON, M. K., OOI, W. L., MORGENSTERN, H., *ET AL* (1990) Women, myocardial infarction and dementia in the very old. *Neurology*, **40**, 1102–1106.

——, COX, D., GUASTADISEGNI, P., *ET AL* (1992) Dementia and the Nursing Home: Association with Care Needs. *Journal of the American Geriatrics Society*, **40**, 27–33.

BAHL, V. (1993) Access to health care for black and ethnic minority people: general principles. In: *Access to Health Care for People from Black and Ethnic Minorities* (eds. A. Hopkins & V. Bahl), pp. 93–96. London: Royal College of Physicians.

BEEKMAN, A. T. F., COPELAND, J. R. M. & PRINCE, M. J. (1999) Review of community prevalence of depression in later life. *British Journal of Psychiatry*, **174**, 307–311.

BERGMANN, K. (1972) The neuroses in old age. In: *Recent Developments in Psychogeriatrics* (eds D. W. K. Kay & A. Walk), pp. 39–50. Ashford: Headley Bros.

BLAKEMORE, K. & BONEHAM, M. (1994) *Age, Race and Ethnicity: A Comparative Approach*. Buckingham: Open University Press.

BREAKEY, W. R., FISCHER, P. J., KRAMER, M., *ET AL* (1989) Health and mental health problems of homeless men and women in Baltimore. *Journal of the American Medical Association*, **262**, 1352–1357.

BREWIN, C. R. & WING, J. K. (1993) The MRC Needs for Care Assessment: Progress and controversies. *Psychological Medicine*, **23**, 837–841.

—— & ——, MANGEN, S. P., *ET AL* (1987) Principles and practice of measuring needs in the long-term mentally ill: the MRC Needs for Care Assessment. *Psychological Medicine*, **17**, 971–981.

BURN, W. K., DAVIES, K. N., MCKENZIE, F. R., *ET AL* (1993) The prevalence of psychiatric illness in acute geriatric admissions. *International Journal of Geriatric Psychiatry*, **8**, 171–174.

CARTER, M. F., CROSBY, C., GEERTSHUIS, S., *ET AL* (1996) Developing reliability in client-centred mental health needs assessment. *Journal of Mental Health*, **5**, 233–243.

CASSEL, C. K. (1994) Researching the health needs of elderly people (editorial). *British Medical Journal*, **308**, 1655–1656.

COCHRANE, R. & BAL, S. S. (1989) Mental hospital admission rates of immigrants to England: a comparison of 1971 and 1981. *Social Psychiatry and Psychiatric Epidemiology*, **24**, 2–12.

COOPER, B. (1987) Psychiatric disorders among elderly patients admitted to hospital wards. *Journal of the Royal Society of Medicine*, **80**, 13–16.

—— (1991) Principles of service provision in old age psychiatry. In: *Psychiatry in the Elderly* (eds R. Jacoby & C. Oppenheimer), pp. 274–300. London: Oxford University Press.

CRANE, M. (1994) The mental health problems of elderly people living on London streets. *International Journal of Geriatric Psychiatry*, **9**, 87–95.

—— (1998) The associations between mental illness and homelessness among older people: an exploratory study. *Aging and Mental Health*, **2**, 171–180.

EVANS, D. A., FUNKENSTEIN, H. H., ALBERT, M. S., *ET AL* (1989) Prevalence of Alzheimer's disease in a community population of older persons. *Journal of the American Medical Association*, **262**, 2551–2556.

FISK, J. (1997) Abuse of the elderly. In: *Psychiatry in the Elderly* (eds R. Jacoby & C. Oppenheimer), pp. 736–748. London: Oxford University Press.

FLEISS, J. L. (1981) The measurement of inter-rater agreement. In: *Statistical Methods for Rates and Proportions* (ed. J. L. Fleiss). New York: John Wiley.

GILLEARD, C. & PATTIE, A. (1979) *Clifton Assessment Procedures for the Elderly.* Windsor: NFER/Nelson.

GORDON, D. S., SPICKER, P., BALLINGER, B. R., *ET AL* (1997) A population needs assessment profile for dementia. *International Journal of Geriatric Psychiatry*, **12**, 642–647.

GOW, L. & CHOW, R. (1989) Survey of the needs of elderly people with mental handicap in Hong Kong. *Australia & New Zealand Journal of Developmental Disabilities*, **15** (Special Issue), 267–275.

GWYTHER, L. P. & STRULOWITZ, S. Y. (1998) Care-giver stress. *Current Opinion in Psychiatry*, **11**, 432–434.

HAMID, W. A. (1997) The elderly homeless men in Bloomsbury hostels: Their needs for services. *International Journal of Geriatric Psychiatry*, **12**, 724–727.

——, HOWARD, R. & SILVERMAN, M. (1995) Needs assessment in old age psychiatry – a need for standardization. *International Journal of Geriatric Psychiatry*, **10**, 533–540.

HOGG, L. I. & MARSHALL, M. (1992) Can we measure needs in the homeless mentally ill? Using the MRC Needs for Care Assessment in hostels for the homeless. *Psychological Medicine*, **22**, 1027–1034.

HOLLAND, T & MOSS, S. (1997) The mental health needs of older people with learning disabilities. In *Psychiatry in the Elderly* (eds. R. Jacoby & C. Oppenheimer), pp. 294–506. London: Oxford University Press.

HOMER, A. C. & GILLEARD, C. (1990) Abuse of elderly people by their carers. *British Medical Journal*, **30**, 1359–1362.

HOUSE OF COMMONS (1990) *The National Health Service and Community Care Act.* London: HMSO.

—— (1993) *The National Health Service and Community Care Act.* London: HMSO.

JACKSON, G. A., & WHYTE, J. (1998) Effects of hospital closure on mortality rates of the over-65 long-stay psychiatric population. *International Journal of Geriatric Psychiatry*, **13**, 836–839.

JORM, A. F., KORTEN, A. E. & HENDERSON, A. F. (1987) The prevalence of dementia: A quantitative integration of the literature. *Acta Psychiatrica Scandinavica*, **76**, 465–479.

KATZMAN, R. (1986) Alzheimer's disease. *New England Journal of Medicine*, **314**, 964–973.

KEIGHER, S. & GREENBLATT, S. (1992) Housing emergencies and the etiology of homelessness among the urban elderly. *Gerontologist*, **32**, 457–465.

KOEGEL, P., BURNAM, A. & FARR, R. K. (1988) The prevalence of specific psychiatric disorders among homeless individuals in the city of Los Angeles. *Archives of General Psychiatry*, **45**, 1085–1092.

LINDESAY, J. (1991) Phobic disorders in the elderly. *British Journal of Psychiatry*, **159**, 531–541.

LINN, M. W., GUREL, L., WILLIFORD, W. O., *ET AL* (1985) Nursing home care as an alternative to psychiatric hospitalization. *Archives of General Psychiatry*, **42**, 544–551.

MARSHALL, M., HOGG, L. I., GATH, D. H., *ET AL* (1995) The Cardinal Needs Schedule – a modified version of the MRC Needs for Care Assessment Schedule. *Psychological Medicine*, **25**, 605–617.

MARTIN, M., PEHRSON, J. & ORRELL, M. (1999) A national survey of social services needs assessments for elderly mentally ill people. *Age and Ageing*, **28**, 575–577.

MASLOW, A. H. (1954) *Motivation and Personality*. New York: Harper and Row.

MATHER, R. (1997) Old age psychiatry in a general hospital. In: *Psychiatry in the Elderly* (eds R. Jacoby & C. Oppenheimer). London: Oxford University Press.

McEWAN, E. (1992) The consumer's perception of need. In: *Long-Term Care for Elderly People*. London: HMSO.

McWALTER, G., TONER, H., McWALTER, A., *ET AL* (1998) A community needs assessment: The Care Needs Assessment Pack for Dementia (Care NAP–D) – its development, reliability and validity. *International Journal of Geriatric Psychiatry*, **13**, 16–22.

MEDICAL RESEARCH COUNCIL (1994) *Topic Review on Care of the Elderly*. London: MRC.

MURPHY, E. (1992) A more ambitious vision for residential long-term care (editorial). *International Journal of Geriatric Psychiatry*, **7**, 851–852.

OFFICE FOR NATIONAL STATISTICS (1999) *Social Trends 29*. London: The Stationery Office.

PHAROAH, C. (1994) *The Provision of Primary Health Care for Elderly People from Black and Minority Ethnic Communities*. London: Age Concern, Institute of Gerontology, King's College.

PHELAN, M., SLADE, M., THORNICROFT, G., *ET AL* (1995) The Camberwell Assessment of Need: the validity and reliability of an instrument to assess the needs of people with severe mental illness. *British Journal of Psychiatry*, **167**, 589–595.

PITT, B. (1993) The liaison psychiatry of old age. In: *Recent Advances in Clinical Psychiatry*, vol. 8 (ed. K. Granville-Grossman), pp. 91–106. Edinburgh: Churchill Livingstone.

PRYCE, I. G., GRIFFITHS, R. D., GENTRY, R. M., *ET AL* (1991) The nature and severity of disabilities in long-stay psychiatric in-patients in South Glamorgan. *British Journal of Psychiatry*, **158**, 817–821.

——, ——, ——, *ET AL* (1993) How important is the assessment of social skills in current long-stay in-patients? An evaluation of clinical response to needs for assessment, treatment and care in a long-stay psychiatric in-patient population. *British Journal of Psychiatry*, **162**, 498–502.

RAMSAY, R., WRIGHT, P., KATZ, A., *ET AL* (1991) The detection of psychiatric morbidity and its effects on outcome in acute elderly medical admissions. *International Journal of Geriatric Psychiatry*, **6**, 861–866.

REGIER, D. A., BOYD, J. H., BURKE, J. D., *ET AL* (1988) One month prevalence of mental disorders in the United States. *Archives of General Psychiatry*, **45**, 977–986.

REYNOLDS, T., THORNICROFT, G., ABAS, M., *ET AL* (2000) Camberwell Assessment of need for the elderly; development, validity and reliability. *British Journal of Psychiatry*, **176**, 444–452.

RICHARDS, T. (1998) Ageing costs. Evidence to Royal Commission emphasises need for explicit standards and funding. *British Medical Journal*, **317**, 896.

ROBINSON, S. (1961) Problems of drug trials in elderly people. *Gerontologia Clinica*, **3**, 247–257.

RODRIGUEZ-FERRERA, S. & VASSILAS, C. A. (1998) Older people with schizophrenia: providing services for a neglected group (editorial). *British Medical Journal*, **317**, 293–294.

ROYAL COLLEGE OF PSYCHIATRISTS & ROYAL COLLEGE OF PHYSICIANS (1998) *The Care of Older People with Mental Illness: Specialist Services and Medical Training*. Council Report CR69. London: Royal College of Psychiatrists & Royal College of Physicians of London.

ROYAL COMMISSION ON THE FUNDING OF LONG TERM CARE (1999) *With Respect to Old Age: Long Term Care – Rights and Responsibilities*. London: The Stationery Office.

SEE, C. J., ELLIS, D. N., SPELLMAN, C. R., *ET AL* (1990) Using needs assessment to develop programs for elderly developmentally disabled persons in a rural setting. *Activities, Adaptation and Aging*, **15**, 53–66.

SKOOG, I., NILSSON, L., PALMERTZ, B., *ET AL* (1993) A population based study of dementia in 85-year olds. *New England Journal of Medicine*, **328**, 153–158.

SLADE, M., PHELAN, M., THORNICROFT, G., *ET AL* (1996) The Camberwell Assessment of Need (CAN): comparison of assessments by staff and patients of needs of the severely mentally ill. *Social Psychiatry and Psychiatric Epidemiology*, **31**, 109–113.

TERI, L. (1999) Training families to provide care: effects on people with dementia. *International Journal of Geriatric Psychiatry*, **14**, 110–119.

TIMKO, C., NGUYEN, A. Q., WILLIFORD, W. O., *ET AL* (1993) Quality of care and outcomes of chronic mentally ill patients in hospital and nursing homes. *Hospital and Community Psychiatry*, **44**, 241–246.

TRIEMAN, N., WILLS, W. & LEFF, J. (1996) TAPS Project 28: does re-provision benefit elderly long-stay mental patients? *Schizophrenia Research*, **21**, 199–208.

UNITED NATIONS (1998) *World Population Projections*. New York: United Nations.

VICTOR, C. R. (1991) *Health and Health Care in Later Life*. Milyon Keynes: Open University Press.

WATTIS, J. P., HOBSON, J. & BARKER, G. (1992) Needs for continuing care of demented people: a model for estimating needs. *Psychiatric Bulletin*, **16**, 465–467.

WYKES, T., CREER, C. & STURT, E. (1982) Needs and the deployment of services. In: *Psychological Medicine Monograph*, Supplement No. 2 (ed. J. K. Wing).

——, STURT, E. & CREER, C. (1985) The assessment of patients' needs for community care. *Social Psychiatry*, **20**, 76–85.

23 Mental health needs in primary care

ANDRE TYLEE

Primary care groups (PCGs) in England came into operation in April 1999 and are expected to assist health authorities in constructing their health improvement programme on health and health care. To do this, they must assess the perspective of the local community, service providers and patients. To assess the mental health needs of their mentally ill patients, they need first to compile registers of their long-term mentally ill using well-tried methods (Strathdee *et al*, 1997; Cohen & Paton, 1999). These methods include: analysing the practice computer database (by diagnosis and prescriptions); viewing the appointment system; asking the practice team; and asking psychiatric services. Once these registers have been constructed, they can be compared with nationally derived figures, such as those of Strathdee & Jenkins (1996) (see Table 23.1), which were extrapolated from the Office for Population Censuses and Surveys (OPCS) Surveys of Psychiatric Morbidity in Great Britain (Meltzer *et al*, 1995) and sought to explain any differences between real and expected prevalence. An inner-city practice might find that it has more patients with schizophrenia than average because of proximity to closing psychiatric hospitals. Inter-practice variation can help services to be targeted appropriately. To assess overall prevalence of common mental health problems (e.g. mixed anxiety and depression), it is best to screen consecutive attenders (Armstrong, 1997).

Eliciting real and perceived needs

The next step is to elicit real and perceived needs of identified patients. One recommendation (Cohen & Paton, 1999) is to analyse Care Programme Approach (CPA) data for needs concerning physical health, mental health and social factors (i.e. housing, benefits,

TABLE 23.1
Distribution of mental health diagnoses in a general practice

Diagnosis	No. of patients per general practice
Schizophrenia	4–12
Bipolar illness	6–7
Organic dementia	4–5
Depression	60–100
Anxiety states and other neuroses	70–80
Situational and bereavement type problems	50–60
Substance misuse problems including alcohol misuse	5–6

Source: Strathdee & Jenkins (1996), assuming an average patient list of 2000.

occupation and activity). Local organisations such as the National Schizophrenia Fellowship (NSF) and Depression Alliance can be canvassed for information about social deprivation, refugees, the homeless, ethnic groups, religious groups, etc. Many non-statutory agencies and faith communities operate in isolation to care for people with mental health needs and will complete the locality picture. Practices with a great interest in psychiatry may attract greater numbers of patients with mental health needs.

Another needs assessment could be undertaken of individuals at high risk of developing mental illness (e.g. the bereaved, unemployed, pregnant/postnatal, single parents, carers, chronically physically ill, refugees, etc). A PCG with a high number of any of these groups may wish to commission a service tailored to their particular needs (e.g. a team to visit the homeless). Other methods of assessing need include looking at the historical use of services for the mentally ill (i.e. referrals). This may be very misleading if there have been high need and low referral patterns. Sometimes, low referral can reflect long waiting lists, so that referrers do not bother referring. Deprivation indices indicate likely need geographically, so that part of a PCG's area may have more needs because of social deprivation. Prescribing analysis will indicate practices that are high prescribers. Another method advocated by Cohen & Paton (1999) is that of comparing practices by the numbers of patients on the three different levels of the CPA (level 3 being the highest and indicating greatest need).

This depends, however, on different community mental health teams (CMHTs) using similar criteria for rating need.

Direct service user measures of need

One of the best ways to find out the likely mental health needs of the population and just how disabled they may be is to ask patients directly. Several studies have indicated what users would like from primary care, notably Rogers *et al* (1993). Generally, they view GPs as helpful, less stigmatising, more local, offering better continuity of care and providing the way in to other services. However, they would like GPs to be more accessible, flexible and friendly. Overall, they would like more time than is available, physical needs to be taken seriously and more information about the problem and its treatment. If they were to suffer from depression, the general public would want to be listened to rather than given a prescription and fear that drugs for depression are addictive (Priest *et al*, 1996). Cohen & Paton (1999) also list the needs of carers and people from ethnic minorities.

There are few instruments designed to assess need in primary care, so the best approach for any reader is to follow Chapter 1 of *A Workbook for Primary Care Groups* (Cohen & Paton, 1999), which can be obtained from the Sainsbury Centre for Mental Health. This chapter provides guidance on how to assess how many patients there are with severe and enduring mental illness and with common mental illness. Methods of assessing the needs (and wants) of individuals using available data-sets within the practice, the mental health service, the public health department and the local authority are also described.

I will now outline findings from a patient satisfaction survey conducted in seven practices in South West London just before the establishment of PCGs. The South West London Total Purchasing Pilot (SWLTPP) previously comprised eight general practices, seven of which have now joined the Nelson PCG and remain within that group as the South London Primary Care Organisation (SWLPCO). This organisation was the first and largest overarching general practice partnership in the UK (subject to the Department of Trade and Industry changing the regulations on size of medical partnerships), with 38 partners. As the Nelson PCG has 75 GP principals, the SWLPCO cares for over half of the 150 000 population within the PCG. The previously unpublished findings are published here in some detail, as the method used may be of use to other PCGs wishing to undertake similar surveys and because this survey, to my knowledge, seems to be the only survey of its kind to date.

User satisfaction survey of primary care mental health services in South West London

Method

This study was a two-stage satisfaction survey of mental health patients in the SWLTPP using two questionnaires. The SWLTPP was one of 50 pilot projects across the UK and allowed groups of GPs to purchase all health care for their patients within the Merton, Sutton and Wandsworth Area Health Authority. Each of the eight practices in the SWLTPP was asked to produce a list of all their long-term mentally ill patients who could be contacted to participate in the study. Long-term mentally ill (LTMI) was defined as patients with a mental health disorder continually present for one year, requiring prophylactic treatment (Strathdee *et al*, 1997) or treatment from the CMHT. One practice (which has now moved to a neighbouring PCG) was excluded from this study as many of its mental health patients were participating in another study. Every third patient was randomly selected from the seven practice-generated LTMI lists, producing 30–40 patients per practice and 245 patients in total.

The first-stage questionnaire (Bosanquet, 1997) assessed which local mental health services were used and overall satisfaction. Respondents were asked if they would be willing to complete the second stage. Non-responders were mailed again after three weeks. This questionnaire had been piloted with three patients (not included in the study) and no changes were necessary.

Patients willing to participate in the second stage completed the Verona Service Satisfaction Scale–54 version for patients (VSSS–54; Ruggeri, 1993). The VSSS–54 measures seven areas of patient satisfaction using a five-point scale: overall satisfaction; access to services; involvement of relatives; types of intervention; professionals' skills and behaviour; information; and efficacy of services. These were completed by the research assistant (K.B.) by telephone or at the practice. Questions were added concerning: whether respondents received treatment from a community psychiatric nurse (CPN) or other keyworker; what else the mental health services could do to help; and whether they attended any voluntary or self-help groups. These questions had been piloted with three LTMI patients (again, not included in the study) and no changes were necessary.

Data analysis

The data were entered, frequencies of responses totalled and the mode and mean satisfaction scores for each question were calculated.

Results

First-stage interview

For the first questionnaire, 113 (40 male, 73 female) usable replies (25 unusable) were received (from 245). Respondents were mainly aged 20–64 years (nine were over 64 years). One-hundred-and-three (91%) were Caucasian (two Indian, one Caribbean, one Iranian, one Eurasian and five left blank). Most respondents said they had a keyworker (71%), defined as "someone they saw regularly to help with their mental health problems"; these were GPs (22%), CPNs (31%), psychiatrists (9%) and psychologists (7%). Some respondents indicated more than one person (the one seen most frequently or cited first was assumed to be the keyworker). Social workers, health visitors, day hospitals/centres and practice nurses were also cited.

Services used most frequently in the past year for mental health problems were GPs (79%), CPNs (37%), psychiatrists (37%), social workers (15%), psychologists (14%), day hospitals/centres (12%), practice nurses (9%), health visitors (6%), and practice counsellors (2%). More respondents expressed satisfaction than dissatisfaction with the services they had received, in terms of obtaining an appointment, time allowed for the appointment and help received. Many respondents stated that they could not have managed without the excellent care and understanding of the GP, CPN or psychiatrist.

Causes of dissatisfaction were as follows (with the frequency of the complaint given in parentheses if more frequent than once): long waiting times (nine); not being seen frequently enough (three); the psychiatrist not arranging follow-up (two); being kept on the telephone by a receptionist; and not being considered an emergency. Other problems included: being rushed (four); the appointment being too short (six); feeling a nuisance; feeling that the GP had given up on them and that they were wasting his or her time; psychiatrists and GPs not understanding the problems (eight); the GP not taking physical problems seriously (three); the GP not being available in times of crisis (two); locum GPs' ignorance of the patient's history; questions from the CPN seeming intrusive rather than helpful; and not being able to find a Christian psychiatrist.

Involvement in care planning, access to psychiatrists/specialist services and the local practice, support for families and carers, help with employment and more social opportunities/day centres were all areas where at least 20% of respondents thought there could be improvement. Written comments included:

- want real understanding of aetiology;
- want to see the psychiatrist when well;

- lack of back-up care or help;
- lack of sympathetic employers;
- difficulty getting job references;
- feel 'written off';
- little need for temporary home help during crises;
- want rapid access to services (two); and
- want help-line for emergencies.

Second-stage interview with VSSS–54

Fifty-five respondents (31 female, 24 male) to the first questionnaire were willing to complete the VSSS–54. Of the other 25 respondents willing to be interviewed, two subsequently changed their minds, two were too unwell, four were considered too unwell by their carers, two were too busy with work, one had given a wrong contact telephone number, and 14 others could not be contacted before the planned target of 30 interviews had been reached. Thirty respondents (13 male) were interviewed. Ages ranged from 28 to 66 years (mean 46 years). Ten interviews were performed at practices and the remaining ones over the telephone.

Respondents rated satisfaction as follows: 5 = extremely satisfied, 4 = mostly satisfied, 3 = neither satisfied nor dissatisfied, 2 = mostly dissatisfied, and 1 = extremely dissatisfied. Other scores were: 6 = exempt, 7 = not applicable, 8 = do not want to answer, and 9 = do not know. Satisfaction scores were averaged to give an overall impression of satisfaction with mental health services.

Below is a summary of the results for items relating to the various areas of patient satisfaction.

Overall satisfaction and professionals' skills and behaviour.   Overall satisfaction and the behaviour and skills of the staff were generally rated highly. Advice on coping between appointments was not rated so highly. Most of the items were rated highly by two-thirds to three-quarters of respondents. Punctuality of professionals was better on home visits than at clinics, with eight respondents being neither satisfied nor dissatisfied/mostly dissatisfied with clinic punctuality. Information about diagnosis and treatment had a mean satisfaction score of <4. Many respondents felt that more could be done to educate the general public.

Access to services.   All questions relating to access had a mean satisfaction score of <4. Regarding the appearance and comfort of the facility, 18 participants were mostly satisfied/extremely satisfied, while two were extremely dissatisfied.

Involvement of relatives. These items were felt to be not relevant by eight respondents who did not want their family to be involved, while others thought this area needed more emphasis within their treatment. All questions relating to this area of satisfaction had a mean score of <4. Twelve respondents were mostly/extremely satisfied with the ability of psychiatrists and psychologists to listen to and understand any worries that relatives might have about the respondent. Nine respondents were mostly/extremely satisfied with the effectiveness of the service in helping relative(s) improve their knowledge and understanding of the respondent's problems.

Types of intervention. Thirteen respondents were mostly/extremely satisfied and six extremely dissatisfied with help received for side-effects from medication. The dissatisfaction expressed related to both how to avoid the side-effects and what to do once they had occurred. The types of intervention mostly received by respondents in the past year were drug prescriptions, individual psychotherapy, referral to a CPN, help from a keyworker and help obtaining welfare benefits. Overall satisfaction was generally high (mode = 4+).

Twenty-five respondents had received drug prescriptions for their mental health problems in the past year and 16 respondents were mostly/extremely satisfied with the treatment (nine were neither satisfied nor dissatisfied/mostly dissatisfied). None of the five respondents not currently taking medication wanted to take it.

Nineteen respondents had received individual psychotherapy, with 15 respondents being mostly/extremely satisfied with the treatment. Of the 11 respondents not having had individual psychotherapy, seven did not want it, one did not know and three would have liked it.

Three respondents had received family therapy and were all mostly satisfied; eight not receiving it would have liked it.

Fifteen were being treated by CPNs and 10 respondents were mostly/extremely satisfied with their CPNs (five were neither satisfied nor dissatisfied/mostly dissatisfied). Of the remaining 15 respondents, five would have liked to see a CPN. Twenty respondents did not have a keyworker, but nine would have liked one. Those who did have one found them to be very good, with 80% being mostly/extremely satisfied.

Nine respondents had received help to obtain welfare benefits and all who received this help were mostly/extremely satisfied. Another 20% (six) of respondents would have liked help. Eleven respondents would have liked participation within recreational activities (both those run by mental health services and those outside of the NHS), help finding a job (more would have liked this outside of a sheltered working environment than within one) and practical help at home.

Group therapy was not very popular with the four people who had received it, and only five others would have liked it. Four respondents had received informal hospital admission and two would have liked this. Two had received compulsory hospital admission and two said they would have liked this. Informal hospital admissions were seen as more preferable than compulsory admissions. No respondents had been offered sheltered accommodation, but two would have liked this. When asked to rate how appropriate their treatment was for them on a scale of 0 to 10, where 0 = not at all and 10 = completely, the mean score was 7 and the mode was 8.

Information.   Ten respondents were neither satisfied nor dissatisfied/ mostly dissatisfied with information given to them on diagnosis, treatment and possible development of their disorder. The availability of public information on mental health services was not felt to be very good, with only one respondent being extremely satisfied and six respondents not knowing what information was available or where to look for it.

Efficacy of services.   The response of the services to emergencies within office hours was rated better than to emergencies out of office hours. Half of respondents were dissatisfied with the help given to them for side-effects from medication (mean satisfaction score = 3.31). Those that did receive help found it to be very good. Twenty respondents were mostly/extremely satisfied with the response within office hours. Fifteen respondents were mostly/extremely satisfied and four extremely dissatisfied with the response out of office hours. Not all respondents had needed to make use of the services during an emergency and their score reflected their confidence in what service they thought would be available.

What else can the mental health services do?
Education of the general public, potential employers and some GPs was seen as important. Respondents would like quicker responses in terms of shorter waiting times for appointments, and wider availability of certain forms of treatment, for example, family therapy.

Voluntary agencies/self-help groups.   Twenty-five respondents did not use voluntary agencies or self-help groups to help them with their mental health problems. Some respondents commented that they did not want to be classed alongside the type of people who went to these places. They also felt that mixing with so many people with mental health problems would only make their own problems worse. The five respondents did use these sources found them helpful.

What service users liked best and least in primary care

Respondents appeared to like the sense of security that their care provided. The sense that someone was there if needed was important. They liked the sympathy offered and being listened to with an open mind, their problems being understood and advice given. Some respondents mentioned medication as being the part of their care that was most satisfying. One respondent said she was fearful of her own safety from the other patients during her hospitalisation and felt it unlikely that she had benefited from the experience. Long waiting times to obtain an appointment and long periods between appointments left respondents feeling insecure. Some doctors (both GPs and psychiatrists) were seen to be unsympathetic towards patients and inattentive towards their physical ailments. Stigmatisation of respondents because of their mental health problems was experienced by respondents from the public, their family, potential employers and sometimes, they felt, their GP.

Discussion

The survey findings largely concur with those of Rogers *et al* (1993). While it is heartening to note the high levels of satisfaction, it is important not to ignore the continuing causes of dissatisfaction still being experienced. In the first-stage questionnaire, most respondents identified a keyworker. The definition of a keyworker used for this survey was very loose, being 'a person who regularly helps you with your mental health problems'. This could account for the instances of GPs and psychiatrists being cited as a keyworker, and so the actual number of keyworkers is lower than that perceived by respondents. More satisfaction was expressed than dissatisfaction, with many respondents annotating their questionnaires with 'excellent' to describe their level of satisfaction with the care they had received.

Problems identified with the services included: long waiting times for appointments; receptionists appearing not to see mental health problems as an emergency; appointments being rushed and too short; and lack of understanding of their problems from their GP/psychiatrist. Much of this may be owing to high numbers of patients and the pressure of time on professionals. Respondents felt there needed to be more back-up care and help after the initial course of treatment, to provide reassurance to respondents that help was there if they needed it quickly; they did not want to have to go to the bottom of the waiting list to be seen again. Care seems to be more reactive than proactive. Many respondents also mentioned the need for sympathetic employers willing to give them a chance to prove themselves capable of holding down a job. This was seen as an important factor in improving their chances of remaining well.

Again, with the second questionnaire there was more satisfaction expressed than dissatisfaction. A high level of satisfaction was found with the behaviour, manners and skills of all levels of staff. Doctors tended to score more highly than nurses and receptionists for behaviour and manners, although only a minority of respondents were not satisfied. Some nurses were perceived as bossy, particularly those making home visits, and some receptionists were not seen to be sympathetic towards patients with mental health problems. Most respondents were satisfied with the level of confidentiality and respect they received and the level of understanding for their problems shown by professionals.

Respondents' main areas of dissatisfaction with the mental health services concerned inadequate information, involvement of their family, side-effects from medication and responses to crises. There was a lack of public information on local mental health services, with many not knowing what there was or where to look. This question attracted the lowest mean satisfaction score for the VSSS–54 (mean score 2.92). Involvement of the respondent's family in treatment was seen as essential by some and unnecessary by others. The former felt there was not enough involvement of their family, while the latter either found this intrusive or did not want their family involved in their treatment. Respondents particularly felt that their families needed more help to improve their knowledge and understanding of their problems. Help with side-effects from drugs was an area that received a mixed response, respondents felling that there was a lack of information about side-effects beforehand and a lack of help to resolve the problem of side-effects after they had occurred. However, most patients who received drug therapy were mostly satisfied with it. Respondents felt that help was not always available in times of crisis. Typically, if the respondent's GP was the main source of intervention, then help during a crisis was not always available. An appointment with his or her GP might not be available for a week or more. As one respondent said, "the problem is here now – it won't wait to come back in two weeks' time for my appointment". Many respondents were sympathetic towards the GP in this situation, realising that they were busy people with a lot of other patients to see as well.

The treatments most commonly received were drug therapy and individual psychotherapy. Half of respondents also received treatment from a CPN and a third had a keyworker. There was some confusion as to what a keyworker was; few respondents had had someone identified to them as such. A third of respondents said they would have liked family therapy and to involve their family more in their treatment. Family therapy (albeit undefined) stands out as an area of imbalance between what the mental health services provide and what people with mental health problems appear to want.

The sense of security that respondents got from the mental health services was very important to their sense of well-being. Long waiting times to obtain appointments and between appointments left them feeling insecure. Hospitalisation was unpopular, although generally accepted as necessary. Stigmatisation because of mental health problems was experienced by many respondents from all sections, including the public, their families, employers and sometimes doctors. Thus, the thing that was seen as most important for the mental health services to do was to educate people about mental health problems. Stigmatisation of people with mental health problems would appear to be evident also among those with mental health problems themselves, more so among those considering themselves not to be severely affected. Surprisingly few respondents used voluntary sector groups or agencies. Interestingly, this seemed to be because of a lack of understanding about what they offered and a reluctance to be associated with the people they thought used those places.

Many of the respondents had been treated for many years for their mental health problems and had had a lot of experience of the local mental health services. It was often difficult for them to isolate their evaluation of the mental health services to the past 12 months. It might have been preferable to interview patients who had been diagnosed and referred for treatment within the past 12 months for the first time. The representativeness of this small sample could be criticised for being self-selected. Thus, the high levels of satisfaction with the mental health services might be because a high proportion of respondents replied because they were happy with and grateful for their treatment. We did not assess in any way our non-responders and we did not corroborate our findings with the respondents' carers or professionals. We note the high proportion of Caucasian respondents (91%) in the study, especially when the ethnic mix of the research setting is considered.

Conclusion

Information is a key issue both for patient services and for public education. If respondents were better informed about what their local voluntary services offered, they might be more inclined to make use of them. However, efficient and coordinated follow-up services would still be important to facilitate respondents contacting the mental health services or vice versa if necessary. It is also of great importance to reduce waiting list times for treatment whenever possible. Continuity of care was important to respondents; informing them well in advance of a change of doctor, for example, owing to job moves, was seen to be important and a sign of respect towards the patient. Increasing overall public awareness of mental health problems was seen as necessary to reduce the stigmatisation experienced by many respondents from the public. This might improve local opportunities for respondents by encouraging employers to offer work to people with a history of mental health problems. The differences, although small, between respondents' perceptions of doctors, nurses and receptionists highlights the interface problems faced by staff and their need to receive training in dealing with patients.

These findings are likely to be largely generalisable to the other practices in the Nelson PCG, as the mental health services are from the same providers. There may be minimal differences in care that arise because some of the practices not surveyed in the PCG are smaller and therefore possibly less likely to have similar numbers of attached staff. These survey findings may be of use to other PCGs and their mental health leads who wish to use similar methods as part of their own mental health needs assessment. As outlined earlier in this chapter, however, the patient survey will only be one part of a whole range of methods necessary to assess the mental health needs of each PCG.

Acknowledgements

The survey described in this paper was undertaken with an unrestricted grant from Janssen Cilag, who funded Kathleen Beresford to undertake the survey under the supervision of myself and Professor Nick Bosanquet. I would also like to acknowledge the assistance of Ian Ayres, who was the chief executive of the SWLTPP at the time (now chief executive of the Nelson PCG and SWLPCO) and Dr Sarah Woropay, who led the mental health special interest group and helped to oversee the project.

References

Armstrong, E. (1997) *The Primary Mental Health Care Toolkit.* Available from NHSE response-line free of charge (0541 555455).

Bosanquet, N. (1997) *Patient Satisfaction with Mental Health Services, A Questionnaire.* London: Department of General Practice, Imperial College London.

COHEN, A. & PATON, J. (1999) *A Workbook for Primary Care Groups*. London: The Sainsbury Centre for Mental Health.

MELTZER, D., GILL, B., PETTICREW, M., *ET AL* (1995) *OPCS Surveys of Psychiatric Morbidity in Great Britain. Report 1: The Prevalence of Psychiatric Morbidity among Adults Living in Private Households.*. London: HMSO.

PRIEST, R. G., VIZE, C., ROBERTS, A., *ET AL* (1996) Lay people's attitudes to treatment of depression: results of opinion poll for Defeat Depression Campaign just before its launch. *British Medical Journal*, **313**, 858–859.

ROGERS, A., PILGRIM, D. & LACEY, R. (1993) *Experiencing Psychiatry, Users' Views of Services.* London: Macmillan/Mind Publications.

RUGGERI, M. (1993) *Verona Service Satisfaction Scale, Patients' Version, Version for use by PRISM*. London: Institute of Psychiatry.

STRATHDEE, G. & JENKINS, R. (1996) Purchasing mental health care for primary care. In: *Commissioning Mental Health Services* (eds G. Thornicroft & G. Strathdee), pp. 71–85. London: HMSO.

——, KENDRICK, T., COHEN, A., *ET AL* (1997) *A Health General Practitioner's Guide to Managing Long-term Mental Disorders*. 2nd edition. London: The Sainsbury Centre for Mental Health.

24 Mental health needs assessment for ethnic and cultural minorities

KAMALDEEP BHUI

The ethnic minority population in the UK has increased rapidly since the Second World War. Minority ethnic people represented 1% of the population in 1961; this had grown to 5.5% of the population at the time of the last census in 1991 (Peach, 1996). In some inner-city areas, minority groups constitute as much as 40% of residents. Ethnic and cultural minorities are diverse in their preferred language, customs and health beliefs. As these groups become more prominent in British society, and as the second and third generations increasingly identify themselves as legitimate 'British' citizens, they are less tolerant of inequalities of health care across ethnic groups. Inequalities in health care received significant attention in the British Government's recent Quality White Paper called *A First Class Service* (Department of Health UK, 1998*a*) and in a public health document called *Our Healthier Nation*:

> "The Government recognises that the social causes of ill health and the inequalities that stem from them must be acknowledged and acted on. Connected problems require joined-up solutions. This means tackling inequality that stems from poverty, poor housing, pollution, low educational standards, joblessness and low pay. Tackling inequalities generally is the best means of tackling health inequalities in particular." (Department of Health UK, 1998*b*)

Ethnic minority groups who suffer from mental illness constitute one 'group' of many that attract attention to reduce variations in access to, and benefit from, health care. The interplay with social deprivation, unemployment, traumatic pre-migration and post-migration experiences and a persistent lack of opportunities to

420

escape social exclusion appear to 'generate' and 'sustain' such inequalities. In this chapter, I do not intend to draw on the considerable literature that sets out the differential rates of disorders, treatment delivery, service utilisation or instances of 'falling out of care' (see Mental Health Foundation, 1995; Cochrane & Shashidharan, 1996; Nazroo, 1997; Bhui & Olajide, 1999). I will begin by briefly discussing the 'needs-based approach' and its conceptual limitations when applied to ethnic and cultural minorities. I will then address needs assessment issues for cultural and ethnic minorities at the level of: (a) surveys of individual and population need; (b) service structural and functional needs; (c) professional needs; and (d) local community need.

Conceptualisation of need

The chapters in this volume present a comprehensive account of the needs-based approach, and its relevance to the provision of high-quality services. These chapters address the mental health needs of differing populations. The main issues that are common to needs assessment among both Black and other ethnic minorities and other special groups are methodologies to measure need, achieving a balance of priorities within cost limitations, the service response, and the information systems required to realise the potential of routine needs assessments. Black and other ethnic minority mental health needs are prioritised in some national polices (Box 24.1), but systematic needs assessments tied to service responses that capture the spirit of these policies remain elusive.

The White paper *Caring for People* (Department of Health, 1989) advocated a greater degree of individual say in how people live their lives, and in determining the services they need to help them to live their lives. It was envisaged that users would be empowered by actively defining their health needs using shared assessment pro formas, access to care plans, and by having a choice of options wherever possible and yet the social services inspectorate practitioner's guide states that the assessing professional is responsible for defining the user's need (Myers & MacDonald, 1996). Need is relative and subjective; it is context-driven irrespective of how we attempt to objectify and operationalise it. It can be defined by users, their carers, service providers and the government. Each of these groups can legitimate certain forms of need and prohibit others. A truly needs-led philosophy accords well with a transfer of power from service provider to service user, and implicitly this should include Black and other ethnic minority users. Myers & MacDonald

---

Box 24.1
*Mental health policies directed at mental health of ethnic minorities or
of direct relevance to future services for ethnic minorities
(adapted from Olajide & Bhui, 1999)*

1993	Mental Health and Britain's Black Communities
1994	Ritchie Report
1994	Mental Health Task Force: London project and regional race programs
1994	Black Mental Health: a dialogue for change
1994	National Health Service (NHS) Executive letter on collection of ethnic group in-patient data EL(94)77
1994	Establishment of Ethnic Health Unit
1995	*Mental Health: Towards a Better Understanding.* Health of the Nation public information booklet for ethnic minorities and their carers
1998/9	*First Class Service* advocates National Service Frameworks for Mental Health to ensure best quality and fairest access; inequalities in health
1999	MacPherson Inquiry on institutionalised racism
1999	National Service Frameworks

(1996) assert the following ingredients as essential for a successful process of empowering users to define their needs:

- an organisational or political context within which the balance of power is located;
- a culture that determines different weighting of this power;
- compatible value systems: user–provider, user–carer and carer–provider; and
- a relationship within which power transfer takes place.

Each of these is heavily constrained by other parallel changes in the re-organisation of health care.

Evidence-based psychiatry

Evidence-based psychiatry is a welcome 'technology' to ensure the informed development of health care systems. Yet 'evidence-based psychiatry' contributes to the illusion that there is an adequate body of evidence that can efficiently and logically determine treatment recommendations and service structures. For example, randomised controlled trials of psychiatric interventions are rarely conducted on ethnic minority populations. Where there are trials, these are conducted on aggregated cultural and ethnic groups, and generalised to those groups who are not at all represented in the trials. Few of the trials of psychotropics include adequate numbers of ethnic minority patients to ensure generalisability, while it is well known that pharmaco-kinetic and pharmacodynamic properties of psychotropics vary across ethnic groups (Lin *et al*, 1995). Similarly, new service developments such as court diversion, or the CPA, are rarely piloted among ethnic minority populations. This means that the fundamental range of interventions that are supposed to address unmet need *may* be flawed when applied to ethnic minority groups.

Professions, society and value systems

Professionals are held to account for fulfilling certain functions on behalf of society, and these functions are determined by dominant value systems, professionalised codes of conduct and ethics, and bodies of law. These constraints are not always sensitive to culturally diverse ways of thinking about distress and mental disorders. Conflict arises between the value systems of carer, provider and user. Each has a different experience of mental illness and particular views about the most appropriate treatments. Among ethnic minority clients, culturally unique health beliefs of carers and users are likely to be more compat-ible with each other than with those of the provider. Thus, even if an optimal individual needs assessment is successfully completed, there are likely to be conflicts. These should be anticipated and addressed at the macro-service level as well for individual patients (Table 24.1).

There is a need to develop a better understanding of lay narratives of illness, to ensure that the evidence-based interventions being advocated by professionals are 'actively' accepted, and that they are appropriate. Common mental disorders are subject to much more diverse 'interpretative' behaviour in a 'search for meaning'. Conse-quently, common mental disorders are likely to be the most difficult to disentangle from normative experiences or transient psychosocial disturbances that do not lead to a persistent state of disability and need. A further complication is that ethnic minorities are subject to higher levels of background distress owing to traumatic pre- and post-migration experiences. Therefore, specific intensities of distress that amount to a 'significant mental disorder' are more difficult to distinguish from normative, transient and non-disabling conditions.

Meeting needs through culturally competent action

Needs assessment should be considered to be more than simply a way of estimating the 'amount' of illness. It is also about investigating

TABLE 24.1
Potential needs assessment conflicts for a 'specific intervention'

Professional judgement[1]	Patient judgement[2]	Carer judgement[3]	Conflict
Unmet need	Unmet need	Unmet need	No
	Met need	Met need	Yes
	Met need	Unmet need	Yes
	Unmet need	Met need	Yes
Met need	Met need	Met need	No
	Unmet need	Unmet need	Yes
	Unmet need	Met need	Yes
	Met need	Unmet need	Yes
No effective intervention	Unmet need	Met need	Yes
	Met need	Unmet need	Yes
	Unmet need	Unmet need	Yes
	Met need	Met need	No

1. Evidence-based intervention sanctioned by the standards of professional practice, clinical governance and the National Institute of Clinical Excellence.
2. Patients' beliefs about intervention are not always research evidence-based, but are determined by health beliefs, experience of services, 'lay epidemiology', religious and social subcultures, and their belief systems.
3. Carer beliefs about appropriate intervention may be the same as patients' but may also be quite different because of generation gap, gender gap, active symptoms affecting patients' judgement, carer disabilities and illness, and other competing responsibilities.

how existing services are delivered, and the effectiveness and cost-effectiveness of interventions intended to meet needs, as there is little point in only estimating the amount of illness if nothing can be done to reduce it (Wright *et al*, 1998). Yet, this is where the existing process seems to fail Black and other ethnic minorities. Care deficits, once identified, are not strategically addressed. Thus, the morass of data indicating an excess of African and Caribbean people with severe and enduring mental illness has not prompted a balanced health service response. In view of differing expectations of health and social care services, some ethnic minority groups prefer a different style of service to deliver these interventions (Wilson, 1993; Francis & Jonathan, 1999). Interventions will, at least, need to be delivered without compromising culture imperatives and beliefs, while nurturing the fragile treatment alliance that providers appear to have with Black and other ethnic minorities (Wilson, 1993; NHS Task Force, 1994).

Ownership and ascription of need

A further consideration is that Black and ethnic minority groups are inevitably not adequately represented in organisations that determine the definitions of health need, or the systems of addressing those needs. There is a potential for the legitimate needs, as perceived by Black and other ethnic minority groups, to be relegated to other 'priorities' that are more closely related to the dominant organisation's views of legitimate need. For example, 'women-only' wards for Muslim patients are essential if the sufferer's existing religious coping strategies are not to be compromised. Similarly, an anti-medication philosophy advocated in some Eastern religions and cultures raises concerns among patients about how best to deal with problems of living without resorting to culturally or religiously prohibited approaches, and without using medication. Such groups are only too respectful of Western medicines and treatment approaches, but the choice they are offered is to abandon their belief systems and adopt unfamiliar professionalised ones. If their confidence in professionals is threatened by disagreements or bad treatment experiences (Parkman *et al*, 1997), then any treatment alliance breaks down, and the intellectual exercise of conducing needs assessments become meaningless. Thus, the sequence of:

$$\text{Distress} \longrightarrow \text{Illness} \longrightarrow \text{Disability} \longrightarrow \text{Unmet need}$$
$$\longrightarrow \text{Specific intervention} \longrightarrow \text{Met need} \longrightarrow \text{Distress resolution}$$

is not so readily transferred to ethnic and cultural groups if beliefs systems and lay views are not compatible across medical, psychiatric or statutory sector responses. Statutory treatment approaches can be introduced to, and considered with, carers and users until agreement is reached. The hurdle is professionals' acceptance of patients' cultural or religious objections. There needs to be a willingness to give time to the development of a shared understanding of need. This helps engagement. A failure of understanding, or a loss of confidence in the statutory response, can be difficult to reconcile.

The cultural context of core needs

The Camberwell Assessment of Need (CAN; Psychiatric Research in Service Measurement (PRiSM), 1998) is one of the most comprehensive needs assessment instruments for use in mental health services. It covers basic core needs (left-hand column in Table 24.2), which I have elaborated (right-hand column) in order to highlight the cultural 'nuance' that must be borne in mind when considering these needs among ethnic minorities. It is clear that the core needs of mentally ill Black and other ethnic minority patients might not differ in terms of a 'label', but they do differ in terms of the origin of the need, the cultural meaning of the need, acceptable and unacceptable interventions, and culturally sanctioned interventions. This means that the 'unmet need' implications for one ethnic group do not translate into the same 'unmet need' implications for another. The specific intervention that is offered, let us say medication, may be identical; but the manner in which it must be delivered, and the manner in which it will be received, are quite different.

Needs that arise from religious, racial, and cultural persecution are daily social realities to minority groups. Racial violence, or racial prejudice, is a disquieting subject that generates defensive and avoidant reactions by service providers and purchasers. Black and other ethnic minority groups are unlikely to raise it themselves when they are in crisis or at a time of acute need, and it is therefore incumbent on the professional to consider these traumas as a legitimate source of distress, and perhaps requiring therapeutic attention.

Research and surveys as assessments of need

The process of needs assessment can be carried out at various levels:

- international
- national
- regional
- health authority-/board-based
- locality
- practice specific
- small neighbourhoods
- individual.

Epidemiologic surveys to assess prevalence and incidence of specific diagnostic groups are one approach to the quantification of need (Cochrane & Shashidharan, 1996; Nazroo, 1997). Specifically, schizophrenia is more common among African–Caribbeans, and has an especially high incidence among second-generation Caribbean patients. This alone does not give a sufficiently complex indication of a needs profile; for example, some studies suggest that the prognosis of schizophrenia is better among African–Caribbean men, therefore the treatment recommendations might be different (McKenzie *et al*, 1995). Similarly, studies that show fewer diagnoses of common mental disorders among 'Asian' patients are interpreted to indicate 'less need'; a putative protective effect of culture is hypothesised (Cochrane

TABLE 24.2
Core needs and cultural contexts

Core needs	Culture and ethnic context
Basic needs	
Accommodation	Poorer using; overcrowding; racism; poverty; local authority policies on ethnic minorities, mental health and housing
Food	Obtaining familiar foods; sense of neighbourhood cultures
Occupation	Ensuring qualifications accepted; training; language schools
Health needs	
Physical health	Higher prevalence of some conditions; changing lifestyle
Psychotic illness	Special emphasis on stigma, value conflict, normalised living
Neurotic illness	Interpersonal and social explanations; alternative traditional remedies; perceptions about drug treatment to treat mind conditions
Drugs and alcohol	Cultural taboos and mores, subcultures; may be a form of self-medication
Safety to self	Cultural perceptions of risk, violence and causes of violence
Safety to others	Cultural and religious meanings of suicide
Social needs	
Company	Dealing with statutory bodies; attuned to gender and religious roles
Intimate relationships	Dealing with condemnation about different values on marriage/dating
Sexual expression	Dealing with a different value system on marriage/dating
Everyday functioning	
Household skills	
Self-care	Racist threats; protecting family; children; leisure; religion
Childcare	Communication with schools; ensuring traditions are not lost
Basic education	Language mastery
Budgeting	Poverty
Service receipt	
Information	Language/illiteracy
Telephone	Poverty
Transport	Poverty
Welfare benefits	Negotiating a system in a different language; rules that are made by the 'better off' for those who are 'worse off'

& Stopes Roes, 1981). There is considerable debate about the validity of diagnostic groups and outcome measures that are developed in a specific ethnic group and applied to others ethnic and cultural groups (Kleinman, 1987; Leff, 1990; Littlewood, 1990). One solution is to include ethnographic work as a means of exploring needs, and sensitising epidemiological surveys to culturally meaningful or 'emic' constructions of mental disorders (Patel & Winston, 1997). Such an approach also contributes to the development of new instruments that are reputed to hold better cultural validity. However, comparative cultural research on needs and 'quality of life' across cultures is in its infancy (Chisholm & Bhugra, 1997).

Nazroo (1997) quite recently completed the fourth national morbidity study on ethnic minorities in the UK. Where English was not the first language, despite careful translation and inter-pretation of questions, the interviewers clearly stated difficulties of comprehension that raised concerns about the validity of the data. Patel & Winston (1997) argue that local and regional surveys yield the highest validity. Local beliefs and values can then be sys-tematically taken into account using ethnographic surveys that precede and run parallel with the main epidemiological surveys (for example, see Fenton & Siddiqui, 1993; Bhugra, 1996; Wilkinson & Murray, 1998).

In order to improve recruitment, Nazroo (1997) matched for language and ethnicity, but there was still an underrepresentation of certain ethnic groups. Recruitment of the chosen 'ethnicities or cultures' becomes a major part of planning surveys as ethnic minority groups are underrepresented in any official statistics except those involving custodial care or imprisonment. Hence, the 1991 census is known to have under-enumerated young men, and especially young Black men. This presents several problems. First, estimates of the base population are flawed and hence estimates of rates of disorders that use these denominators are likely to overestimate rates. This is one reason often advanced to explain the apparently higher rates of conspicuous psychosis among minority groups; this alone cannot explain the findings, but might magnify the excess risk of schizophrenia among Africans and Caribbeans, making it appear to be greater than it is. A second implication is that the recruitment of specific cultural and ethnic groups is hindered where unreliable local demographic data make study sites difficult to identify.

Survey estimates are dependent on referral filters and help-seeking behaviour. For example, Lloyd (1993) showed that African and Caribbean people were underrepresented among general practitioner (GP) attenders identified to have a psychiatric disorder, although ethnic minorities do attend their GP as often, if not more often, than the White population for physical disorders (Gillam *et al*, 1980). Yet, Nazroo (1997) demonstrated that the population prevalence of depressive symptoms among African–Caribbeans is higher than that of local White populations. Therefore, the study base population must be carefully selected to include the target 'ethnic or cultural group' in sufficient numbers to enable the hypotheses to be tested with sufficient power. Meaningful research must ensure that:

(a) the methodology, and the researchers, are informed about the cultures and ethnicities under study;

(b) the subjects of research have a say in the way the findings are interpreted;

(c) the study design must be scientifically rigorous and maximally efficient to answer a research question;

(d) the research question must be relevant to the 'needs profiles' of the ethnic minority groups under study; and

(e) the findings must be linked into an adequate service response in order to address new unmet needs.

Service needs

Although studies on the prevalence and incidence of diagnoses, and variations in treatment interventions and outcomes, are now increasingly common, there are practically no studies looking systematically at the 'service needs' pertaining to the development of culturally competent services. Bhui *et al* (1995) identified domains of service need (Box 24.2).

Each of these domains can be operationalised into quality standards that can serve as a measure of 'service need' in order to ensure a high-quality culturally competent service (see Bhui, 1997). For example, under 'information/advice', one might consider the following quality standards:

- knowledge of Black mental health organisations operating in your area;
- 'cultures' (cultures, ethnicities, religions and languages) they serve;
- opening times and referral or attendance criteria;
- 24-hour crisis service;
- 'cultures' of statutory service providers; and
- the quality and extent of links between Black organisations and the local health/social care services (case conferences, educational meetings, business meetings and training meetings).

Box 24.2
Domains of service need for culturally competent services (Bhui et al, 1995)

Service information
Public information campaigns
Information/advice facilities
Interpreting services
Multi-professional and user fora
Directories of mental health agencies

Range of health care services
Mechanisms to define local minority group needs
Range of locally available and flexible treatment packages
Addressing the needs of minority groups: specialist services
Religious and cultural imperatives
Psychotherapy services
Family care
Culturally congruent rehabilitation programmes
Service policies

New service models and evaluation
Monitoring take-up and success rates across groups
Black mental health teams
Specialist teams or generic teams with specialist training

Social care
Application of policy to minority groups
Ensure quick and effective access
Housing organisations/strategy
Benefits/systems to ensure quick processing
Families/comprehensive care

Staff and institutions
Training in culture and psychiatry
Multi-professional 'in-service' training
Black-led research pertinent to consumer views
Equal opportunities policies; audit of use

Sathyamoorthy & Ford (1998) have developed an audit tool to assess the prominence of service characteristics that are essential for competent cultural practice. In the context of rapidly reorganising health services, audit can be used to identify service development needs for a specific service serving specific cultural and ethnic groups. The difficulty here is that of identifying a suitable intervention when service models have not been evaluated among ethnic minority groups to an extent that these models, or any innovations, are considered culturally competent. Advice from culturally grounded voluntary and independent agencies is helpful. Indeed, such agencies might be the most appropriate to provide needs assessment in this specialist area of practice. Special attention must be given to clinical and managerial procedures where these might inadvertently compromise the optimal care being offered to specific cultural groups (Chandra, 1999). For example, some women may prefer not to be seen by a male doctor, or appointments may clash with specific prayer times or religious and cultural festivals.

Professional needs

Much is made of improving the cultural sensitivity of psychiatric practice, and yet there is little training of professionals that constructively attends to working within a multicultural society. Professional multi-disciplinary training as part of routine service provision is essential for all (Bhui & Bhugra, 1998). This, I suggest, should be one component of a 'service need'. The Royal College of Psychiatrists (1996) published recommendations for education of psychiatrists in a multicultural society. Furthermore, the Medical Protection Society, a prominent defence union for doctors, recently published guidance on cultural issues in general medical assessments (Medical Protection Society, 1997), making cultural competence a basic requirement for professionals working in multicultural societies. Clinical Governance also makes it a responsibility of providers to ensure that employees are all competent to provide a service to local patients, and this must also include cultural competence. For example, the simple act of communication, even in the same language, can be riddled with prejudicial and stereotypical contexts that are used to make poor and prejudicial sense of information provided by a patient (Robinson, 1998).

Local community needs

'Transcultural psychiatry' has grown as a sub-speciality of social psychiatry, yet its identity as a discipline and its boundaries with other disciplines are unclear. This difficulty is partly born of the inherent contradictions of a categorical system that aims to classify people according to racial, cultural or ethnic characteristics, where these are dynamic and not fixed entities (Jenkins, 1997). Indeed, the relationship between health behaviours and racial/ethnic category is undergoing constant change. The second and third generations absorb the cultural milieu of their parents' host country as well as of their parents' culture of origin. Communities that are identified as 'ethnic minorities' in any single locality at any one time will vary. There is therefore no national source of data to facilitate 'rapid local profiling' of cultural need. Providers need to systematically, and at regular intervals, identify what cultures, religions, health beliefs, expectations and risk factors are present in their locality and how these are associated with core mental health needs. Rapid appraisal of health needs in new communities is not a new concept (Wilkinson & Murray, 1998), but systematic routine application of these methodologies to ethnic minority populations is not common practice. Jordan *et al* (1999) identify a 'democratic deficit' in NHS provision, and suggest a template for taking into account community views:

- formal governance, including the election of health authority members and transferring NHS function to localities;
- consultation with the general public; and
- consultation with service users.

Consultation can consist of a single survey, meetings where participants are given no information, or consultations where participants are informed and encouraged to contribute by deliberating and discussing the issues. Within this framework, citizens' juries, user panels, focus groups, and questionnaire and opinion surveys are valuable. Focus groups in particular are a useful way of establishing significant qualitative insights grounded in the culture, language and experience of ethnic minority groups. Questionnaire surveys are quick and cheap, but are likely to suffer poor response rates as they represent the disclosure of information about 'personal' issues and time spent completing forms, with no direct or immediate benefit to subjects. Rapid appraisal using focus groups appears to be the most appropriate option. If information obtained in this way is carefully channelled, the yield will be the least constrained view of services rich in detailed cultural expectations and health beliefs. With the advent of primary care trusts (PCTs), an ongoing process of consultation with ethnic minority groups is essential. Otherwise, PCTs will repeat the errors of every NHS reorganisation, where the needs of ethnic minorities are assumed to be represented by the needs of the majority. Culture-specific needs and interventions can be discussed with the public using one of these processes to produce 'statements' or treatment protocols about which disorders and what sorts of problems will be addressed by primary and secondary care services, and which problems might be better taken to traditional sources of help and/or to the voluntary sector. The voluntary and independent sector provide a great deal of culturally competent work, but this remains organisationally separate from statutory sector responses (Francis & Jonathan, 1999).

Conclusions

Needs assessment of the mental health of Black and other ethnic minorities is gaining some prominence as a research area. The methodological implications warrant more attention; however, more practical rapid assessment procedures and the use of routinely collected data are rarely resourced to provide urgently needed measures of need. The assessment of need, without an awareness of the conceptual limitations of the concept, and the failure to consider the service and professional implications of newly defined areas of need, illustrate inequalities but have not mobilised an adequate strategic response to address ethnic and cultural variations of need. Local action at the provider level appears to be the most promising way of assessing need and addressing professional and service implications.

References

BHUGRA, D. (1996) Depression across cultures. *Primary Care Psychiatry*, **2**, 155–165.

BHUI, K. (1997) Addressing the mental health needs of minority ethnic groups. In: *Mental Health Service Development Skills Workbook* (eds K. Thompson, G. Strathdee & H. Wood). London: Sainsbury Centre for Mental Health.

—— & BHUGRA, D. (1998) Training and supervision in effective cross cultural mental health services. *British Journal of Hospital Medicine*, **59**, 861–865.

—— & OLAJIDE, D. (1999) *Mental Health Service Provision for a Multi-Cultural Society*. London: Saunders.

——, CHRISTIE, Y., BHUGRA, D., *ET AL* (1995) Essential elements of culturally sensitive psychiatric services. *International Journal of Social Psychiatry*, **41**, 242–256.

CHANDRA, J. (1999) Managing for cultural competence. In: *Mental Health Service Provision for a Multi-Cultural Society* (eds K. Bhui & D. Olajide), pp. 225–237. London: Saunders.

CHISHOLM, D. & BHUGRA, D. (1997) Socio-cultural and economic aspects of quality of life measurements. *European Psychiatry*, **12**, 210–215.

COCHRANE, R. & SHASHIDHARAN, S. P. (1996) Mental health and ethnic minorities: a review of the literature and service implications. In: *Ethnicity and Health: Reviews of Literature and Guidance for Purchasers in the Areas of Cardiovascular Disease, Mental Health and Haemoglobinopathies*. CRD Report 5. York: NHS Centre for Reviews and Dissemination Social Policy Research Unit, University of York.

—— & STOPES ROES, M. (1981) Psychological symptom level in Indian immigrants to Britain: A community survey. *Social Psychiatry*, **12**, 195–206.

DEPARTMENT OF HEALTH (1989) *Caring for People: Community Care in the Next Decade and Beyond.* Cmnd 849. London: HMSO.

—— (1998a) *A First Class Service. Quality in the new NHS.* London: Department of Health.

—— (1998b) *Our Healthier Nation. A Contract for Health.* Presented to Parliament by the Secretary of State for Health by Command of Her Majesty. London: The Stationery Office.

FENTON, S. & SIDDIQUI, A. (1993) *The Sorrow in my Heart.* London: Commission for Racial Equality..

FRANCIS, J. & JONATHAN, D. (1999) The voluntary sector. In: *Mental Health Service Provision for a Multi-Cultural Society* (eds K. Bhui & D. Olajide), pp. 118–134. London: Saunders.

GILLAM, S., JARMAN, B., WHITE, P., *ET AL* (1980) Ethnic differences in consultation rates in urban general practice. *British Medical Journal*, **289**, 953–957.

JENKINS, R. (1997) *Rethinking Ethnicity. Arguments and Explorations.* London: Sage.

JORDAN, J., DOWSWELL, T., HARRISON, S., *ET AL* (1999) Health needs assessment. Whose priorities? Listening to users and the public. *British Medical Journal*, **316**, 1668–1670.

KLEINMAN, A. (1987) Anthropology and psychiatry. The role of culture in cross-cultural research on illness. *British Journal of Psychiatry*, **151**, 447–454.

LEFF, J. (1990) The 'new cross-cultural psychiatry'. A case of the baby and the bath water. *British Journal of Psychiatry*, **156**, 305–307.

LIN, K., POLAND, R. & ANDERSON, D. (1995) Psychopharmacology, ethnicity and culture. *Transcultural Research Review*, **32**, 3–40.

LITTLEWOOD, R. (1990) From categories to contexts: a decade of the 'new cross-cultural psychiatry'. *British Journal of Psychiatry*, **156**, 308–327.

LLOYD, K. (1993) Depression and Anxiety among Afro-Caribbean general practice attenders in Britain. *International Journal of Social Psychiatry*, **39**, 1–9.

MCKENZIE, K., VAN OS, J., FAHY, T., *ET AL* (1995) Psychosis with good prognosis in Afro-Caribbean people now living in the United Kingdom. *British Medical Journal*, **311**, 1325–1328.

MEDICAL PROTECTION SOCIETY (1997) *Problems of Medical Practice in a Multi-Cultural Society.* London: Medical Protection Society.

MENTAL HEALTH FOUNDATION (1995*) "Towards a Strategy", Proceedings of a Seminar on Race and Mental Health.* London: Mental health Foundation.

MYERS, F. & MACDONALD, C. (1996) Power to the people? Involving users and carers in needs assessment and care planning – views from the practitioner. *Health and Social Care in the Community*, **4**, 86–95.

NAZROO, J. (1997) *The Mental Health of Ethnic Minorities in Britain.* London: Policy Studies Institute.

NHS TASK FORCE (1994) *Black Mental Health: a Dialogue for Change.* London: Mental Health Task Force, NHS Management Executive.

OLAJIDE, D. & BHUI, K. (1999) Government policy and ethnic minority mental health. In: *Mental Health Service Provision for a Multi-Cultural Society* (eds K. Bhui & D. Olajide), pp. 67–81. London: Saunders.

PARKMAN, S., DAVIES, S., LEESE, M., *ET AL* (1997) Ethnic differencs in satisfaction with mental health services among representative people with psychosis in a south London study. *British Journal of Psychiatry*, **171**, 260–264.

PATEL, V. & WINSTON, M. (1997) 'Universality of mental illness' revisited: assumptions, artefacts and new directions. *British Journal of Psychiatry*, **165**, 437–440.

PEACH, C. (1996) Introduction to Ethnicity in the 1991 Census, vol. 2. In: *The Ethnic Minority Populations of Great Britain* (ed. C. Peach). Office for National Surveys. London: HMSO.

PRISM (1998) *Camberwell Assessment of Need..* London: PRISM, Institute of Psychiatry.

ROBINSON, L. (1998) Interpersonal perception and inter-ethnic communication. In: *Race, Communication and the Caring Profession.* Milton Keynes: Open University Press.

ROYAL COLLEGE OF PSYCHIATRISTS (1996) *Report of the Working Party to Review Psychiatric Practice and Training in a Multi-Ethnic Society.* Council Report CR48. London: Royal College of Psychiatrists.

SATHYAMOORTHY, G. & FORD, R. (1998) *Audit Tool to Assess the Cultural Sensitivity of Mental Health Services: Staff and User Interview Schedules.* London: Sainsbury Centre for Mental Health.

WILKINSON, J. & MURRAY, S. (1998) Health needs assessment. Assessment in primary care: practical issues and possible approaches. *British Medical Journal*, **316**, 1524.

WILSON, M. (1993) *Britain's Black Communities.* London: Mental Health Task Force & King's Fund Centre, NHS Management Executive.

WRIGHT, J., WILLIAMS, R. & WILKINSON, J. (1998) Health needs assessment. Development and importance of health needs assessment. *British Medical Journal*, **316**, 1310–1313.

25 Needs assessment for rural mental health services

ALAIN GREGOIRE

Rurality is a diffuse concept about which most people hold clear stereo-typical beliefs. An idealised view of rural life has been fashionable in Western society for two or three centuries and continues to be a powerful sales image in many industries, most obviously exemplified by magazines based on a country theme that are produced in towns and sell most to urban dwellers. This stereotype is of a peaceful, unpressurised existence led by economically advantaged people with simple needs living in supportive communities. It is somewhat surprising, given this commonly held view, that 80% of the population of the UK choose not to live in rural areas. This may be because the stereotype is often at odds with the facts.

The nature of rural areas

Because what is meant by rurality varies according to the context in which it is being considered, it can encompass a number of different parameters such as population density, physical environment, social characteristics and land use. It is therefore impossible to arrive at a universally agreed definition of rurality, and care must be taken to clarify the definition being used when examining available data or undertaking research. Furthermore, one must be cautious when single indices are used for definition, as these can be severely misleading. Thus, a definition dependent on the nature of land use could falsely label as 'urban' a motorway corridor and service stations or an oil refinery, whereas a definition relying on population density could label the area covered by New York Central Park or parishes in the City of London as rural. However, the use of complex indices (e.g. Cloke, 1977) can pose insurmountable practical difficulties; in most areas of the literature, simple indices such as population density or size of settlement have been used (Shucksmith, 1990; Countryside Agency, 1999), but others have abandoned any attempt to formalise a definition and have relied on the arbitrary definition of research workers' impressions of the area (Meltzer *et al*, 1995).

Another complicating factor in assessing and understanding the characteristics of rural areas is the wide variation in these characteristics across different locations. This variation is obviously very dramatic between nations; for example, what is considered to be a rural area in Australia will differ markedly from a rural area in southern England. Thus, a starting point for any assessment of mental health needs must be an appraisal of the national, regional and local background rural characteristics. Such statistics are often available from official bodies, and the data for rural areas is sometimes specifically extracted, as exemplified by the Countryside Agency in England. To use England as an example, the available data provide a useful general background against which to understand the context for an analysis of needs and the planning of services (Countryside Agency, 1999).

Rural areas in England

Twenty per cent of the population of England and 88% of the land are in areas outside settlements of 10 000 or more people. Compared with the national averages, the proportion of young people is lower and that of people over the age of 65 years is higher. There are thus proportionately fewer people of working age, but, with some exceptions, most rural areas of England have lower rates of unemployment than urban areas. However, incomes tend to be low, with the lowest wage levels nationally in peripheral rural counties such as Cornwall and the Isle of Wight, and a greater proportion of both men and women in rural areas earn low wages (Countryside Agency, 1999). Rates of part-time employment, self-employment and home employment are also higher in rural areas. There has been a very substantial loss of land-based employment (there was a 14% decrease in agricultural jobs from 1987 to 1997) in the past two decades, but more recently there has been an increase in employment in the service sector, and the mix of industry and service employment in rural areas is now very similar to that found nationally. In the past 10 years, the income from farming in England has dropped by about half. The changing nature of the work has now made it a very lonely, isolated occupation. These employment characteristics of rural areas are likely to be particularly disadvantageous to people with mental health problems, who may need levels

Box 25.1
Effects of low population density on clients

Geographical isolation
- Complete inability to travel to services
- Inconvenience travelling to services
- Time travelling to services
- Unwillingness to travel to services
- Costs of transport

Social isolation
- Perceived or actual stigma
- Reduced community supports
- Reduced opportunity for social contact

Poor availability of services
- Chemists
- Shops/post offices
- Local employment
- Leisure facilities
- Primary health care
- Social services
- Specialist mental health services

of support not available in self-employment or home employment, particularly in the absence of locally based employment support schemes.

People living in rural areas in England can expect poorer access to most types of services (Box 25.1). In addition to this general paucity of amenities such as shops, buses, health centres and leisure facilities, which affects the whole population, the young, the old and people with disabilities and health problems are particularly disadvantaged. For example, 96% of rural parishes have no form of day care for people with disabilities and 91% have no residential care of any sort. The special nature of rural poverty and social exclusion is often unacknowledged, but is none the less very real (Cox, 1998).

The government's standard spending assessments in the rural shires of England allows for only 60% of the spending per head of population on public services that is available in inner London. The result in shire areas is that there is less access to adult education, fewer sports and leisure facilities and reduced concessionary travel schemes. Public transport in rural areas is characteristically very poor and there is a much greater dependency on cars, including by those people with low incomes for whom the financial burden of car ownership is particularly intense. There is considerably less social housing available in rural areas, where it accounts for only 15% of the housing stock, compared with 23% nationally. Rural Development Commission figures indicate that less than a quarter of the additional affordable housing required in rural areas between 1990 and 1995 was actually built. The homelessness problem, which had been growing faster in rural areas than anywhere else, therefore remains substantial. The impact of the lack of amenities and services in rural areas is particularly keenly felt by people with mental health problems, who are so often dependent on public sector services, affordable rented housing and supported or supportive employment.

Rural services for people with mental illness

Large centres of clinical excellence, academic departments that often support them and the sub-speciality services associated with them are to be found almost exclusively in urban areas, mainly in the centres of large cities. This seems an inevitable consequence of population density and transport, which facilitate the co-location or efficient collaboration of institutions and professionals. Unlike physical health care resources, this pattern is a relatively recent one for mental health services in most Western countries. It replaces the large Victorian asylums that concentrated almost all the mental health care resources in isolated rural institutions. However, rural populations were even more poorly served by these institutions, as they were not founded on any principle of local service provision.

The concentration of secondary and tertiary resources and expertise in urban areas is often considered necessary in order to achieve a critical mass of patients and staff, and justifiable as the urban location will be accessible to the greatest majority of patients. The validity of these arguments is widely assumed, but service planners and providers for rural populations would be right to question such assumptions. Indeed, it is very likely that the needs of rural populations are poorly met by this model, particularly in the context of mental health services, which are increasingly geographically defined.

A small number of UK studies have examined rural service provision. Smith & Ramana (1998) demonstrated the absence of rehabilitation services and facilities in rural Cambridgeshire, which resulted from historical differences in provision and unquestioning urban focus, rather than any analysis of the needs of the local population. This had resulted in rural clients only being able to access urban-based facilities. As rehabilitation services are particularly aimed at maximising patients' ability to live independently in their community, such a situation must surely be a disincentive to accessing such services and may compromise the quality of service offered to rural clients. In a study conducted in Nottingham and surrounding areas, Seivewright *et al* (1991) found that patients with mental illnesses in urban areas had more frequent contact with psychiatrists than those in rural areas. This included a greater number of contacts that resulted from physical complaints rather than mental health ones. Use of psychotropic drugs and admission rates were also higher in the urban sample. It is not clear from this study whether these differences are related to greater severity of illness in urban areas or lower service provision in rural areas. However, other findings suggest that lower service provision in rural areas is at least an important factor. Rural patients in this study had more contacts with their general practitioner (GP) than those in urban areas, and other studies have demonstrated findings that support this conclusion. For example, studies have demonstrated later first presentation of schizophrenia (Keatinge, 1988), underreporting of neurotic symptoms and a more negative attitude to psychiatric facilities (Keatinge, 1987), and higher thresholds for admission to psychiatric hospital in rural areas (Cuffel, 1994). Distance from services is a significant predictor of use of mental health services (Hall, 1998). Gyllenhammar *et al* (1988) were able to compare rural and urban areas in Sweden with equally accessible emergency psychiatric services, finding that in these circumstances the number and nature of emergency presentations of rural and urban clients were the same. A UK survey of GPs demonstrated perceived inaccessibility of mental health services in rural areas (Stansfield *et al*, 1992). Although poorly documented, there is no doubt that the same difficulties with access also apply to social services (Bentham & Haynes, 1986; Fearn, 1987).

With the establishment of community-based mental health care, the importance of primary care in providing services to people with mental illnesses at all levels of severity is increasingly acknowledged. This role appears to be particularly important for mentally ill people in rural areas, who have more contact with their GPs (Seivewright *et al*, 1991) and are more dependent on them as a result of the relative inaccessibility of secondary and tertiary mental health services. However, access to primary care also presents problems in rural areas, particularly in more isolated areas (Bentham & Haynes, 1986). Furthermore, excessive dependency on GPs for the provision of mental health care in rural areas may compromise the quality of care to patients: the role of primary care in the assessment and treatment of severe mental illness should be a shared one.

Non-governmental organisations are playing an increasing role in providing support, advocacy and sometimes direct care for people with

---

Box 25.2
UK rural mental health organisations

RuralMinds
Arthur Rank Centre, Stoneleigh Park, Warwickshire CV8 2LZ
Website: www.mind.org.uk/ruralminds

Rural Stress Information Network
Arthur Rank Centre, Stoneleigh Park, Warwickshire CV8 2LZ
Website: www.ruralnet.org.uk/~rusin

The Samaritans
17 Uxbridge Road, Slough SL1 1SN

Institute of Rural Health
Gregynog, Newtown, Powys, Wales SY16 3PW
Website: www.rural-health.ac.uk

---

mental illness and their families. Access to a range of such services is now the norm in most urban areas, but still rare in rural areas. Some of these organisations are beginning to address the lack of community facilities for the rural mentally ill with a range of initiatives. Most of these are local, small-scale projects (see below), but others, such as RuralMinds, The Samaritans and the Rural Stress Information Network, are national initiatives focusing on particular issues (The Samaritans, 1997; see Box 25.2).

For many people with mental illness, the greatest burden of care falls on friends or relatives. This may be particularly true in rural areas that have a lack of residential or day support facilities (Smith & Ramana, 1998) and where the severely mentally ill are more likely to be living with informal carers. The needs of carers of people with severe mental illness in rural areas have been described (e.g. Tucker *et al*, 1998), but very few resources exist to support them (Sherlock, 1994).

It is well documented that people with mental illnesses have worse physical health than the rest of the population and are less likely to access or receive adequate medical care (e.g. Bartsch *et al*, 1990). This disadvantage for the mentally ill is compounded in rural areas by poor accessibility to primary and secondary medical care (Fearn, 1987; Watt *et al*, 1993).

Studies of mental health services in other parts of the world show remarkably similar patterns of poor service provision and access problems, despite widely differing socio-economic and demographic patterns. Murthy (1998) has reviewed mental health strategies and services in developing countries. The author points to the need for national policy and programmes in developing countries and cites examples of considerable progress where these exist. Successful strategies invariably rely on close integration of limited specialist provision with primary care and adopt community-based models. Consistent features of the populations they serve include greater community acceptance of mentally ill people, cohesive and supportive families and the absence of large numbers of institutionalised patients. However, in most parts of the developing world, the family has been the substitute for any form of mental health care rather than a component of it. Mental health often remains a low priority of many governments, despite its clear importance to their population's disability and their economies (Desjarlais *et al*, 1995). Furthermore, rural populations in developing countries are generally in the majority; for example, in India, 70% of the population of 960 million is rural. The largest body of rural service research comes from the USA, where the National Institute of Mental Health has given this priority. Findings are broadly comparable with those in the UK, despite a different service and demographic context, but offer greater detail. Various authors have described US rural mental health services as fragmented, costly and ineffective (Fox *et al*, 1994). Studies examining current US rural mental health service provision highlight the limited community resource, client access problems, poor education of staff, family and clients (Human & Wasem, 1991; Murray & Keller, 1991; Sullivan *et al*, 1996), and inadequate numbers of psychiatrists, particularly relative to urban areas (Eveland *et al*, 1998). More research is needed for evidence-based rural service planning and provision, as these are currently dependent on "the idiosyncratic beliefs of policy makers and administrators about what constitutes good care in rural areas". Much the same could be said about the UK.

Unmet need is an obvious result of shortfalls in certain services. Another important though less obvious result is the resource-led drift of patients from rural to urban areas. People are drawn into towns as a result of housing and employment shortages in rural areas (Rural Development Commission, 1992). Smith & Ramana (1998) have described this effect with patients needing rehabilitation services. This type of drift not only takes people away from their own local areas, family and social networks, but it also drains resources and clinical experience from the rural services and increases the burden on urban services. It could, of course, be assumed that adequate access to a full range of mental health services is not necessary in rural areas because of an absence of need, which could result from peculiarities in either the epidemiology or the nature of mental illnesses in rural areas. These factors will therefore be considered.

Nature and epidemiology of mental illness in rural areas

There is no convincing evidence to suggest any differences in the nature or severity of mental illnesses between rural and non-rural areas. Particular caution must be exercised in interpreting any occasional apparent differences that may emerge, such as higher rates of suicide attempts in rural, compared with urban, depression (Rost *et al*, 1998), as these are at least as likely to be related to differences in help-seeking behaviour or service utilisation and availability as the nature or severity of the disorders. For example, Keatinge (1987, 1988) has described the tendency in rural areas to underreport neurotic symptoms and for first admission for psychotic illness to be delayed and to occur at a more chronic stage. In the previously mentioned study by Rost *et al* (1998), participants with depression had significantly fewer out-patient contacts in rural areas and, apparently related to this, tended to have a greater number of in-patient admissions, the latter effect disappearing when the number of out-patient contacts was controlled for. Another measure of severity of mental illness is the disability that results from it. Studies that have examined levels of disability related to mental illness in community, primary care and secondary care samples have demonstrated that people in rural areas are not in any way immune from the serious impact of mental illnesses on their functioning (McCreadie *et al*, 1997; Clayer *et al*, 1998; Thurston-Hicks *et al*, 1998).

The few studies that have been carried out examining rates of mental illness in rural areas, sometimes compared with urban or national data, vary widely in their findings (see Table 25.1 and Gregoire & Thornicroft, 1998). The findings from these studies indicate that no generalised international rural/urban patterns emerge in the epidemiology of mental illnesses. It is unlikely that there is some unidentified core-defining characteristic of rurality that is a direct determinant of rates of mental illness, but rather that other factors are operating that determine such rates. Such factors may be differentially distributed across urban and rural areas, may act differently or indeed may be peculiar to some rural or urban areas. Studies examining such factors have contributed to the development of proxy indicators of need and indices of deprivation, now frequently applied in resource allocation. However, all these indices have been developed in urban areas and their validity in rural areas has been challenged (Jessop, 1992). The relationship between these indices and psychiatric morbidity may disappear or be different in rural areas (Thornicroft *et al*, 1993). Indeed, urban and rural areas may differ in

TABLE 25.1
Studies of rural psychiatric morbidity

Author	Location	Disorders (if specified)	Findings
Cheng (1989)	Taiwan	–	Rural = urban
McGee *et al* (1991)	New Zealand	–	Rural = urban
Romans-Clarkson *et al* (1990)	New Zealand	–	Rural = urban
Romans *et al* (1992)	New Zealand	–	Rural = urban
Gyllenhammar *et al* (1988)	Sweden	–	Rural = urban
Keatinge (1988)	Eire	Schizophrenia	Rural = urban
Brown & Prudo (1981)	UK: Hebrides *v.* Camberwell	Depression	Rural = urban
Meltzer *et al* (1995)	UK: Community Survey	Obsessive–compusive disorder/panic psychosis[1]	Rural = urban
Bowling & Farquhar (1991)	UK	–	Rural < urban
Lewis & Booth (1994)	UK	–	Rural < urban
McCreadie *et al* (1997)	UK: Dumphries *v.* Camberwell	Schizophrenia	Rural < urban[2]
Meltzer *et al* (1995)	UK: Community Survey	Anxiety/ depression/ phobia	Rural < urban
Keatinge (1988)	Eire	Neuroses	Rural < urban
Crowell *et al* (1986)	USA	Anxiety/ depression	Rural < urban
Lee *et al* (1990)	Korea	–	Rural > urban
Guinness (1992)	Swaziland	–	Rural > urban
Thornicroft *et al* (1993)	Italy	Schizophrenia	Rural > urban
Orley & Wing (1979)	Uganda *v.* Camberwell	Depression	Rural > urban

1. Numbers are very small.
2. The increased prevalence of schizophrenia in Camberwell was almost entirely accounted for by racial differences, the rates in the White population being similar in both areas.

the relationships found between mental illness and a number of other factors, such as social support, life events and physical illness (Brown & Prudo, 1981; Campiniello *et al*, 1989; Romans-Clarkson *et al*, 1990;

Bowling & Farquhar, 1991). Thus, from a theoretical point of view, the factors determining levels of psychiatric morbidity in rural areas are yet to be established and therefore the impact of rurality on the epidemiology of mental illness cannot, in the absence of reliable proxy indicators, be ignored. However, from a practical point of view, the literature can inform the process of evaluating the nature and extent of psychiatric morbidity in a given rural area. Thus, as the features of the area that need to be taken into account (Gregoire & Thornicroft, 1998) include racial distribution and poverty, the strong possibility of significant local variation in rates of various disorders needs to be allowed for (Torrey, 1987; Youssef *et al*, 1991), the various psychiatric disorders must be distinguished when examining morbidity and not estimates for mental illness or severe mental illness as a whole, or indeed estimates relating to one disorder alone, and, finally, occupational characteristics of the population may be very relevant.

Particular attention has recently been paid to farmers, an occupational group almost exclusively found in rural areas, who suffer high rates of suicide, stress and isolation. The risk of suicide in farmers in the UK between 1979 and 1990 ranked fourth in order of risk by occupation, but since 1991, the rate appears to have decreased and farmers are now the seventh highest-risk occupational group, along with farm managers and horticulturists (Kelly & Bunting, 1998). However, suicide accounts for the second most common cause of death in male farmers under the age of 45 years and in terms of total numbers of suicides, farmers have the highest numbers of any occupational group in the UK. The risk of suicide among farmers' wives is also high (Kelly & Charlton, 1995). The key factors associated with suicide in farmers appear to be the presence of mental illness, low rates of treatment, the lack of a close confiding relationship, work and financial problems, and the availability of firearms (Malmberg *et al*, 1999). These factors suggest various possibilities for suicide prevention strategies, and indeed various local and national organisations have in recent years been trying to target farmers with support, advice and improved access to treatment. The slight decrease in suicide rates over the past few years, despite increases in stress, isolation and reductions in income, suggests the possibility that targeted measures such as these may have been beneficial.

A possible source of neuropsychological morbidity giving rise to concern is exposure to agricultural chemicals, notably organophosphates, principally by agricultural workers, although at present there is too little research to support any firm conclusions on the scale and nature of the effects (Royal College of Physicians and Royal College of Psychiatrists, 1998).

Meeting mental health needs of rural populations

Evaluations or even descriptions of services that are particularly adapted to rural areas are very rare, even internationally. This is not surprising as the culture that fosters evaluation and dissemination usually arises from academic centres that are located in urban areas. However, some general principles can be derived from the literature, and a number of descriptions of specific services illustrate ways in which these principles have been successfully applied.

Many aspects of urban service models are poorly suited to rural areas as they do not address the challenges or utilise the opportunities that are peculiar to rural populations. All too often, models of care based on experiences or beliefs developed in influential urban centres are declared as national gold standards. It is likely that the difficulties in applying such urban models will have led to some of the inadequacies of services for rural populations.

To develop more effective services, the challenges and opportunities need to be considered alongside the available evidence and experience about rural service provision.

The challenges

A key characteristic of rural areas from which many challenges flow is low population density, which reduces the cost-effectiveness of a whole range of local services (Box 25.3). The resulting limited public transport

---

Box 25.3
Effects of low population density on services

Low patient density
- Transport costs for clients and staff
- Staff travel time

Low staff density
- Professional isolation
- Limited educational opportunities
- Limited peer supervision and support
- Limited exchange of clinical experience
- Limited cross cover, work sharing and flexibility

Poor availability of service
- Fewer specialist services to refer to
- Fewer services to share care with

provision in turn compounds the problems of the dispersed population. This is particularly felt by the mentally ill, who are already disadvantaged socio-economically, and are less likely to own a car or to be able to drive. People with mental illness living in rural areas also often describe use of public transport (and attendance at known mental health facilities) as particularly intimidating because of the lack of anonymity. Unless services can be provided locally across rural areas, it is inevitable that service utilisation and cooperation with care plans, particularly those involving leisure or occupational activities, will be reduced.

Local provision requires staff to be geographically spread out and highly mobile. This will limit opportunities for joint activities such as peer support, formal networking and education. This can compromise staff knowledge, skills, specialist expertise and, therefore, quality of services to patients. Staff in small isolated service units are less able to cross-cover or share work and can suffer considerably from fluctuations in workload or staffing levels. Furthermore, safety of staff can be very difficult to ensure because of the size and staffing of local rural units and services.

The limited availability of the range of statutory and non-statutory resources in rural areas, coupled with limited staff training and experience, makes the brokerage or care management model of mental health provision difficult to apply in rural areas (Rohland *et al*, 1998). A model that relies more upon assertive outreach, with most elements of care being provided directly by mental health professionals, is probably more appropriate in most rural areas, but this has implications for staff time, training and resources (Santos *et al*, 1993).

The opportunities

There is little empirical evidence to support assertions about the positive aspects of rural environments in relation to psychiatric disorder. Nevertheless, one can postulate several features that have face validity. For example, the rural aesthetic environment would be considered positive by most people, at least in developed countries, although there are some exceptions, such as disused coal-fields.

The author's experience suggests that the recruitment of skilled mental health staff can be very difficult, but staff turnover tends to be low. In the UK, attracting good staff to primary care, at least in the less isolated areas, does not appear to be difficult. However, in many countries and in more isolated rural areas everywhere, staffing presents such problems that some governments have had to introduce incentives or even directives to ensure minimum staffing.

The stereotype of small, supportive communities may partially reflect reality. However, this is a complex and very poorly documented issue.

One of the few studies of rural networks of formal and informal care of people with mental illness, carried out in the USA, indicates that networks in rural areas are in fact often very large, that they appear to function within discreet geographical areas (counties) rather than across them, and that formal methods of interaction and communication within networks are very difficult, with informal interaction providing important channels of communication (Fried *et al*, 1998). These findings suggest that opportunities for informal communication should be fostered rather than relying on formal procedures, which are probably more efficient and effective in urban areas, and that services in rural areas should operate locally within natural population boundaries rather than across them. Local provision is particularly important for certain groups of clients for whom community networks are central to therapeutic aims. For example, the care of people with chronic severe mental illness with impaired functioning (traditionally known as rehabilitation) cannot hope to engage them into their community networks from a distance.

Examples of local solutions

Rural services all over the world have evolved or been designed to provide local solutions to the sorts of challenges and opportunities described above. Unlike urban services, published evaluation of the outcomes of such services is almost completely lacking, but a number of qualitative descriptions are available. Examples from the UK can be used to illustrate the scope and experiences of such services. Some of these have been published (e.g. Sherlock, 1995) and others have been described in local reports made available to the author by some of the organisations listed at the end of the chapter, or through personal communication to the author.

Although the services described enable clients with severe mental illnesses to access what should be considered essential components of good-quality modern mental health care, a common theme in most of these services is the temporary grant-based funding and, in some areas, particularly provision of transport, funding relies on charity or payment by the clients themselves.

Assessment and treatment of mental illness

These have mainly been developed by statutory services in primary care, secondary care mental health services and social services. Schemes include: education and support programmes aimed at increasing early detection and intervention of mental illness in primary care involving GPs and practice nurses; named mental health teamworkers allocated to specific general practices; regular opportunities for primary care/ secondary care communication; and community mental health teams (CMHTs) using rural community facilities, delivering home-based care, 24-hour crisis intervention and shared care with GPs. Features common to these services include: making use of local unstigmatised community facilities such as village or church halls and GP surgeries; fostering and using local knowledge by allocating staff to particular areas or GP practices; working closely with the few organisations operating in rural areas (e.g. The Samaritans, Farmers Union, Young Farmers' clubs, MIND, Women's Royal Voluntary Service, etc); and a very strong emphasis on the provision of transport for patients.

Information, advocacy and advice

The need for information and advice, often unmet, emerges consistently in studies or surveys of users and carers in rural areas (Sherlock, 1995; Tucker *et al*, 1998). It is inevitable that when services are small and dispersed over a wide geographical area awareness among professionals, carers and clients will be hampered. Valuable models for improving this situation in rural areas include the use of telephone help- and support-lines, printed newsletters, directories of services, intercommunicating networks of information, advice centres and programmes of regular informal gatherings in decentralised locations. Regular meetings for users, carers and professionals and all combinations of these three groups appear to be an effective and widely adopted component of local rural services.

Counselling and therapy

The successful delivery of psychological services in rural areas by both statutory and non-statutory organisations relies on flexible local delivery of a range of services. Most of the organisations that deliver such services, including Citizens' Advice Bureaux, counselling organisations, telephone counselling services, farmers' counselling services, the Samaritans, NHS mental health services and Social Services departments have in various places successfully developed outreach or peripatetic psychological therapy services. However, these still tend to be isolated examples rather than organisation-wide strategies.

Supported and crisis accommodation

A growing number of examples demonstrate that it is possible to provide the full range of supported accommodation from 24-hour nursed care for high-dependency chronically mentally ill patients through to low-support crisis flats even in quite isolated rural areas. Most such services operate with great flexibility in order to derive maximum benefit from very limited infrastructure, for example, attaching crisis beds to supported accommodation provision or using spare beds for that purpose and spare rooms above drop-in centres as crisis flats. Day care services are being used to provide support to people in crisis accommodated in a network of 'time-out' beds made available in every district of a large rural area in Wales.

Day care services and drop-ins

Centralised day hospital or day care and drop-in services provided in a single fixed location in or outside a rural area tend to be unsuccessful in providing accessible services to the population. More successful models involve services provided in local village facilities or in mobile facilities, such as buses or trailers. To ensure that such facilities can be flexible to clients' needs, it is essential to also provide transport to back up such services. Even with such resources, users are likely to only have access to very part-time day services.

Leisure and occupational services

The keystone of successful services for daytime occupation in rural areas is the employment of staff with transport and access to facilitating funds rather than buildings or other facilities. Successful projects have developed as a result of the energy and enthusiasm of workers, users and carers and of the local individuals or organisations they have managed to inspire into providing support and facilities. This type of development in rural areas depends on local knowledge and initiative, with central organisations providing encouragement, support and funding rather than directions. Successful projects are also characterised by great flexibility, allowing adaptation to individual client needs and opportunities available in the local rural area.

Conclusions

The provision of adequate and appropriate mental health resources and services in any area requires a reliable understanding of mental health needs. Current research evidence on rural mental issues is limited and cannot be relied upon as the basis for assumptions about needs in any particular rural area. However, some important generalisations emerge that should inform the needs evaluation process. First, the nature, prevalence and distribution of mental illnesses in different rural areas can vary substantially, as can the demographic characteristics of rural populations. Conjecture or estimations based on national norms are therefore likely to be inaccurate and the validity of currently available proxy indicators in rural areas is questionable. Furthermore, hidden or unmet need, inadequate provision of services and service-led drift of populations from rural areas compromise the accuracy of assessments based on currently accessed services. There is therefore no current substitute for local evaluation of prevalence of severe mental illness and local socio-demographic factors.

Second, the literature consistently identifies a number of factors that affect mental health needs and service delivery in rural areas. These include poor access to statutory, non-statutory and commercial services, social and functional isolation, inadequate educational and occupational opportunities, and stigma without the protection of urban anonymity. There is a high level of dependency on primary care services and on carers. Accessible care must therefore be locally delivered and be home-based, which presents particular problems in rural areas, given the travelling distances and professional isolation faced by staff.

Third, the range of services accessible to rural populations is likely to be incomplete, although the gaps in provision described in the literature differ from those which typify deficiencies in urban services – notably, lack of access to specialised services and facilities, and poor levels of education, expertise, support and safety for mental health staff. Fourth, opportunities offered by the higher levels of involvement with family as carers, the greater input of primary care, the higher level of connectivity of social networks and the intimate local knowledge of professionals should be fostered for the benefit of clients. These may be some of the factors that contribute to the potential for a better quality of life for people with mental illnesses in rural areas. A well-conducted needs assessment process that takes into account these rural characteristics should provide the foundations for an improvement in the mental health care for the local population. Rural issues and described models will then also need to be reflected in the design of services aimed at meeting the identified needs. Finally, just as metropolitan areas in the UK argue for fairer distribution of resources, which are so heavily centred in the capital (Mahoney & Sashidharan, 1999), mental health services in rural areas must use the increased understanding of their needs to argue more vigorously for equitable access to mental health services for their populations.

References

BARTSCH, D. A., SHERN, E. L., FEINBERG, L. E., *ET AL* (1990) Screening CMHC outpatients for physical illness. *Hospital and Community Psychiatry*, **41**, 786–790.

BENTHAM, G. & HAYNES, R. (1986) A raw deal in remoter rural areas? *Family Practitioner Services*, **13**, 84–87.

BOWLING, A. & FARQUHAR, M. (1991) Associations with social networks, social support, health status and psychiatric morbidity in three samples of elderly people. *Social Psychiatry and Psychiatric Epidemiology*, **26**, 115–126.

BROWN, G. W. & PRUDO, R. (1981) Psychiatric disorder in a rural and an urban population: 1. Aetiology of depression. *Psychological Medicine*, **11**, 581–599.

CAMPINIELLO, B., CARTA, M. G. & RUDAS, N. (1989) Depression among elderly people. *Acta Psychiatrica Scandinavica*, **80**, 445–450.

CHENG, T. A. (1989) Urbanisation and minor psychiatric morbidity. *Social Psychiatry and Psychiatric Epidemiology*, **24**, 309–316.

CLAYER, J., BOOKLESS, C., AIR, T., *ET AL* (1998) Psychiatric disorder and disability in a rural community. *Social Psychiatry and Psychiatric Epidemiology*, **33**, 269–273.

CLOKE, P. (1977) An index of rurality for England and Wales. *Regional Studies 1977*, **11**, 31–46.

COUNTRYSIDE AGENCY (1999) *The State of the Countryside*. Cheltenham: Countryside Agency.

COX, J. (1998) Poverty in rural areas – is more hidden but no less real than in urban areas. *British Medical Journal*, **316**, 722.

CROWELL, B. A., GEORGE, JR, L. K., BLAZER, D., *ET AL* (1986) Psychosocial risk factors and urban/rural differences in the prevalence of major depression. *British Journal of Psychiatry*, **149**, 307–314.

CUFFEL, B. J. (1994) Violent and destructive behaviour among the severely mentally ill in rural areas: evidence from Arkansas' Community Mental Health System. *Community Mental Health Journal*, **30**, 495–504.

DESJARLAIS, R., EISENBERG, L., GOOD, B., *ET AL* (1995) Conclusions and agenda for action. In: *World Mental Health* (eds R. Desjarbis, L. Eisenberg, B. Good, *et al*), pp. 259–278. Oxford: Oxford University Press.

EVELAND, A. P., DEVER, G. E. A., SCHAFER, E., *ET AL* (1998) Analysis of health service areas: another piece of the psychiatric workforce puzzle. *Psychiatric Services*, **49**, 956–960.

FEARN, R. (1987) Rural health care: a British success or a tale of unmet need? *Social Science Medicine*, **24**, 263–274.

FOX, J. C, BLANK, M. B. & KANE, C. F. (1994) Balance theory as a model for co-ordinating delivery of rural mental health services. *Applied and Preventive Psychology*, **3**, 121–129.

FRIED, B. J., JOHNSON, M. C., STARRETT, B.E., *ET AL* (1998) An empirical assessment of rural community support networks for individuals with severe mental disorders. *Community Mental Health Journal*, **34**, 39–56.

GREGOIRE, A. & THORNICROFT, G. (1998) Rural mental health. *Psychiatric Bulletin*, **22**, 273–277.

GUINNESS, E. A. (1992) Patterns of mental illness in the early stages of urbanisation. *British Journal of Psychiatry*, **160** (Suppl. 16).

GYLLENHAMMAR, C., LUNDIN, T., OTTO, U., *ET AL* (1988) The panorama of psychiatric emergencies in three different parts of Sweden. *European Archives in Psychiatry and Neurological Science*, **237**, 61–64.

HALL, G. (1988) Monitoring and predicting community mental health centre utilisation in Auckland, New Zealand. *Social Science and Medicine*, **26**, 55–70.

HUMAN, J. & WASEM, C. (1991) Rural mental health in America. *American Psychologist*, **46**, 232–239.

JESSOP, E. G. (1992) Individual morbidity and neighbourhood deprivation in a non-metropolitan area. *Journal of Epidemiology and Community Health*, **46**, 543–546.

KEATINGE, C. (1987) Community factors influencing psychiatric hospital utilisation in rural and urban Ireland. *Community Mental Health Journal*, **23**, 192–203,

—— (1988) Psychiatric admissions for alcoholism, neuroses and schizophrenia in rural and urban Ireland. *International Journal of Social Psychiatry*, **34**, 58–69.

KELLY, S. & BUNTING, J. (1998) Trends in suicide in England and Wales, 1982–1996. *Population Trends*, **92**, 29–41.

—— & CHARLTON, J. (1995) Suicide deaths in England and Wales 1982–1992: The contribution of occupation and geography. *Population Trends*, **80**, 16–25.

LEE, C. K., KWAK, Y. S., YAMAMOTA, J., *ET AL* (1990) Psychiatric epidemiology in Korea – Part II: Urban and rural differences. *Journal of Nervous and Mental Disease*, **178**, 247–252.

LEWIS, G. & BOOTH, M. (1994) Are cities bad for your mental health? *Psychological Medicine*, **24**, 913–915.

MAHONEY, J. & SASHIDHARAN, S. (1999) Mental health services – poor relations. *Health Service Journal*, April 1999, 24–26.

MALMBERG, A., SIMKIN, S. & HAWTON, K. (1999) Suicide in farmers. *British Journal of Psychiatry*, **175**, 103–105.

McCREADIE, R. G., LEESE, M., TILAK-SINGH, D., *ET AL* (1997) Nithsdale, Nunhead and Norwood: similarities and differences in prevalence of schizophrenia and utilisation of services in rural and urban areas. *British Journal of Psychiatry*, **170**, 31–36.

McGEE, R., STANDTON, W. & FEEHAN, M. (1991) Big cities, small towns and adolescent mental health in New Zealand. *Australian and New Zealand Journal of Psychiatry*, **25**, 338–342.

MELTZER, H., GILL, B., PETTICREW, M., *ET AL* (1995) *The Prevalence of Psychiatric Morbidity among Adults Living in Private Households*. London: Office of Population Censuses and Surveys.

MURRAY, J. D. & KELLER, P. A. (1991) Psychology and rural America. *American Psychologist*, **46**, 220–231.

MURTHY, S. R. (1998) Rural psychiatry in developing countries. *Psychiatric Services*, **49**, 967–969.

ORLEY, J. & WING, J. K. (1979) Psychiatric disorders in two African villages. *Archives of General Psychiatry*, **36**, 513–520.

ROHLAND, B. M., ROHRER, J. E., & TZOU, H. (1998) Broker model of case management for persons with serious mental illness in rural areas. *Administration and Policy in Mental Health*, **25**, 549–553.

ROMANS, S. E., WALTON, V. A., HERBISON, G. P., *ET AL* (1992) Social networks and psychiatric morbidity in New Zealand women. *Australian and New Zealand Journal of Psychiatry*, **26**, 485–492.

ROMANS-CLARKSON, S., WALTON, V. A., HERBISON, G. P., *ET AL* (1990) Psychiatric morbidity and women in urban and rural New Zealand: psycho-social correlates. *British Journal of Psychiarty*, **156**, 84–91.

ROST, K., ZHANG, M., FORTNEY, J., *ET AL* (1998) Rural–urban differences in depression treatment and suicidality. *Medical Care*, **36**, 1098–1107.

ROYAL COLLEGE OF PHYSICIANS AND ROYAL COLLEGE OF PSYCHIATRISTS (1998) *Organophosphate Sheep Dip – Clinical Aspects of Long-Term Low-Dose Exposure*. London: Royal College of Physicians and Royal College of Psychiatrists.

RURAL DEVELOPMENT COMMISSION (1992) *Homelessness in Rural Areas*. Salisbury: Rural Development Commission.

—— (1994) *Rural Development Areas 1994*. London: Department of the Environment.

THE SAMARITANS (1997) *County Rural Initiatives – Reaching Out to Rural People*. Slough: The Samaritans.

SANTOS, A. B, DEVI, P. A., LACHANCE, K. R., *ET AL* (1993) Providing assertive community treatment for severely mentally ill patients in a rural area. *Hospital and Community Psychiatry*, **44**, 34–38.

SEIVEWRIGHT, H., TYRER, P., CASEY, P., *ET AL* (1991) A three-year follow-up of psychiatric morbidity in urban and rural primary care. *Psychological Medicine*, **21**, 495–503.

SHERLOCK, J. (1994) *Through the Rural Magnifying Glass*. London: Good Practices in Mental Health.

—— (1995) *Magnifying Rural Mental Health. Examples of Good Practice*. London: Good Practices in Mental Health.

SHUCKSMITH, M. (1990) *The Definition of Rural Areas and Rural Deprivation. Report to Scottish Homes*. Aberdeen: Department of Land Economy, University of Aberdeen.

SMITH, A. J. & RAMANA, R. (1998) Mental health in rural areas: experience in south Cambridgeshire. *Psychiatric Bulletin*, **22**, 280–284.

STANSFIELD, S. A., LEEK, C. A., TRAVERS, W., *ET AL* (1992) Attitudes to community psychiatry among urban and rural general practitioners. *British Journal of General Practice*, **42**, 322–325.

SULLIVAN, G., JACKSON, C. A, SPRITZER, K. L., *ET AL* (1996) Characteristics and service use of seriously mentally ill persons living in rural areas. *Psychiatric Services*, **47**, 57–61.

THORNICROFT, G., BISOFFI, G., DE SALVIA, D., *ET AL* (1993) Urban–rural differences in the associations between social deprivation and psychiatric service utilisation in schizophrenia and all diagnoses: a case-register study in Northern Italy. *Psychological Medicine*, **23**, 487–496.

THURSTON-HICKS, A., PAINE, S. & HOLLIFIELD, M. (1998) Functional impairment associated with psychological distress and medical severity in rural primary care patients. *Psychiatric Services*, **49**, 951–955.

TORREY, E. F. (1987) Prevalence studies in schizophrenia. *British Journal of Psychiatry*, **150**, 598–608.

TUCKER, C. J., GREGOIRE, A. & BARKER, A. (1998) Living with schizophrenia: caring for a person with a mental illness. *Social Psychiatry and Psychiatric Epidemiology*, **33**, 305–309.

WATT, I. S., FRANKS, A. J. & SHELDON, T. A. (1993) Rural health and health care – unjustifiably neglected in Britain. *British Medical Journal*, **306**, 1358–1359.

——, —— & —— (1994) Health and health care of rural populations in the UK: is it better or worse? *Journal of Epidemiology and Community Health*, **48**, 16–21.

YOUSSEF, H. A., KINSELLA, A. & WADDINGTON, J. L. (1991) Evidence for geographical variations in the prevalence of schizophrenia in rural Ireland. *Archives in General Psychiatry*, **48**, 254–258.

26 Needs assessment and drug misuse services

JOHN MARSDEN and JOHN STRANG

This chapter applies an epidemiologically based framework to conceptualise drug misuse problems and the effective services available; it does not address the question of how to assess the needs of individuals who misuse drugs. In the UK, there is considerable concern about illicit drugs and a national 10-year strategy is underway to tackle the problem (UK Anti-Drugs Coordinating Unit, 1998). Health authorities have primary responsibility for the provision of treatment services for drug misusers, while local authorities are primarily responsible for meeting the physical and social care needs of drug misusers in their areas. The drug action team (DAT) constitutes the critical body to assess local treatment needs and coordinate a response for its resident population. The present discussion is structured as follows: the nature of drug misuse, its prevalence and the nature of specific population sub-groups are described first, followed by a brief review of treatment services and a summary of research evidence for their effectiveness. The structure of the current treatment system is then described together with a discussion of contemporary needs assessment and performance monitoring issues.

Nature and extent of the problem

Estimating the number of illicit users – particularly users of heroin – is notoriously difficult given the stigmatised nature of drug use and the marginalised position in society that many drug users occupy. This makes contact and accurate reporting using household survey methods problematic. Problem drug users are often described as a hidden population, meaning that a major proportion of the target population are not in contact with services or included in routine sources of data on drug users. In England and Wales, the latest British Crime Survey conducted in 1998 with 10 000 participants aged 16–59 years revealed that around one-third of the population have used an illicit drug at some point in their lives (Ramsay & Partridge, 1999). Approximately 1.2 million people aged 16–24 years have consumed an illicit drug in the past month. Cannabis is the most widely used drug (used by almost half of 20–24-year-olds) and cocaine hydrochloride has been used on at least one occasion by some 6% of the 16–29-year-old group and by 9% of the 20–24-year-old subgroup.

During 1997–1998, the Department of Health's Regional Drug Misuse Databases reported some 52 515 new treatment episodes of drug misuse (Department of Health, 1999). The majority present for treatment with opiate problems, with around 56% citing heroin as their main problem drug. The overall ratio of males to females is 3:1 and 52% are in their 20s. For the six months ending September 1998, the estimated number of cases entering treatment in England was 58 per 100 000 population (estimated on 1991 census-based population estimates for mid-year 1997). The rates by age band are as follows: under 20 years (33 per 100 000); 20–24 years (250 per 100 000); 25–29 years (195 per 100 000); and 30 years and over (32 per 100 000).

Types of drugs

Drug misuse control strategies mainly target the following classes of psychoactive substance: opioids, cocaine, amphetamine-type stimulants, sedatives/hypnotics and hallucinogens. The most common population to have health and social care needs people with primary opioid dependence (usually illicit heroin). A significant proportion of these individuals have histories that include problematic use of cocaine, sedatives/hypnotics (chiefly the benzodiazepines) and alcohol. The treatment needs of some primary users of cocaine have also received increased attention in recent years (Strang *et al*, 1993; Marsden *et al*, 1998a). Special consideration is additionally required for a variety of other drugs, including synthetic hallucinogenic amphetamines (e.g. MDMA) and other hallucinogens, cannabis and inhalants (glues, gases and solvents).

Drug-related risks and harms

The population of drug misusers is heterogeneous. Understanding the risks and harmful consequences of drug use and drug dependence demands consideration of a range of personal, health, social, economic and legal risks and harms, which can be experienced at the individual, familial and community level. Specific harms from drug misuse range from minor adverse physical or psychological morbidities that are directly induced by an illicit substance to acute and chronic health disorders (e.g. circulatory problems) to overdose and death. Heroin misusers have an elevated risk of mortality and drug-related deaths in comparison with users of other drugs and the general population. A long-term follow-up study of heroin users estimated that compared with the general population, this population has a 12-fold increased risk of mortality (Oppenheimer *et al*, 1994). There has been a nine-fold increase in mortality from self-poisoning with opiates over the past two decades (Neeleman & Farrell, 1997) and between 1985 and 1995 accidental deaths among young people aged 15–19 years recorded as owing to drug poisoning showed a marked increase (Roberts *et al*, 1997).

Individuals with drug use disorders are more likely to experience physical health symptoms and medical complications (Wartenberg, 1994; Rubin & Benzer, 1997).

Substance use disorders also covary with other psychiatric disorders, and comorbidity is prevalent for substance use and dependence and anxiety, affective and antisocial and other personality disorders (Regier *et al*, 1990; Kessler *et al*, 1994; Farrell *et al*, 1998).

There is also widespread recognition of the importance of improving clinical treatments and support services, particularly for people with severe mental illness who have drug misuse problems (Johnson, 1997). There is currently no research and clinical evidence base for the effective management and care of patients with psychoactive substance misuse comorbidity in psychiatric in-patient units, and this is an important development area. There is some evidence that people with substance use problems and comorbid psychiatric disorders appear to have a relatively high contact with medical services and may require more intensive treatment (Alterman *et al*, 1993).

Injecting drug users (IDUs) may be exposed to blood-borne infections through the sharing of infected needles/syringes and, potentially, through the sharing of other injecting paraphernalia (Gossop *et al*, 1998*a,b*). Since many substance users are sexually active, penetrative sexual behaviour without condom use (and several other behaviours) also increases the risk of viral exposure (Magura *et al*, 1990; Donoghoe, 1992). Injecting use is a major risk factor for the transmission and acquisition of human immunodeficiency virus (HIV), hepatitis B (HBV) and hepatitis C (HCV). For example, a recent study of IDUs in a London National Health Service (NHS) clinic found an 86% rate of HCV seropositive and a 55% rate of HBV (Best *et al*, 1999). In many places, the high prevalence and incidence rates of HCV infection among IDUs are in sharp contrast to trends in HIV infection in the past decade (Bloor *et al*, 1994; van Beek *et al*, 1998).

In the social functioning area, drug misuse is linked with problems of varying intensity, and these are often chronic in nature. Many drug users report conflict in their personal relationships with family and friends and this has been shown to be a negative predictor of treatment outcome (Moos *et al*, 1988). Equally, many users have enduring problems with obtaining and retaining paid employment. Involvement in work has been found to be a predictor of retention in treatment and good outcome (Simpson *et al*, 1986). Although the ability of a treatment programme to secure a job for a client may be limited, community services will usually seek to support a client to improve employment opportunities, and securing or maintaining a job is recognised to be an important goal (French *et al*, 1992). There is also concern about drug use, and criminal behaviour has been a major factor in the priorities for action set by the government's national drugs strategy. Police surveillance estimates suggest that half of all recorded crimes are drug-related, with associated costs to the criminal justice system totalling some 1 billion pounds per annum (UK Anti-Drugs Coordinating Unit, 1998). There is long-standing awareness of links between drug use and social and economic deprivation and that some individuals (particularly those dependent on opiates) become involved in crime to support their dependence (Nurco *et al*, 1984). The link between crime and drug use may also be related to lifestyle aspects of criminality, which lead some individuals to become deviant in other areas (Hammersley *et al*, 1989); moreover, drug use and criminal involvement may be a cultural fact of life in areas of economic and social deprivation (Pearson & Gillman, 1994).

Diagnostic definitions of drug misuse

Two core concepts relevant to assessment are dependence and misuse (or hazardous use). Based on the original conception of alcohol dependence, illicit drug dependence is incorporated within both the World Health Organization's disease classification ICD–10 and the APA's DSM–IV (World Health Organization (WHO), 1992; American Psychiatric Association (APA), 1994). The ICD and DSM classifications include diagnostic criteria that view impairment of control over drug use and negative consequences as primary problems. ICD–10 seeks to provide diagnostic guidelines that distinguish a range of disorders that vary depending on severity of intoxication, hazardous, harmful use and dependence dimensions. ICD–10 also makes a distinction between harmful use (discernible psychological and/or physical health damage to an individual) and dependence. DSM diagnoses misuse of a particular substance following the endorsement of one or more of the following: (a) use leading to neglect of personal, social or occupational roles; (b) use in an unsafe or dangerous situation; (c) use leading to repeated problems with the law; and (d) continued use despite relationship, domestic, occupation or educational problems.

Sub-categories of drug misuse

The heterogeneous population of drug users in the UK can be divided into subgroups in a variety of ways. In terms of the individual drug misuser, the following factors are important in considering the nature of each case encountered: age, gender, race, culture and religion; pregnancy; familial pattern; type of drug(s) used, including quantity and frequency of administration; acute intoxication (overdose liability); extent of impairment and complications; route of administration (oral, inhalation, intramuscular or intravenous); and nature of living situation and social environmental supports and stressors. Complex cases will usually (but not always) be characterised by drug-related impairment, dependence, regular injecting, high tolerance levels and comorbid problems across the physical, psychological and social functioning domains. Seven subgroups of non-independent (overlapping) drug misuser can be identified that have specific ramifications for the assessment of health care needs and the commissioning and purchasing of treatment services. These are as follows: (A) the drug misuser (non-dependent); (B) the injecting drug user (IDU); (C) the dependent user; (D) the acutely intoxicated drug misuser; (E) the drug user with comorbidity; (F) the user in withdrawal; and (G) the drug user in recovery.

The non-dependent drug misuser (subgroup A) is included to describe those individuals who have begun to use drugs relatively recently, may have drug-related problems, but do not meet the criteria for drug dependence at the point of contact with the treatment system. These individuals (both adults and particularly young people) are at risk of advancing their drug involvement to more serious levels and may be ideal candidates for early intervention services. These sorts of intervention are usually based on a comprehensive assessment of need, a functional analysis concerning drug involvement and a programme of brief counselling and support. This may then trigger the identification of other health and social care needs.

Services available and their effectiveness

Treatment for drug misuse may be discreet or may involve several stages and provision by different providers and community/out-patient or residential settings. The seven subgroups may come into contact (through self- or family-referral or referral by a professional agency) with a wide range of agencies and service providers who are either predominantly drug specialist or predominantly generic. The probation service is an important point of referral into community treatment; there is now limited provision of detoxification and methadone reduction treatment within prisons, but this is poised for considerable expansion. There may be additional contact and screening points that can be identified, including schools/colleges and employment settings. Effective coordination and joint working between primary health care, specialist treatment agencies and social support agencies is considered essential to manage the needs of a majority of people with established drug misuse problems. As with other heath problems, services are summarised in terms of the different service agencies concerned, but it is stressed that many individuals require treatment and support from several different types of provider and over a protracted period. The Social Services Department occupies a key role in the assessment of need for drug users, particularly complex cases such as those requiring residential rehabilitation, those with drug-using parents, pregnant drug users, and children and young people.

Treatment tiers

Treatment of drug misusers ranges from brief interventions by primary health care teams (PHCTs) through to intensive services delivered in a controlled medical (or criminal justice) environment. Many individuals may require the provision of several different types of service over time (i.e. a continuum of care). It is quite common for an individual receiving treatment from one provider to receive additional support services from other agencies (e.g. housing support and legal advice). These supports are important elements in an effective package of care services that evolves over the course of an individual's treatment. Fig. 26.1 illustrates a four-tier structure of current treatment services.

These tiers represent a continuum of care in which providers can refer both up and down the levels to access an appropriate treatment or support service. A thorough assessment of a drug use disorder spans personal demographic features, health status, health symptoms and social functioning considerations, together with an appraisal of the

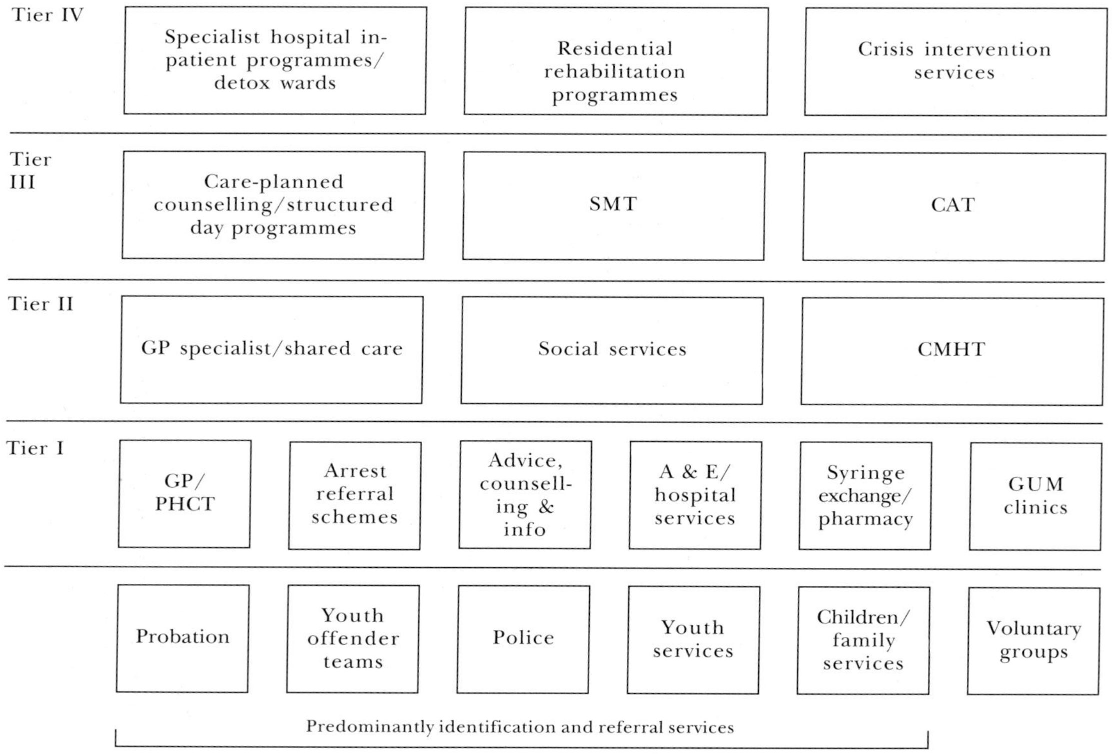

Tier IV

- Specialist hospital in-patient programmes/detox wards
- Residential rehabilitation programmes
- Crisis intervention services

Tier III

- Care-planned counselling/structured day programmes
- SMT
- CAT

Tier II

- GP specialist/shared care
- Social services
- CMHT

Tier I

- GP/PHCT
- Arrest referral schemes
- Advice, counselling & info
- A & E/hospital services
- Syringe exchange/pharmacy
- GUM clinics
- Probation
- Youth offender teams
- Police
- Youth services
- Children/family services
- Voluntary groups

Predominantly identification and referral services

Fig. 26.1 *Tiered care delivery system for treatment of drug misuse*

specific psychological and social functions that drug use serves the individual. An important principle is that services in Tier IV, which are by definition of higher unit costs than treatment in Tiers I–III, should be reserved for cases of significant treatment need that cannot be managed safely or effectively in a non-residential setting. Other health and social care services that provide services to drug misusers span sexual health and allied services, and maternity and dentistry. Table 2.6.1 summarises, in a simplified fashion, the general broad sweep of treatment providers and services that are available. The various specific interventions that are currently funded by the public health and social care system are now described.

Syringe exchange services

There are currently in excess of 300 dedicated syringe exchange schemes in England (Department of Health, 1997*b*). Specialist agencies and community pharmacists constitute important services that aim to reduce the extent of harm caused by injecting, by promoting improved hygiene during intravenous drug use and encouraging the use of new needles and syringes and the disposal of used equipment. The main outcome measure for evaluating the impact of specialist and community syringe exchange programmes is the frequency of needle and syringe sharing incidents during the month prior to interview. There is evidence from observational studies that, on average, participation in some exchanges is linked to some decrease in HIV-related risks among drug injectors (Stimson, 1996). Collectively, syringe exchange and distribution services may have achieved a measurable effect in the UK in declining prevalence of markers of exposure to HBV in some areas, which is currently estimated at around 20–30% among London IDUs (Hunter *et al*, 1998; Judd *et al*, 1999). Nevertheless, the research evaluation literature on the specific impact of the syringe exchange schemes is mixed.

Prescribing services

A 1994 census of treatment programmes (MacGregor *et al*, 1994) identified a total of 163 specialist community drug teams and other specialist prescribing services. Between September 1997 and September 1998, new episodes reported by substance misuse teams (SMTs) accounted for some 48.8% of the total reported (Department of Health, 1999). These services aim to reach drug users who are usually dependent on heroin and are current users of several other illicit substances. Specialist prescribing services provide opioid substitution treatment, usually with oral methadone hydrochloride in either a

TABLE 26.1

Drug misuse services and treatment providers

Provider	Potential service functions
General practitioners (GPs)/PHCTs (Tier I)[1]	Open access: brief counselling; illness screening; vaccination; health care information; prescribing; referral to specialist services, stand-alone or shared-care provider
Specialist and community syringe exchange schemes (Tier II)	Open access: syringe and injecting equipment distribution; condom availability; harm minimisation information; referral advice and information
Community-based advice and information	Open access: drop-in facilities; assessment; education; referral; advocacy; outreach; advice and counselling; telephone help-lines; individual support; specialist counselling; shared-care prescribing with local GPs
Structured individual/ group counselling/ programmes (Tier II)	Usually referral-based: comprehensive needs assessment; individualised counselling and/or psychotherapy; referral to other specialist providers; after-care support, active work with relapsing clients; job skills and work experience
Non-statutory community-based drugs services (Tier II)	Usually open access: assessment and referral; shared-care prescribing with local GPs; counselling and support
Substance misuse teams (SMTs) (Tier III)[2]	Usually open access: specialist assessment; vaccination; health care information; agonist prescribing (maintenance and reduction/detoxification regimes); management of complex cases; prescribing for psychosocial and physical comorbidity; education; general support; onward referral
Specialist hospital in-patient units (Tier IV)[2]	Referral-based: medically supervised drug withdrawal management; screening for illnesses; vaccination and provision of health care information; education, general health care; relapse prevention counselling; onward referral
Crisis intervention and detoxification units (Tier IV)[2]	Usually open access: rapid access for users in crisis; medically supervised withdrawal via agonist prescribing; primary health care; onward referral
Residential rehabilitation programmes (Tier IV)	Referral-based: comprehensive assessment; medically supervised withdrawal management (in some units); group and individual counselling and support; training; after-care

1. Medical practitioners in Tier I, correspond to generalist practitioners in drug misuse treatment teams (Level I: generalist) and specialised generalist practitioners (Level 2: the specialised generalist) who have a special interest in treating drug misusers (see Department of Health, 1997*a*; Department of Health *et al*, 1999).
2. Specialist medical practitioners in this tier are usually those whose main clinical activity is the provision of expertise, training and competence in drug misuse treatment. Most specialists (Level 3: specialists) are consultant psychiatrists.

reducing or a maintenance regimen (Farrell *et al*, 1994; Marsden *et al*, 1998*b*). Two broad types of substitution programme are delivered, each with distinct goals and with in excess of 25 000 individuals receiving methadone at any one time (Sheridan *et al*, 1996). In abstinence-oriented *opioid reduction*, community-treated clients are first stabilised on methadone and then gradually withdrawn over a period ranging from several weeks to many months. There is limited use of other pharmacological agents to manage withdrawal, notably the α_2-adrenergic agonist lofexidine (prescribed either singly or in combination with methadone). In *opioid maintenance*, where retention in treatment is a priority, the substitute is administered at a stable level for a period of several months or sometimes years.

In addition to heroin use, community treatment providers must also deal with dependent use of other drugs. An increase in cocaine distribution and prevalence in Britain since the late 1980s has been accompanied by growing concerns to ensure that services can respond to the treatment needs of dependent cocaine users. A survey of 318 treatment services in England in 1995 revealed that 53% had received referrals for primary cocaine hydrochloride or crack users in the previous six months and that the majority had provided some form of planned treatment for these clients (Donmall *et al*, 1995). Consumption of another common illicit stimulant – amphetamine – is also rising in the UK and internationally. There is evidence that the prescribing of dexamphetamine sulphate may be quite widely undertaken by physicians providing treatment for dependent users (Strang & Sheridan, 1997). There is currently only the most limited research evidence base for treatments for dependent amphetamine users (Fleming & Roberts, 1994). Contemporary treatment approaches combine counselling, health care for physical and psychological symptoms and substitution prescribing.

Nationally, GPs have a substantial overall level of treatment involvement with drug misusers. GPs issue some two-fifths of methadone prescriptions to the subgroup of dependent heroin users and these are dispensed by retail pharmacists (Strang *et al*, 1996). Between September 1997 and September 1998, a total of 3052 patient episodes were reported by general practice workers (some 5.7% of the total numbers recorded by returning agencies). Health authorities are expected to continue to develop a shared care arrangement for the treatment of drug misusers at the primary care level. In the case of methadone prescribing to a dependent heroin user, a specialist agency and GP usually agree who has overall clinical responsibility for a client. Guidelines on the effective clinical management of drug users has been recently revised by the UK Department of Health (1999). In some instances, the agency will undertake the initial client assessment and institute methadone induction and stabilisation. After this phase of treatment is completed, the client may be transferred to the GP at an appropriate point (Waller, 1997). In 1996, some 53% of all health authorities reported specified arrangements for shared care, of which one-third met the criteria set out by the Department of Health. Returns in 1996 from 24 health authorities indicated that an average of 40 GPs per district were participating in shared-care arrangements; however, the level of participation varied widely from 1% to over 50% of all GPs in the area (Department of Health, 1997a).

Internationally, there is a well-established research and clinical evidence base for substitution treatment with oral methadone (Ward *et al*, 1992). On average, methadone maintenance is associated with lower rates of heroin consumption, reduced levels of crime and improved social functioning. A lower risk of premature mortality among maintained patients has been reported, and substitution programmes have also contributed to the prevention of the spread of HIV infection, by encouraging change in injection risk-taking practices. In the UK, results from the National Treatment Outcomes Research Study (NTORS; Gossop *et al*, 1999) suggests that, on average, post-treatment outcomes from opioid substitution treatments are positive across a broad range of substance use, injecting and needle-/syringe-sharing behaviours, health symptoms and crime measures.

Counselling services

The provision of counselling and support for drug misusers, dependent users and users in recovery is quite widespread but remains under-researched in the UK. Almost all treatment programmes for opiate users contain some form of counselling that tends to be aimed at enhancing personal motivation for change and oriented to problem-solving and to providing ongoing support to clients. In the 1994 agency survey (MacGregor *et al*, 1994), 112 drug misuse advice and counselling centres were recorded. In recent years, there has been growing interest in commissioning high-quality individually structured day programmes (Standing Conference on Drug Abuse, 1996). These services are designed to provide an intensive programme of counselling, tailored to the needs of the individual. Counselling is of a finite duration and is intended to be subject to high-quality monitoring of progress against objectives. There is widespread belief in the importance and value of counselling for opiate addicts in the UK and internationally (Task Force to Review Services for Drug Misusers, 1996). However, the evidence-base for the effectiveness of counselling with this population is sparse. Of all the psychosocial counselling approaches, relapse prevention-oriented cognitive–behavioural therapies have received the most frequent evaluation in other countries (US General Accounting Office, 1996). Cognitive–behavioural coping skills training approaches have been used successfully with heroin users in assisting the prevention of relapse (Saunders *et al*, 1995). Several psychological treatments that incorporate behavioural elements have also produced encouraging results, notably contingency reinforcement therapy (Higgins *et al*, 1995). Some 24 randomised controlled trials of cognitive–behavioural therapy (CBT) have been conducted among adult users of tobacco, alcohol, cocaine, marijuana, opiates and other types of substances (Carroll, 1996). These studies indicate that there is good evidence for the effectiveness of CBT compared with no-treatment controls. The most rigorous tests of cognitive–behavioural therapies are comparisons with existing treatments and here results to date have been more varied.

Residential services

The main types of residential treatment services currently provided are drug-free rehabilitation programmes, crisis intervention services and hospital in-patient programmes. These programmes serve the subgroups of users in withdrawal and users in recovery. Rehabilitation programmes are largely community care-funded, and abstinence-based services that have been pioneered and sustained largely by the voluntary sector. There are approximately 70 programmes operating in England, and some 1200 beds are available (Cook, 1995). In England in 1994, there were some 16 specialist units providing about 100 such beds (MacGregor *et al*, 1994). There were also a small number of crisis intervention facilities in several cities across the country that could be rapidly accessed and which provided a withdrawal management and support service.

A relatively small number of studies have evaluated the impact of hospital in-patient units and residential rehabilitation programmes. One follow-up study of patients who were treated by a specialist in-patient unit found that 51% of patients were drug-free at a six months follow-up (Gossop *et al*, 1989). The only controlled study of in-patient and out-patient treatment of opiate withdrawal in the UK found in-patient withdrawal to be four times more effective (in terms of the proportion of patients who completed the withdrawal regime (Gossop *et al*, 1986). For residential rehabilitation programmes, both US and UK studies have shown positive psychosocial benefits after treatment (DeLeon & Jainchill, 1982; Bennett & Rigby, 1990). In the UK, NTORS examined outcomes after discharge from eight in-patient units and 16

TABLE 26.2
Evidence-base for drug misuse treatment services

Treatment service	Effectiveness rating	Comment
Syringe exchange schemes	*	Evidence is mixed
Specialist community prescribing[1]	**	
Shared-care prescribing	***	
Counselling	****	CBT[2]
Hospital in-patient units	***	
Residential programmes	***	

1. Using oral methadone with dependent opiate misusers
2. Cognitive behavioural therapy (international research evidence)

* Evidence obtained from well-designed cohort or case control analytic studies (service has a measurable beneficial effect)
** Evidence from several consistent randomised controlled trials (service has a moderate beneficial effect)
*** Evidence obtained from well-designed cohort or case control analytic study (service has a moderate beneficial effect)
****Evidence from at least one properly designed randomised controlled trial (service has a moderate beneficial effect)

residential rehabilitation programmes. One-year follow-up results indicated that abstinence rates increased from 22% to 50% for opioids, and from 30% to 68% for stimulants (Gossop *et al,* 1999). The available research evidence for the effectiveness of treatment is summarised in Table 26.2.

Towards more integrated services

Given the broad range of health, social and economic harms that are associated with drug misuse, an integrated and partnership-based approach is required to underpin commissioning and service delivery. Partnership arrangements are now seen as essential between agencies spanning specialist drug treatment services, general medical and general practice, and across health authorities, social services, non-statutory agencies and criminal justice services. It is important for local planners to ensure that the full range of drug-related interventions – drug education, prevention and treatment (counselling, detoxification, prescribing, etc) – is available. Meeting the needs of certain care groups (e.g. young drug misusers and drug misusing rough sleepers) may be undertaken efficiently through the sharing of resources across several local areas. Problems may arise if only a partial network of coverage of the four tiers is available for a local area, for example, commissioning advice and information services without more specialist treatment services.

Contact and referral through the treatment tiers

In Figure 26.1, a fully integrated treatment system is described that contains an array of mainly generic, predominantly drugs specialist providers, together with feeder agencies and services that may come into contact with drug users in the course of their work and which can provide brief advice and referral (e.g. voluntary agencies and telephone help-lines) of individuals into the treatment system as appropriate. In the near future, the probation service and police may well undertake direct referrals and make specific placements for drug misusers at an appropriate point in the tiered system. Generic and specialist providers are likely to make referrals to a higher tier as well as to a lower one, according to the presenting or current needs of their case-loads. To an extent, the unit costs of treatment services increase from Tier I to Tier IV as access to each service moves from being open to referral-based.

In this tier system, all agencies have a role to play in staging a coordinated response. We see the SMT as occupying a critical role as the hub of the specialist treatment system. The SMT should serve important functions across client assessment, direct treatment provision, onward referral, community liaison, promotion of users groups, professional and volunteer training and service development areas. The kinds of professional linkages initiated by an SMT in a locality for specific client needs are as follows:

(a) shared-care management with the community alcohol team (CAT) in cases of significant alcohol-related problems;
(b) referral to general hospitals in cases of significant physical illness;
(c) liaison and referral to general psychiatric services in cases of drug misuse and psychiatric comorbidity;
(d) liaison with other community service providers in the voluntary sector;
(e) active participation in performance monitoring (in concert with the DAT); and
(f) liaison with local criminal justice services (police, probation, courts and prisons).

The commissioning and organisation arrangements for the services in the tiered system vary substantially across and sometimes within the treatment systems in many countries. Additionally, special initiatives are required alongside targeted prevention and treatment

TABLE 26.3
Likely required level of contact by drug misusers with the treatment system

Subgroup	Treatment system tier			
	I	II	III	IV
A Drug misuser	***	**	***	*
B IDU	***	***	***	*
C Dependent user	*	**	***	***
D Intoxicated user	***	*	*	*
E User with comorbidity	*	***	**	*
F User with withdrawal	*	*	**	***
G User in recovery	*	***	*	***

Likely extent of contact: * = low; ** = medium; *** = high

interventions aimed at priority client groups. The seven population-level subgroups are identified in Section 2 of the four tiers of treatment. These can be combined into a matrix. Table 26.3 indicates the likely extent of contact of each subgroup at each level of the tiered treatment system.

Conclusions

The provision of effective and well-organised treatment services for drug misusers is a priority within the national drug misuse strategy. Drug use disorders are diverse and are characterised and influenced by individual, social and environmental factors. There are a variety of access points into treatment in the public health and social care systems, and to an increasing extent in the criminal justice system. There is a growing evidence base for the effectiveness of several types of well-delivered harm minimisation, substitute prescribing, and detoxification and rehabilitation services, and there should be appropriate access or direct provision of these services. Partnership is vital between agencies spanning specialist drug treatment services, general medicine and general practice, and across health authorities, social services, non-statutory agencies, and criminal justice agencies. There is great variability in the scope and effectiveness of commissioning and purchasing arrangements for drug misuse services across the

UK. To date, there are no nationally agreed standards for single or joint commissioning and purchasing, and there are no universally agreed specifications for drug misuse treatment, although valuable work has been undertaken in recent years on clinical management, quality standards and audit, together with major advances in strategic planning by drug action teams. Commissioning arrangements are also in a state of flux, with the emergence of the primary care groups (PCGs) as commissioning bodies in this area. Against this background, the Government's White Paper on the NHS (Department of Health, 1997*b*) heralded significant changes to the structure of health care commissioning. While health authorities continue to have responsibility for alcohol and drug services, an emergent commissioning role is envisaged for PCGs.

References

ALTERMAN, A. I., McLELLAN, T. & SHIFMAN, R. B. (1993) Do substance patients with more psychopathology receive more treatment? *Journal of Nervous and Mental Disease*, **181**, 576–582.

AMERICAN PSYCHIATRIC ASSOCIATION (1994) *Diagnostic and Statistical Manual of Mental Disorders* (4th edn). Washington, DC: APA.

BENNETT, G. & RIGBY, K. (1990) Psychological change during residence in a rehabilitation centre for female drug misusers. Part I. Drug misusers. *Drug and Alcohol Dependence*, **27**, 149–157.

BEST, D., NOBLE, A., FINCH, E., *ET AL* (1999) Accuracy of perceptions of hepatitis B and C status: a cross-sectional investigation of opiate addicts in treatment. *British Medical Journal*, **319**, 290–291.

BLOOR, M., FRISCHER, M., TAYLOR, A., *ET AL* (1994) Tideline and turn: possible reasons for the continuing low HIV prevalence among Glasgow's injecting drug users. *Sociological Review*, **42**, 738–757.

CARROLL, K. M. (1996) Relapse prevention as a psychosocial treatment approach: A review of controlled clinical trials. *Experimental and Clinical Psychopharmacology*, **4**, 46–54.

COOK, C. (1995) *Residential Rehabilitation. A report prepared for the Department of Health's Task Force to Review Services for Drug Misusers*. London: Department of Health.

DELEON, G. & JAINCHILL, N. (1982) Male and female drug abusers: Social and psychological status two years after treatment in a therapeutic community. *American Journal of Drug and Alcohol Abuse*, **8**, 465–497.

DEPARTMENT OF HEALTH (1997*a*) *Purchasing Effective Treatment and Care for Drug Misusers: Guidance for Health and Social Services Departments*. London: Stationery Office.

—— (1997*b*) *Purchasing Effective Treatment and Care for Drug Misusers: Guidance for Health and Social Services Departments*. London: Stationery Office.

—— (1997*c*) *The New NHS: Modern, Dependable*. London: Stationery Office.

—— (1999) *Drug Misuse Statistics*. London: Department of Health.

——, THE SCOTTISH OFFICE DEPARTMENT OF HEALTH, WELSH OFFICE AND DEPARTMENT OF HEALTH AND SOCIAL SECURITY IN NORTHERN IRELAND (1999) *Drug Misuse and Dependence – Guidelines on Clinical Management*. London: Stationery Office.

DONMALL, M., SEIVEWRIGHT, N., DOUGLAS, J., *ET AL* (1995) *National Cocaine Treatment Study: The Effectiveness of Treatments Offered to Cocaine/Crack Users. A report prepared for the Department of Healths Task Force to Review Services for Drug Misusers*. London: Department of Health.

DONOGHOE, M. C. (1992) Sex, HIV and the injecting drug user. *British Journal of Addiction*, **87**, 405–416.

FARRELL, M. J., WARD, R., MATTICK, W., *ET AL* (1994) Methadone maintenance treatment in opiate dependence: a review. *British Medical Journal*, **309**, 997–1001.

——, HOWES, S., TAYLOR, C., *ET AL* (1998) Substance misuse and psychiatric comorbidity: an overview of the OPCS national psychiatric morbidity survey. *Addictive Behaviors*, **23**, 909–918.

FLEMING, P. M. & ROBERTS, D. (1994) Is the prescription of amphetamine justified as a harm reduction measure? *Journal of the Royal Society of Health*, **114**, 127–131.

FRENCH, M. T., DENNIS, M., McDOUGAL, G. L., *ET AL* (1992) Training and employment programs in methadone treatment: Client needs and desires. *Journal of Substance Abuse Treatment*, **9**, 293–303.

GOSSOP, M., JOHNS, A. & GREEN, L. (1986) Opiate withdrawal: in-patient versus outpatient programmes and preferred versus random assignment to treatment. *British Medical Journal*, **293**, 697–699.

——, GREEN, L., PHILLIPS, G., *ET AL* (1989) Lapse, relapse and survival among opiate addicts after treatment. A prospective follow-up study. *British Journal of Psychiatry*, **154**, 348–353.

——, MARSDEN, J. & STEWART, D. (1998*a*) *National Treatment Outcome Research Study: NTORS at One-Year*. London: Department of Health.

——, ——, ——, *ET AL* (1998*b*) Substance use, health and social problems of clients at 54 drug treatment agencies. Intake data from the National Treatment Outcome Research Study. *British Journal of Psychiatry*, **173**, 166–171.

——, ——, ——, *ET AL* (1999) Treatment retention and 1 year outcomes for residential programmes in England. *Drug and Alcohol Dependence*, **57**, 89–98.

HAMMERSLEY, R., FORSYTH, A., MORRISON, V., *ET AL* (1989) The relationship between crime and opioid use. *British Journal of Addiction*, **84**, 1029–1043.

HIGGINS, S. T., BUDNEY, A. J., BICKEL, W. K., *ET AL* (1995) Outpatient behavioural treatment for cocaine dependence, *Experimental and Clinical Psychopharmacology*, **3**, 205–212.

HUNTER, G., STIMSON, G. V., JONES, S., *ET AL* (1998) *Survey of Prevalence of Sharing by Injecting Drug Users Not in Contact with Services: An Independent Study Carried out on Behalf of the Department of Health*. London: Centre for Research on Drugs and Health Behaviour.

JOHNSON, S. (1997) Dual diagnosis of severe mental illness and substance misuse: a case for specialist services. *British Journal of Psychiatry*, **171**, 205–208.

JUDD, A., HUNTER, G., MACONOCHIE, N., *ET AL* (1999) HIV prevalence and risk behaviour among female injecting drug users in London, 1990 to 1996. *AIDS*, **13**, 833–837.

KESSLER, R. C., McGONAGLE, K. A., ZHAO, S., *ET AL* (1994) Lifetime and 12 month prevalence of DSM–III–R psychiatric disorders in the United States: Results from the National Comorbidity Survey. *Archives of General Psychiatry*, **51**, 8–19.

MACGREGOR, S., SMITH, L. E. & FLORY, P. (1994) *The Drugs Treatment System in England*. Middlesex University: School of Sociology and Social Policy.

MAGURA, S., SHAPIRO, J. L., SIDDIQI, Q., *ET AL* (1990) Variables influencing condom use among intravenous drug users. *American Journal of Public Health*, **80**, 82–84.

MARSDEN, J., GRIFFITHS, P., FARRELL, M., *ET AL* (1998*a*) Cocaine in Britain: Prevalence, problems and treatment responses. *Journal of Drug Issues*, **28**, 225–242.

——, ——, ——, *ET AL* (1998*b*) Opioid substitution: critical issues and future directions. *Journal of Drug Issues*, **28**, 231–248.

MOOS, R. H., FENN, C. & BILLINGS, A. (1988) Life stressors and social resources: an integrated assessment approach. *Social Science and Medicine*, **27**, 999–1002.

NEELEMAN, J. & FARRELL, M. (1997) Fatal methadone and heroin overdoses: time trends in England and Wales. *Journal of Epidemiological Community Health*, **51**, 435–437.

NURCO, D. N., SHAFFER, J. W., & CISIN, I. H. (1984) An ecological analysis of the interrelationships among drug abuse and other indices of social pathology. *International Journal of the Addictions*, **19**, 441–451.

OPPENHEIMER, E., TOBBUTT, C., TAYLOR, C., *ET AL* (1994) Death and survival in a cohort of heroin addicts from London clinics. *Addiction*, **89**, 1299–1308.

PEARSON, G. & GILLMAN, M. (1994) Local and regional variations in drug misuse: the British heroin epidemic of the 1980s. In: *Heroin Addiction and Drug Policy: The British System* (eds J. Strang & M. Gossop), pp. 102–120. Oxford: Oxford University Press.

RAMSAY, M. & PARTRIDGE, S. (1999) *Drug Misuse Declared in 1998: Results from the British Crime Survey. Home Office Research Study 197.* London: Home Office.

REGIER, D. A., FARMER, M. E., RAE, D. S., *ET AL* (1990) Comorbidity of mental disorders with alcohol and other drug abuse: Results from the Epidemiologic Catchment Area (ECA) study. *Journal of the American Medical Association*, **264**, 2511–2518.

ROBERTS, I., BARKER, M. & LI, L. (1997) Analysis of trends in deaths from accidental drug poisoning in teenagers 1985–1995. *British Medical Journal*, **315**, 289.

RUBIN, J. M. & BENZER, D. G. (1997) Treatment of comorbid medical complications. In: *Manual of Therapeutics for Addictions* (eds N. S. Miller, M. S. Gold & D. E. Smith), pp. 149–158. New York: Wiley-Liss.

SAUNDERS, B., WILKINSON, C. & PHILLIPS, M. (1995) The impact of a brief motivational intervention with opiate users attending a methadone programme, *Addiction*, **90**, 415–424.

SHERIDAN, J., STRANG, J., BARBER, N., *ET AL* (1996) Role of community pharmacists in relation to HIV prevention and drug misuse: findings from the 1995 national survey in England and Wales. *British Medical Journal*, **313**, 270–274.

SIMPSON, D. D., JOE, G. W., & LEHMAN, W. E. K. (1986) *Addiction Careers: Summary of Studies Based on the DARP 12-year Follow-up.* NIDA Treatment Research Report, DHHS Publication No. (AMD) 86-1420. Rockville, MD: National Institute of Drug Abuse.

STANDING CONFERENCE ON DRUG ABUSE (1996) *Structured Day Programmes: New Options in Community Care for Drug Users.* London: SCODA.

STIMSON, G. V. (1996) Has the United Kingdom averted an epidemic of HIV-1 infection among drug injectors? *Addiction*, **91**, 1085–1088.

STRANG, J. & SHERIDAN, J. (1997) Prescribing amphetamines to drug misusers: data from the 1995 national survey of community pharmacists. *Addiction*, **92**, 833–838.

——, JOHNS, A. & CAAN, W. (1993) Cocaine in the UK – 1991. *British Journal of Psychiatry*, **162**, 1–13.

——, SHERIDAN, J. & BARBER, N. (1996) Prescribing injectable and oral methadone to opiate addicts: results from the 1995 national postal survey of community pharmacists in England and Wales. *British Medical Journal*, **313**, 270–274.

TASK FORCE TO REVIEW SERVICES FOR DRUG MISUSERS (1996) *Report of an Independent Review of Drug Treatment Services in England.* London: Department of Health.

UNITED KINGDOM ANTI-DRUGS COORDINATING UNIT (1998) *Tackling Drugs to Build a Better Britain: The Government's 10 Year Strategy for Tackling Drug Misuse.* London: Stationery Office.

US GENERAL ACCOUNTING OFFICE (1996) *Cocaine Treatment: Early Results From Various Approaches.* Washington, DC: GAO.

VAN BEEK, I., DWYER, R., DORE, G. J., *ET AL* (1998) Infection with HIV and hepatitis C virus among injecting drug users in a prevention setting: retrospective cohort study. *British Medical Journal*, **317**, 433–437.

WALLER, T. (1997) A GP's role: past present and future. In: *Care of Drug Users in General Practice: A Harm Minimisation Approach* (ed. B. Beaumont). Oxford: Radcliffe Medical Press.

WARD, J., MATTICK, R. P. & HALL W. (1992) *Key Issues in Methadone Maintenance Treatment.* Sydney: New South Wales University Press.

WARTENBERG, A. A. (1994) Management of common medical problems. In: *Manual of Therapeutics for Addictions* (eds N. S. Miller, M. S. Gold & D. E. Smith), pp. 168–180. Chevy Chase, MD: American Society of Addiction Medicine.

WORLD HEALTH ORGANIZATION (1992) *International Classification of Diseases and Related Health Problems. Tenth revision (ICD–10).* Geneva: WHO.

27 Needs assessment and eating disorders

JANET TREASURE and ULRIKE SCHMIDT

Many people fail to appreciate that anorexia nervosa is a severe mental illness, as defined by Goldberg & Gourney (1997). The mortality rate of anorexia nervosa is 20 times, and the suicide rate 200 times, that of the general population. The mortality rate is twice that of other psychiatric in-patients (Sullivan, 1995; Nielsen *et al*, 1998). In addition, there are high levels of medical and psychological comorbidity. Drug treatment for severe eating disorders is largely ineffective and the results of psychotherapy, even in specialist hands, are only fair to good, so a large proportion of patients have chronic disability. On average, the median duration of illness is six years (Herzog *et al*, 1997), which accounts for the high prevalence in young women. Furthermore, there is some evidence that the course of the illness has become more severe in the past few decades. For example, case register data from Denmark demonstrate that the admission rates for eating disorder have increased over the past decade (Munk-Jorgensen *et al*, 1995). This increase has occurred in the context of a reduction in the admissions for all other psychiatric illnesses. Information from this database also suggests that the mortality from anorexia nervosa may be rising (Moller-Madsen *et al*, 1996). While bulimia nervosa is not associated with high mortality, it is often a chronic disorder and the quality of life of sufferers is markedly impaired (Keilen *et al*, 1994). This chapter describes methods to undertake needs assessments for eating disorder treatments and services at the population level; it will not address the question of how affected individuals can be assessed.

History of services for patients with eating disorders

It was an eminent physician, Sir William Gull, who defined and named the condition anorexia nervosa in 1873 (Gull, 1873). He recognised the importance of psychosocial factors in the aetiology of the disorder. None the less, its management remained in the hands of physicians for the greater part of the 20th century and cases of anorexia nervosa were nursed on general medical wards. As academic psychiatrists, such as Arthur Crisp and Gerald Russell, developed an interest in the condition, its management began to transfer from general medicine to psychiatry. This transfer was probably expedited by the 'discovery' of bulimia nervosa by Russell in 1979, a condition with more overt psychosocial overtones and less overt physical morbidity. Eating disorders began to feature in psychiatric textbooks written in the 1980s, and specialist psychiatric services were developed more fully in the 1990s.

Several reports have commented on either quantitative or qualitative aspects of eating disorder services over the past decade. The first of these was the Royal College of Psychiatrists report in 1992, which documented the paucity of services available. Conservative policies promoted an unplanned proliferation of in-patient services initially in the private sector. Large amounts of National Health Service (NHS) money were used to treat a few patients in such private settings, neglecting the needs of many others. Indeed, private insurers pay for only short admissions to the private sector and so a large proportion of the income to private eating disorder facilities comes from the NHS. The Eating Disorders Association, a charitable self-help organisation, produced guidelines for purchasers and for primary care that made recommendations about models of service provision (Eating Disorders Association, 1995). The Health Advisory Service (HAS) produced a report reviewing services for eating disorders in the West Midlands (1996). This report arose because of the growing awareness of the special needs of people who have an eating disorder and increasing anxiety about the capability and capacity of services to meet those needs. It suggested that the need for in-patient units should be decided on a collaborative basis at a supra-district level and that teams of community-based staff should be available for each district. The Audit Commission document *Higher Purchasing*, published in 1997, included in-patient treatment of anorexia nervosa as one of the examples of specialised services that needed to be planned at a supra-district level. Their conclusions in many ways echoed those of the HAS in that their 'hub and spoke' model suggests that specialised services be linked to clinics within the community.

In 1998, a further survey of UK eating disorder services was undertaken, this time jointly funded by the Royal College of Psychiatrists and the Consumers Association (Robinson, 1999). The report found that although there had been an expansion of the number of NHS and private units since 1992, many of the recommendations of the 1992 report had not been achieved. In particular, there are still few specialist local services. The needs of children and adolescents with eating disorders are often not considered. Only 50% of services have training facilities for junior psychiatrists. Many health authorities underestimate the number of patients with eating disorders in their area. Outside the South East of England, provision of services is poor.

A large study sponsored by COST (Co-operation in the field of scientific and technological research) in progress in 20 European countries is evaluating the outcome of treatment for eating disorders from various types of services and should yield important information about cross-cultural differences in service provision (Treasure, 1995; Kordy & Treasure, 1997).

The predicted demand for services

A variety of epidemiological studies throughout the world have been undertaken to assess the demand for eating disorder services. Several reviews summarise this data (Fairburn & Beglin, 1990; Hoek, 1991, 1993; Van Hoeken *et al*, 1998). There are several basic difficulties that confound this research. For example, one strategy that has been used very successfully in epidemiological research is the two-stage survey, with initial screening for cases considered to be at high-risk, followed up later by a clinical interview. It is interesting that in all studies that have used this methodology, cases of anorexia nervosa have been missed (see Shoemaker (1998) for a review). The screening instruments are insensitive and cases known to professionals are not detected. One reason for this may be that anorexia nervosa is an overt disorder in terms of physical sequelae and so families and teachers can be aware of a problem before the subject herself is prepared to admit to any difficulties. The converse is found in bulimia nervosa, where the patient is ashamed and humiliated by her behaviour and keeps it a secret from family and professionals, but feels safer admitting her difficulties to an anonymous questionnaire.

If the demand for help is assessed, the balance of inaccuracy shifts the other way. Sufferers of bulimia nervosa avoid asking for help, whereas sufferers of anorexia nervosa are taken, often against their wishes, for medical help. The type of medical help that is sought varies; a large number present with the physical complications rather than seeking help for managing the psychosocial aspects of their disorder. Furthermore, diagnostic criteria have been in a state of flux. Bulimia nervosa was only introduced into the ICD system of classification in 1992 (World health Organization (WHO), 1992). The weight criteria for anorexia nervosa have become less stringent and the body image criteria has been dropped (Hsu & Sobkiewicz, 1991). Conversely, for bulimia nervosa, the criteria relating to the frequency of symptoms and the definition of a binge have become tighter and the forms of weight control behaviour have become more explicit.

The incidence of new cases of anorexia nervosa presenting for any type of medical care is 4–8 per 100 000 of the total population (Hoek *et al*, 1991, 1995; Lucas *et al*, 1991; Turnbull *et al*, 1996), whereas the figures that have been reported from psychiatric case registers have been 1–5 per 100 000 population. The majority of the case register studies were conducted in the sixties and seventies, and it is possible that with time more cases have been referred for psychiatric rather than general medical help. The incidence in males is lower than 0.5 per 100 000. The proportion of males detected in primary care is lower than that of those presenting to all forms of medical care, which suggests that GPs may not diagnose cases in males as readily as in females. The incidence rate falls off rapidly by a factor of 10 in women over the age of 25 years.

The short history of bulimia nervosa means that there has been much less epidemiological data available. The incidence of cases presenting to primary care in the UK and Holland is 12 per 100 000 population and 11 per 100 000 population respectively (Hoek *et al*, 1995; Turnbull *et al*, 1996). The incidence of cases presenting to any form of medical care in the USA is 13.5 per 100 000 of the total population (Soundy *et al*, 1995). There is the suggestion that the incidence of bulimia nervosa presenting for medical care increased during the eighties (Turnbull *et al*, 1996). This may be owing in part to a combination of increased recognition by both patient and doctor. The data from a study examining the lifetime psychiatric history of a cohort of twins suggests that there is an age cohort effect with a marked increase in the risk in those women born after the 1950s (Kendler *et al*, 1991).

Both bulimia nervosa and, in particular, anorexia nervosa run a protracted course, which increases the prevalence figures. Lucas and colleagues (1991) estimated the point prevalence of anorexia nervosa to be 0.15% for the total population and 0.48% for 15–19-year-old girls. Drawing from these figures, he suggests that anorexia nervosa is the third most common medical condition of adolescence. A similar figure (0.47%) was found in a study of 15-year-old schoolgirls that used weight as a screening device (probably more sensitive than questionnaires for anorexia nervosa) (Råstam *et al*, 1989). In other studies, the prevalence rate has been found to be slightly lower, but the sensitivity of the first-stage screening was overtly seen to be poor (Meadows *et al*, 1986; Johnson-Sabine *et al*, 1988). Pagsberg & Wang (1994) detected all cases presenting to

TABLE 27.1
Matching services to need: anorexia nervosa

2–3:100 000	*Mild anorexia nervosa* Out-patient treatment; on average, 20–40 sessions For patients <17 years old, parental counselling is helpful Specialised centres are usually needed
1–2:100 000	*Acute severe anorexia nervosa* In-patient admission 3–4 months followed by intensive after-care Many practitioners recommend a year of psychotherapy after discharge
0.5–1:100 000	*Severe chronic anorexia nervosa* Repeated hospitalisations to preserve life are common in this group

medical care on the island of Bornholm, Denmark. They reported a one-year prevalence rate of anorexia nervosa of 23 per 100 000 females. Table 27.1 outlines the epidemiology of service needs of individuals with anorexia nervosa.

The prevalence rate of bulimia nervosa in young women has consistently been found to be about 1% in studies that have used the most sophisticated methodology (Drewnowski *et al*, 1988; Johnson-Sabine *et al*, 1988; Whitehouse *et al*, 1992; Rathner & Messner, 1993). The point prevalence in the total population is 20 per 100 000 (Hoek 1991) and the lifetime prevalence was found to be 1% (Garfinkel *et al*, 1995). Table 27.2 outlines the epidemiology of service needs of individuals with bulimia nervosa.

Treatments for eating disorders

There is no definitive treatment for anorexia nervosa. In-patient treatment is regarded as standard practice (American Psychiatric Association (APA), 1992) despite its high cost and its debatable efficacy (McKenzie & Joyce, 1990; Crisp *et al*, 1991). In the short term, in-patient treatment leads to full recovery of weight, but in the majority of cases these changes are not maintained. Several studies have addressed the issue of additional out-patient therapy to prevent relapse after in-patient treatment. In adolescents, family therapy given during the year following in-patient treatment prevented relapse, whereas individual therapy was more effective in older patients (Russell *et al*, 1987). There was a trend for the effect after one year to persist over five years of follow-up (Eisler *et al*, 1997).

TABLE 27.2
Matching services to need: bulimia nervosa

5:100 000	Short-term therapy in primary care by counsellors, psychologists, etc. Guided self-care, motivational enhancement therapy using resources such as self-care books
5:100 000	Medium-term therapy in more specialised units, primary mental health care teams. Specialised therapy, cognitive–behavioural therapy, cognitive–analytical therapy and interpersonal therapy
3:100 000	Long-term psychotherapy in particular for those with personality disorder
0.5:100 000	In-patient treatment for those with severe personality disorder and severe comorbidity

Simultaneously with these developments in relapse prevention, there has been an interest in developing treatments to prevent admission. The types of therapy and patients considered eligible for out-patient therapy vary widely. In the USA, the threshold for resorting to in-patient care is low, that is, a body mass index (BMI) of less than $16 \, kg/m^2$ (Garner & Needleman, 1997) or 20% weight loss (APA, 1992). In contrast, in the UK and some other European countries, admission is reserved for the severely ill with a BMI of less than $13 \, kg/m^2$ (Treasure & Szmukler, 1995; Van Furth, 1998). Not only are out-patient approaches cheaper, but it has been suggested that they may lead to better long-term outcomes (Morgan *et al*, 1983; Beumont *et al*, 1993).

There have been very few clinical trials that evaluate out-patient psychotherapies for this debilitating disorder. Those that have been accomplished have had very low power and selected samples. Crisp and colleagues (1991) attempted to compare the effectiveness of in-patient care with out-patient treatment. The interpretation of the study is difficult, as 60% of those allocated to in-patient treatment refused this approach despite being offered no other form of treatment. Nevertheless, the outcome of all patients and the subgroup who complied with treatment was no better in those allocated to in-patient treatment than for those given out-patient treatment. These results need to be tempered by the fact that those allocated to in-patient treatment were older and had a longer duration of illness and a lower mean weight, all of which are factors known to be associated with a poor prognosis. An important conclusion to be drawn from these results is that patients with good prognostic features can be managed with out-patient treatment.

Several small studies complement the findings of Crisp and colleagues reported above in that they have shown that out-patient treatment alone can be effective in adult anorexia nervosa (Hall & Crisp, 1987; Channon *et al*, 1989; Brambilla *et al*, 1995*a*,*b*; Treasure *et al*, 1995*b*). A variety of models of treatment were used: nutritional counselling, dynamic psychotherapy, cognitive–behavioural therapy (CBT), behavioural therapy, cognitive–analytical therapy and pharmacotherapy. New models of treatment, such as motivational enhancement therapy, have been developed (Treasure & Ward, 1997). A recent study found that specialised out-patient therapy (family, short-term dynamic or cognitive analytical therapy) was more effective at one year than treatment as usual (Dare *et al*, 2001).

Adolescents aged 17 years and under account for about a quarter of the cases of anorexia nervosa and bulimia nervosa. In anorexia nervosa, the outcome is better for this group and the need for admission is lower. In adolescent anorexia nervosa, either family therapy or a form of parental counselling plus individual therapy can be effective (Le Grange *et al*, 1992; Robin *et al*, 1994, 1999; Eisler *et al*, 2000). Books that detail some of the educational elements have been developed (Crisp *et al*, 1996; Treasure, 1997*a*). Patients with severe chronic unstable anorexia nervosa pose a difficult management problem. All too often, they relapse immediately after discharge and require repeated admission. As yet, there are no satisfactory rehabilitation facilities for this group. If hostels are to be used, staff need to ensure that they have the specific skills needed for managing patients with eating disorders, such as support around meals.

In contrast to anorexia nervosa, there has been a cornucopia of randomised controlled trials evaluating treatment for bulimia nervosa. There is confidence that cognitive–behavioural treatment is effective for approximately half of the patients treated (Wilson, 1996; Schmidt, 1998). However, the standard research designs leave many questions unanswered. How many of the 50% who responded could have been managed with fewer resources? What could have been done for the 50% who did not respond to short-term therapy? It is also uncertain whether the conclusions drawn from randomised controlled trials can be generalised to service delivery, as many of the patients who present for treatment are complex and would be excluded from many such trials (the percentage range of exclusion from psychotherapy trials is 0–39% and from drug trials 0–47%; Mitchell *et al*, 1997).

A sequential model of care for bulimia nervosa was recommended in the Royal College of Psychiatrists report (1992) and several alternative models have been described (Garner *et al*, 1986; Fairburn

& Peveler, 1990; Fairburn *et al*, 1992; Tiller *et al*, 1993; Garner & Needleman, 1997). A series of treatments increasing in intensity can be offered. One advantage of such an approach is that it does not waste resources, because those who respond to a minimal intervention are 'filtered out'. One possible adverse effect of sequential treatment is that it can lead to the experience of failure, which may lower the already fragile self-esteem of the patient and damage the therapeutic alliance.

A variety of low-intensity models of treatment have been developed and evaluated. These involve a variety of methods for disseminating knowledge and skills, while fostering a degree of self-help and therapeutic collaboration.

A group psychoeducational intervention of five 90-minute lectures (total of 7.5 hours) with an emphasis on symptom management was developed in Canada and examined in a quasi-experimental design (Davis *et al*, 1990; Olmsted *et al*, 1991). This produced a 20% abstinence rate from binge eating. The minimal intervention was as effective as a more intensive treatment in the less severely affected subgroup.

Huon (1985) evaluated an intervention that involved sending seven monthly instalments from a self-help programme to 90 subjects with DSM–III bulimia. The group receiving active treatment showed more improvement than the waiting list group. This approach has been continued using books that include education, with cognitive, behavioural and motivational elements, for example, *Getting Better Bit(e) by Bit(e)* (Schmidt & Treasure, 1993). These have been found to be effective (Schmidt *et al*, 1993; Treasure *et al*, 1994) and can reduce the number of therapy sessions given either in sequential models of care (Treasure *et al*, 1996) or as adjuncts in models of guided self (Thiels *et al*, 1998). A different self-care manual as part of guided self-care has also been found to be effective in an open study of bulimia nervosa (Cooper *et al*, 1996). These forms of minimal treatment appear to be of particular use in the treatment of binge eating disorder (Carter & Fairburn, 1998).

Medication with antidepressants is less effective (with abstinence rates of 20–30%) and therapeutic gains are less well maintained than those of psychotherapy for bulimia nervosa (for a review, see Mayer & Walsh (1998)). There is, however, some evidence to suggest that combinations of the two summate.

Many of the individuals who fail to respond to short-term therapy have personality difficulties and may require longer forms of psychotherapy. There is work in progress, evaluating models of staged care, for example, giving CBT as the first step, followed by interpersonal therapy or drug therapy.

Diagnosis and pathways to care

Referrals from primary care

General practitioners (GPs) can reliably diagnose eating disorders. Approximately 70% of GP-diagnosed cases fulfil research diagnostic criteria for an eating disorder (Turnbull *et al*, 1996). Anorexia nervosa presents soon after onset and 90% of cases are referred on for secondary care. The diagnosis and presentation of bulimia nervosa is more delayed. Approximately 75% of cases are referred on for secondary care.

Tertiary referrals

Eating disorders often present to medical specialists, for example endocrinologists or gynaecologists. The risk of developing an eating disorder is increased twofold in women with diabetes mellitus (Rodin *et al*, personal communication). Moreover, the complication rate is multiplied (Rydall *et al*, 1997; Williams & Gill, 1997), with the mortality rate from the combined problem increasing twelvefold (Nielsen & Molbak, 1998). Cases such as these require specialist treatment.

Other referrals

Schools, colleges and occupational physicians also ascertain cases of eating disorders.

Conclusions

There has been a gradual transfer of the management of anorexia nervosa from general physicians to psychiatrists over the last century. This may be owing in part to an implicit recognition that maintaining factors such as cultural and family beliefs are playing an ever-increasing role in the course of the illness. For although the incidence rate of anorexia nervosa appears to be stable over time, there is some evidence to suggest that the prevalence has increased. Also, bulimia nervosa has emerged as a new form of psychiatric disorder that is more common than anorexia nervosa. It is uncertain how many cases are new, arising from the cultural fashion for leanness within an environment of plenty, or whether many cases represent the pathoplastic changes within the expression of psychological distress replacing some forms of depression, substance misuse and personality disorder (Russell & Treasure, 1989).

Eating disorders are not self-limiting conditions. Remission from bulimia nervosa does not occur on the waiting list; indeed, the opposite is the case in that the longer cases are left untreated the more severe the disorder and the poorer the final outcome. Repeated assessments and failed attempts at treatment lower self-esteem and result in a perception of failure. What has clearly emerged from all the research into the treatment of eating disorders is that specific skills are needed. Treatment is not a question of prescribing medication but requires skilled psychotherapy. However, some aspects of treatment can be delivered with minimalist therapist input using self-treatment books or group psychoeducation. Approximately 50% of patients with bulimia nervosa respond to a short-term intervention. The remainder (which includes patients with comorbidity such as borderline personality disorder and diabetes mellitus) require longer-term psychotherapy. Many of the specialised treatments developed for the management of bulimia nervosa require specific training, which is limited. However, manuals for therapists are available (Treasure & Schmidt, 1997).

Much of the treatment for anorexia nervosa is not evidence-based. In particular, adolescents can respond to low intensity of care such as out-patient treatment, especially if specific skills and education are included. However, a proportion of cases (approximately a third) will require higher levels of intensity, such as day patient or in-patient care. Approximately 10% require long-term care.

Reports on services recommend that each district has access to a specialist psychiatrist (someone to provide a minimum of three sessions a week) and that there is a tiered system of service provision with a few supra-district centres that provide high-intensity care such as day patient and in-patient treatment.

References

AMERICAN PSYCHIATRIC ASSOCIATION (1992) Practice guidelines for eating disorders. *American Journal of Psychiatry*, **150**, 208–228.

AUDIT COMMISSION (1997) *Higher Purchasing.* London: HMSO.

BEUMONT, P. J. V., RUSSELL, J. D. & TOUYZ, S. (1993) Treatment of anorexia nervosa. *Lancet*, **341**, 1635–1640.

BRAMBILLA, F., DRAISCI, A., PEIRONE, A., *ET AL* (1995*a*) Combined cognitive behavioral, psychopharmacological and nutritional therapy in eating disorders. 1. Anorexia nervosa – restricted type. *Neuropsychobiology*, **32**, 59–63.

——, ——, ——, *ET AL* (1995*b*) Combined cognitive behavioral, psychopharmacological and nutritional therapy in eating disorders. 2. Anorexia nervosa – binge-eating purging type. *Neuropsychobiology*, **32**, 64–67.

CARTER, J. C. & FAIRBURN, C. G. (1998) Cognitive behavioural self help for binge eating disorder: a controlled effectiveness study. *Journal of Consulting and Clinical Psychology*, **66**, 616–623.

CHANNON, S., DE SILVA, P., HEMSLEY, D., *ET AL* (1989) A controlled trial of cognitive behavioural and behavioural treatment of anorexia nervosa. *Behaviour Research and Therapy*, **27**, 529–535.

COOPER, P. J., COKER, S. & FLEMING, C. (1996) An evaluation of the efficacy of supervised cognitive behavioural self-help for bulimia nervosa. *Journal of Psychosomatic Research*, **40**, 281–287.

CRISP, A. H., NORTON, K., GOWERS, S., *ET AL* (1991) A controlled study of the effect of therapies aimed at adolescent and family psychopathology in anorexia nervosa. *British Journal of Psychiatry*, **159**, 325–333.

——, JOUGHIN, N., HALEK, C., *ET AL* (1996) *Anorexia Nervosa. The Wish to Change.* Hove: Psychology Press.

DARE, C., EISLER, I., RUSSELL, G., ET AL (2001) Psychological therapies for adults with anorexia nervosa. Randomised controlled trial of out-patient treatments. *British Journal of Psychiatry*, **178**, 216–222.

DAVIS, R., OLMSTED, M. P. & ROCKERT, W. (1990) Brief group psychoeducation for bulimia nervosa: assessing the clinical significance of change. *Journal of Consulting and Clinical Psychology*, **58**, 882–885.

DREWNOWSKI, A., YEE, D. K. & KRAHN, D. D. (1988) Bulimia nervosa in college women: incidence and recovery rates. *American Journal of Psychiatry*, **145**, 753–755.

EATING DISORDERS ASSOCIATION (1995) *Guide for Purchasers of Services for Eating Disorders.* Norwich: Eating Disorders Association.

EISLER, I., DARE, C., RUSSELL, G. F. M., *ET AL* (1997) A five year follow-up of a controlled trial of family therapy in severe eating disorder. *Archives of General Psychiatry*, **54**, 1025–1030.

——, ——, HODES, M., *ET AL* (2000) Family therapy for adolescent anorexia nervosa. The results of a controlled comparison of two family interventions. *Journal of Child Psychology and Psychiatry*, **41**, 727–736.

FAIRBURN, C. G. & BEGLIN, S. J. (1990) Studies of the epidemiology of bulimia nervosa. *American Journal of Psychiatry*, **147**, 401–408.

—— & PEVELER, R. C. (1990) Bulimia nervosa and a stepped care approach to management. *Gut*, **31**, 1220–1222.

——, AGRAS, W. S. & WILSON, G. T. (1992) The research on the treatment of bulimia nervosa. Practical & theoretical implications. In: *Biology of Feast and Famine* (eds G. H. Anderson & S. H. Kennedy), pp. 317–340. San Diego: San Diego Academic Press.

GARFINKEL, P. E., LIN, E., GOERING, P., *ET AL* (1995) Bulimia nervosa in a Canadian community sample: prevalence and comparison of subgroups. *American Journal of Psychiatry*, **152**, 1052–1058.

GARNER, D. M. & NEEDLEMAN, L. D. (1997) Sequencing and integration of treatments. In: *Handbook of Treatment of Eating Disorders* (eds D. M. Garner & P. E. Garfinkel), pp. 50–66. New York: Guilford Press.

——, GARFINKEL, P. E. & IRVINE, M. J. (1986) Integration and sequencing of treatment approaches for eating disorders. *Psychotherapy and Psychosomatics*, **46**, 67–75.

GOLDBERG, D. & GOURNEY, K. (1997) *The General Practitioner, the Psychiatrist and the Burden of Mental Health Care.* Maudsley Discussion Paper No. 1. London: Institute of Psychiatry.

GULL, W. W. (1873) Proceedings of the Clinical Society of London. *British Medical Journal*, **1**, 527–529.

HALL, A. & CRISP, A. H. (1987) Brief psychotherapy in the treatment of anorexia nervosa. Outcome at one year. *British Journal of Psychiatry*, **151**, 185–191.

HEALTH ADVISORY SERVICE (1996) *A Review of Services for People with Eating Disorders in the West Midlands.* London: Health Advisory Service.

HERZOG, W., DETER, H. C., FIEHN, W., *ET AL* (1997) Medical findings and predictors of long-term physical outcome in anorexia nervosa: a prospective, 12-year follow-up study. *Psychological Medicine*, **27**, 269–279.

Hoek, H. W. (1991) The incidence and prevalence of anorexia nervosa and bulimia nervosa in primary care. *Psychological Medicine*, **21**, 455–460.

—— (1993) Review of the epidemiological studies of eating disorders. *International Review of Psychiatry*, **5**, 61–74.

——, Bartelds, A. I. M., Bosveld, J. J. F., *et al* (1995) The impact of urbanization on the detection rates of eating disorders. *American Journal of Psychiatry*, **152**, 1272–1278.

Huon, G. (1985) An initial validation of a self help program for bulimia. *International Journal of Eating Disorders*, **4**, 573–588.

Hsu, L. K. G. & Sobkiewicz, T. A. (1991) Body image disturbance: Time to abandon the concept for eating disorders. *International Journal of Eating Disorders*, **10**, 15–30.

Johnson-Sabine,E., Wood, K., Patton, G., *et al* (1988) Abnormal eating attitudes in London school-girls – a prospective epidemiological study: factors associated with abnormal response on screening questionnaires. *Psychological Medicine*, **18**, 615–622.

Keilen, M., Treasure, T., Schmidt, U., *et al* (1994) Quality of life measurements in eating disorders, angina, and transplant candidates: are they comparable? *Journal of the Royal Society of Medicine*, **87**, 441–444.

Kendler, K. S., McLean, C., Neale, M., *et al* (1991) The genetic epidemiology of bulimia nervosa. *American Journal of Psychiatry*, **148**, 1627–1637.

Kordy, H. & Treasure, J. (1997) Effectiveness and efficiency of psychotherapy treatment programmes – The European Collaborative Longitudinal Observational Study on Eating Disorders (ECLOS–ED). In: *Psychotherapeutic Issues in Eating Disorders: Models, Methods and Results* (eds P. Bria, A. Ciocca & S. De Rissio), pp. 1–8. Rome: Socula Editrice Universo.

Le Grange, D., Eisler, I., Dare, C., *et al* (1992) Evaluation of family therapy in anorexia nervosa: a pilot study. *International Journal of Eating Disorders*, **12**, 347–357.

Lucas, A. R., Beard, C. M., O'Fallon, W. M., *et al* (1991) 50-year trends in the incidence of anorexia nervosa in Rochester, Minnesota: A population based study. *American Journal of Psychiatry*, **148**, 917–922.

Mayer, L. E. S. & Walsh, B. T. (1998) Pharmacotherapy of eating disorders. In: *Neurobiology in the Treatment of Eating Disorders* (eds H. W. Hoek, J. L. Treasure & M. A. Katzman), pp. 395–397. Chichester: John Wiley & Sons.

McKenzie, J. M. & Joyce, P. R. (1990) Hospitalisation for anorexia nervosa. *International Journal of Eating Disorders*, **11**, 235–241.

Meadows, G., Palmer, R., Newball, E., *et al* (1986) Eating attitudes and disorder in young women: a general practice based survey. *Psychological Medicine*, **16**, 351–357.

Mitchell, J. E., Maki, D. D., Adson, D. E., *et al* (1997) The selectivity of inclusion and exclusion criteria in bulimia nervosa treatment studies. *International Journal of Eating Disorders*, **22**, 243–252.

Moller-Madsen, S. & Nystrup, J. (1992) Incidence of anorexia nervosa in Denmark. *Acta Psychiatrica Scandinavica*, **86**, 197–200.

——, & Nielsen, S. (1996) Mortality of anorexia nervosa in Denmark 1970–1987. *Acta Psychiatrica Scandinavica*, **94**, 454–459.

Morgan, H. G., Purgold, J. & Welbourne, J. (1983) Management and outcome in anorexia nervosa. A standardised prognostic study. *British Journal of Psychiatry*, **143**, 282–287.

Munk-Jorgensen, P., Moller-Madson, S., Nielsen, S., *et al* (1995) Incidence of eating disorders in psychiatric hospitals and wards in Denmark 1970–1993. *Acta Psychiatrica Scandinavica*, **92**, 91–96.

Nielsen, S. & Molbak, A. G. (1998) Eating disorders and type1 diabetes: Overview and summing up. *European Eating Disorders Review*, **6**, 4–27.

——, Moller-Madsen, S., Isager, T., *et al* (1998) Standardised mortality in eating disorders – a quantitative summary of previously published and new evidence. *Journal of Psychosomatic Research*, **44**, 413–434.

Olmsted, M. P, Davis, R., Rockert, W., *et al* (1991) Efficacy of a brief group psycho-educational intervention for bulimia nervosa. *Behavioural Research Therapy*, **29**, 71–83.

PAGSBERG, A. K. & WANG, A. R. (1994) Epidemiology of anorexia nervosa and bulimia nervosa in Bornholm County, Denmark 1970–1989. *Acta Psychiatrica Scandinavica*, **90**, 259–265.

RÅSTAM, M., GILLBERG, C. & GARTON, M. (1989) Anorexia nervosa in a Swedish urban region. Population-based study. *British Journal of Psychiatry*, **155**, 642–646.

RATHNER, G. & MESSNER, K. (1993) Detection of eating disorders in a small rural town: an epidemiological survey. *Psychological Medicine*, **23**, 175–184.

ROBIN, A. L., SIEGEL, P. T., KOEPKE, T., *ET AL* (1994) Family therapy versus individual therapy for adolescent females with anorexia nervosa. *Developmental and Behavioral Pediatrics*, **15**, 111–116.

——, ——, MOYE, A. W., ET AL (1999) A controlled comparison of family versus individual therapy for adolescents with anorexia nervosa. *Journal of the American Academy for Child and Adolescent Psychiatry*, **38**, 1482–1489.

ROBINSON, P. (1999) *The 1998 UK Survey of Specialist Eating Disorder Services.* Paper given at the Eating Disorders Special Interest Group. Grovelands Priory Hospital, London. February, 1999.

ROYAL COLLEGE OF PSYCHIATRISTS (1992) *Eating Disorders.* Council Report CR14. London: Royal College of Psychiatrists.

RUSSELL, G. F. M. (1979) Bulimia nervosa: an ominous variant of anorexia nervosa. *Psychological Medicine*, **9**, 429–448.

—— & TREASURE, J. (1989) The modern history of anorexia nervosa: an interpretation of why the illness has changed. In: *The Psychobiology of Human Eating Disorders: Preclinical and Clinical Perspectives* (eds L. A. Schneider, S. J. Cooper & K. A. Halmi). *Annals of the New York Academy of Sciences*, **575**, 13–30.

——, SZMUKLER, G. I., DARE, C., *ET AL* (1987) An evaluation of family therapy in anorexia nervosa and bulimia nervosa. *Archives of General Psychiatry*, **44**, 1047–1056.

RYDALL, A. C., RODIN, G. M., OLMSTED, M. P., *ET AL* (1997) Disordered eating behaviour and microvascular complications in young women with insulin-dependent diabetes mellitus. *New England Journal of Medicine*, **336**, 1849–1854.

SCHMIDT, U. (1998) Treatment of bulimia nervosa. In: *The Integration of Neurobiology in the Treatment of Eating Disorders* (eds H. W. Hoek, J. L. Treasure & M. A. Katzman). New York: John Wiley & Sons.

—— & TREASURE, J. (1993) *Getting Better Bit(e) by Bit(e). A Survival Kit for Sufferers of Bulimia Nervosa and Binge Eating Disorder.* Hove: Lawrence Erlbaum.

——, TILLER, J. & TREASURE, J. (1993) Self-treatment of bulimia nervosa: A pilot study. *International Journal of Eating Disorders*, **13**, 273–277.

SHOEMAKER, C. (1998) The principles of screening for eating disorders In: *The Prevention of Eating Disorders* (eds W. Vandereycken & G. Noordenbos), pp. 187–213. London: Athlone Press.

SOUNDY, T. J., LUCAS, A. R., SUMAN, V. J., *ET AL* (1995) Bulimia nervosa in Rochester, Minnesota from 1980 to 1990. *Psychological Medicine*, **25**, 1065–1071.

SULLIVAN, P. F. (1995) Mortality in anorexia nervosa. *American Journal of Psychiatry*, **152**, 1073–1074.

THIELS, C., SCHMIDT, U., TREASURE, J., *ET AL* (1998) Guided self change for bulimia nervosa incorporating a self care manual. *American Journal of Psychiatry*, **155**, 947–953.

TILLER, J., SCHMIDT, U. & TREASURE, J. (1993) Treatment of bulimia nervosa. *International Review of Psychiatry*, **5**, 75–86.

TREASURE, J. L. (1995) European Co-operation in the Fields of Scientific and Technical Research COST B6. Psychotherapeutic treatment of eating disorders. *European Eating Disorders Review*, **3**, 119–120.

—— (1997*a*) *Anorexia Nervosa. A Survival Guide for Sufferers and those Caring for Someone with an Eating Disorder.* Hove: Psychology Press.

—— (1997*b*) *Motivational Enhancement Therapy for Anorexia Nervosa. A Companion Version to Escaping from Anorexia Nervosa.* Hove: Psychology Press.

—— & SCHMIDT, U. (1997) *A Clinician's Guide to Management of Bulimia Nervosa (Motivational Enhancement Therapy for Bulimia Nervosa)*. Hove: Psychology Press.

—— & SZMUKLER, G. I. (1995) Medical complications of chronic anorexia nervosa. In: *Handbook of Eating Disorders. Theory, Treatment & Research* (eds G. Szmukler, C. Dare & J. L. Treasure), pp. 197–220. Chichester: John Wiley & Sons.

—— & WARD, A. (1997) A practical guide to the use of motivational interviewing in anorexia nervosa. *European Eating Disorders Review*, **5**, 102–114.

——, SCHMIDT, U., TROOP, N., *ET AL* (1994) The first step in the management of bulimia nervosa. A controlled trial of a therapeutic manual. *British Medical Journal*, **308**, 686–689.

——, ——, ——, *ET AL* (1995*a*) Sequential treatment for bulimia nervosa incorporating a self care manual. *British Journal of Psychiatry*, **168**, 94–98.

——, TODD, G., BROLLEY, M., *ET AL* (1995*b*) A pilot study of a randomised trial of cognitive analytic therapy vs educational behavioural therapy for adult anorexia nervosa. *Behaviour Research and Therapy*, **33**, 363–367.

——, —— & SZMUKLER, G. (1995*c*) The in-patient treatment of anorexia nervosa. In: *Handbook of Eating Disorders. Theory, Treatment & Research* (eds G. Szmukler, C. Dare & J. L. Treasure), pp. 275–293. Chichester: John Wiley & Sons.

——, TROOP, N. A. & WARD, A. (1996) An approach to planning services for bulimia nervosa. *British Journal of Psychiatry*, **169**, 551–554.

TURNBULL, S. J., SCHMIDT, U., TROOP, N., *ET AL* (1995) Predictors of outcome for bulimia nervosa. *International Journal of Eating Disorders*, **21**,17–22.

——, WARD, A., TREASURE, J., *ET AL* (1996) The demand for eating disorder care. An epidemiological study using the general practice research database. *British Journal of Psychiatry*, **169**, 705–712.

VAN FURTH, E. F. (1998) The treatment of anorexia nervosa. In: *The Integration of Neurobiology in the Treatment of Eating Disorders* (eds H. W. Hoek, J. L. Treasure & M. A. Katzman), pp. 307–322. Chichester: John Wiley & Sons.

VAN HOEKEN, D., LUCAS, A. R. & HOEK, H. W. (1998) Epidemiology. In: *The Integration of Neurobiology in the Treatment of Eating Disorders* (eds H. W. Hoek, J. L. Treasure & M. A. Katzman), pp. 97–126. Chichester: John Wiley & Sons.

WHITEHOUSE, A. M., COOPER, P. J., VIZE, C. V., *ET AL* (1992) Prevalence of eating disorders in three Cambridge general practices: Hidden and conspicuous morbidity. *British Journal General Practice*, **42**, 57–60.

WILLIAMS, G. & GILL, G. V. (1997) Eating disorders and diabetic complications. *New England Journal of Medicine*, **336**, 1905–1906.

WILSON, T. G. (1996) Treatment of bulimia nervosa: when CBT fails. *Behaviour Research and Therapy*, **34**, 197–212.

WORLD HEALTH ORGANIZATION (1992) *International Classification of Diseases and Related Health Problems. Tenth revision (ICD–10)*. Geneva: WHO.

28 Needs assessment and alcohol

E. JANE MARSHALL

Alcohol has been described as 'our favourite drug' (Royal College of Psychiatrists, 1986). It is a legal and universally available substance that gives great pleasure when consumed in moderate quantities. Most people drink without problems. However, excessive consumption has the potential to cause significant physical, psychological and social problems at the individual level. It is estimated that 33 000 deaths per year in Great Britain are alcohol-related (Alcohol Concern, 1997). Alcohol is a risk factor for many disorders, including hypertension, cardiac arrhythmias, stroke, coronary heart disease, cancers of the oesophagus, pharynx and larynx and the female breast, and liver cirrhosis (Anderson, 1995). Alcohol may also have a protective effect against coronary heart disease, but much of this effect can be achieved at consumption levels of less than 10 g (1 unit)[1] daily, and is only relevant to men over 40 years and post-menopausal women.

Alcohol contributes to a wide range of problems in society. It is involved in all types of accidents and contributes to 15% of traffic deaths. Road traffic accidents in which alcohol is involved are more serious than accidents in which it is not (Glucksman, 1994). Alcohol is also implicated in 26–54% of home and leisure injuries (Edwards *et al*, 1994). It is associated with domestic violence, child abuse, crime, homicide and suicide. Up to 14 million working days are lost annually to alcohol-related problems, and annual costs to the National Health Service (NHS) are in the region of £150 million (Alcohol Concern, 1997). The cost in terms of human suffering is incalculable.

Alcohol-related problems are not confined to individuals with chronic excessive alcohol consumption, or those with alcohol dependence. Heavy social drinkers, particularly binge drinkers are also at risk. Indeed, epidemiological evidence supports the view that most

---

[1] A unit of alcohol is defined as a standard pub measure of spirits, a glass of wine or a half-pint of ordinary strength beer.

alcohol-related harm in the general population occurs in heavy drinkers who might not be considered to have an alcohol problem.

Heavy drinkers experience high rates of alcohol-related problems, but only make a small contribution to the overall level of such problems. Most alcohol problems occur in light and moderate drinkers, although such drinkers have low rates of problems (Kreitman, 1986). This underlies the so-called 'preventive paradox', which states that reducing consumption among moderate drinkers will have a greater impact on improving health and social conditions in the whole population than reducing consumption among heavy drinkers.

For the purposes of this chapter, the term 'alcohol misuse' is defined as a level or pattern of alcohol consumption likely to damage the physical and psychological health or social adjustment of the individual drinker, or others directly affected by his or her drinking (Edwards & Unnithan, 1994).

In the mid-1980s, the Royal Colleges recommended 'sensible limits' of 21 units per week for men and 14 units per week for women (Royal College of Psychiatrists, 1986). These guidelines were re-affirmed in 1995 (Royal College of Physicians, Psychiatrists & General Practitioners, 1995). However, in the same year, a Department of Health working party recommended moving to a 'daily benchmark' of 3–4 units per day for men and 2–3 units per day for women (Department of Health, 1995*a*). Although the Department of Health's advice on sensible drinking is now based on these daily benchmarks, the previously recommended weekly maximum levels will be retained in this chapter. There is no consumption limit for dependence, but men drinking above 51 units per week and women drinking above 36 units per week are likely to experience problems with their drinking.

Alcohol misuse is not a neatly circumscribed 'disease' entity. It is a heterogeneous problem that presents itself on several fronts in the health and social services arena. It is often associated with misuse of other substances, and service planning needs to take account of this in order to develop an "integrated, interactive, multi-level and sustained response system targeted at multiple types and degrees of problem" (Edwards & Unnithan, 1994).

Consideration of the various classification systems that demarcate the broad base of alcohol misuse is central to an understanding of what is being treated. Official classification systems include ICD–10 (World Health Organization (WHO), 1992) and DSM–IV (American Psychiatric Association (APA), 1994). Efforts to integrate the two major classification systems have been successful with respect to the definition of alcohol dependence. ICD–10 includes six symptoms under the syndrome of alcohol dependence (Table 28.1). For a diagnosis of dependence, three or more symptoms should have occurred in the past year.

TABLE 28.1
ICD–10 definition of alcohol dependence (components a–f; WHO, 1992)

Criteria	Three or more of a–f at some time in the previous 12 months
Features	
Compulsion	a A strong desire or sense of compulsion to drink
Impaired control	b Difficulty controlling onset, termination and/or amount of drinking
Withdrawal Relief drinking	c Physiological withdrawal symptoms and signs Alcohol used to relieve or avoid withdrawal symptoms
Tolerance	d Evidence of tolerance such that increased doses are required to achieve effects originally produced by lower doses
Salience	e Progressive neglect of alternative pursuits or interests because of drinking, increased use of time spent drinking or seeking alcohol or to recover from its effects
	f Persisting in drinking despite clear evidence of overtly harmful consequences
	(Narrowing of the personal repertoire of patterns of drinking has also been described as a characteristic)

The ICD–10 diagnosis of 'harmful use of alcohol' requires a pattern of drinking that has caused actual physical or psychological harm to the user (Table 28.2).

In recent survey work, the Office for National Statistics (ONS, 1998*a*) – formerly the Office of Population Censuses and Surveys – distinguished between the following weekly levels of consumption in units: 'fairly high' (22–35 units for men; 15–25 units for women); 'high' (36–50 units for men; 26–35 units for women); and 'very high' (51+ units for men; 36+ units for women).

TABLE 28.2
ICD–10 definition of alcohol abuse (WHO, 1992)

Criteria	Acute intoxification or 'hangover' not sufficient in itself Not diagnosed if dependence syndrome is present
Features	Actual damage to the mental or physical health of the drinker

The current diagnostic system can be considered to have three dimensions: 'heavy drinking', 'alcohol problems' and 'dependence'. The relationship between these three is shown in Figure 28.1.

Sub-categories (as target populations)

The assessment of health care needs and demands in the alcohol field is facilitated by the following classification adapted from Edwards & Unnithan (1994):

The 'at-risk' (or hazardous) drinker

This category includes anyone drinking over safe limits (21 units per week for men or 14 units per week for women) who has not developed any alcohol-related problems or dependence. These individuals may experience alcohol-related harm as a result of the pattern of their drinking (binge drinking) or drinking combined with driving.

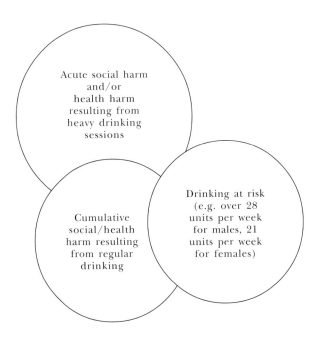

Fig. 28.1 Relationship between excessive drinking, problems and dependence (adapted from Chick et al, 1997)

The problem (or harmful) drinker

This includes excessive drinking associated with alcohol-related problems but without established dependence. Individuals may have acute or chronic problems. Acute problems may be one-off (an alcohol-related road traffic accident or pancreatitis). Chronic problems include hypertension, cirrhosis, alcohol-related brain impairment, and domestic violence. Such problems typically present to the primary care team, but also to the general hospital.

The dependent drinker

This includes excessive drinking with problems and dependence. Although alcohol-related problems and dependence are conceptualised along different and distinct dimensions, dependent individuals almost always have alcohol-related problems as well. This group will present to a range of services, ranging from primary care to general hospitals (for treatment of physical complications) to psychiatric hospitals (for psychological complications such as depression) and/or to specialised alcohol services, either statutory or non-statutory.

It may also be helpful to consider other groups in addition to this three-point system.

Women

Women drink considerably less than men but are more vulnerable to some of the adverse consequences of alcohol, particularly liver and brain damage. In Britain, the proportion of women drinking more than the recommended sensible limits (14 units per week) increased from 9% in 1984 to 15% in 1998, with the largest increase occurring among the 18–24 age group. This has implications for women who might become pregnant, because alcohol consumption in pregnancy is associated with increased risks of complications during both the pregnancy and the delivery and with harm to the developing foetus (foetal alcohol syndrome).

Ethnic minorities

Individuals from ethnic minorities are underrepresented in specialist alcohol misuse services. Surveys suggest that the prevalence of heavy drinking in the Afro-Caribbean community is about half the national average. However, younger Black people may be drinking at levels closer to the national average.

Young people

Evidence suggests that most young people have tasted alcohol by the age of 13 years, with boys drinking more than girls and older adolescents more than younger ones (Raistrick *et al*, 1999). The pattern of alcohol consumption has also changed, with young people drinking more alcohol on one occasion (Newcombe *et al*, 1995). A recent study of second-year university students from 10 universities in the UK found that 61% of men and 48% of women were drinking above the recommended levels (Webb *et al*, 1996). Binge drinking was also common.

Older people

Older people generally drink less than younger members of the population. However, General Household Surveys suggest that an increasing proportion of individuals over the age of 65 years are drinking more than the recommended limits. Older people are more susceptible to the adverse effects of alcohol as a result of reduced tolerance, greater risk of interactions with prescribed medication and a greater vulnerability to falls and other injuries. Unfortunately, problem drinking is often overlooked in older people, and their needs should be taken into account in the development of services and training.

The homeless population

The homeless population has changed over the past 30 years and is now younger and more heterogeneous. There is a drinking subculture among some groups of homeless people, with a significant proportion of those using night shelters and sleeping rough being alcohol dependent: 44% and 51% respectively (OPCS, 1996). A study of 96 homeless men admitted from the streets to a cold weather shelter in January 1991 reported high levels of alcohol problems (53%) and alcohol dependence (25%) (Reed *et al*, 1992). Homeless drinkers are often excluded from generic services for the homeless and also from community and specialist services set up for drinkers.

Individuals with mental health problems

Prevalence rates of alcohol misuse disorders in psychiatric populations are higher than in the general population, ranging from 10% to 65% (Osher & Drake, 1996), and may be on the increase (Cuffel, 1992). Menezes *et al* (1996) reported a one-year prevalence rate for alcohol problems of 32% in 171 subjects with a lifetime history of psychosis. The prevalence rates of psychiatric disorders in individuals attending alcohol services are also high – 30–40% in one study (Glass & Jackson, 1988). Services for this very disadvantaged 'dual (often multiple) diagnosis' group must be considered in any needs assessment.

Prisoners

Research on alcohol use among prisoners shows that a high proportion (about 30%) are heavy drinkers (Heather, 1982). Between 30% and 60% claim to have offended while under the influence of alcohol.

Polydrug use

Polydrug use has become increasingly prevalent over recent decades. Although the combination and pattern of drugs used continues to change, alcohol is almost always implicated. Treatment services must have a capacity to integrate alcohol and drug treatment if the challenge of polydrug use is to be successfully tackled.

Estimating the levels of need

Ideally, any local needs assessment should be population-based. This requires relevant information to be available. However, there is little population-based information on alcohol use in local populations, and data from other sources has to be adapted.

National estimates of drinking among the general population – the General Household Survey

Questions about drinking alcohol have been included in the General Household Survey (GHS) every two years since 1978. Data from the 1996 survey (ONS, 1998*a*) is summarised in Table 28.3. This shows that the average weekly consumption by men was 16 units, compared with six units for women. The overall population levels conceal wide variations by age. It is notable that 35% of men and 21% of women in the 16–24 age group were exceeding the recommended sensible levels.

Geographical variation in alcohol consumption

Regional differences in reported alcohol consumption can also be examined. Table 28.4 presents data from the 1996 General Household Survey by gender and region, and shows that men in the North and North West of England report the highest mean alcohol consumption levels.

Table 28.3

Alcohol consumption levels as units of alcohol by gender and age

	16–24 years (%)		25–44 years (%)		45–64 years (%)		>65 years (%)		Total (%)	
	M	F	M	F	M	F	M	F	M	F
Non-drinker	8.0	9.0	5.0	8.0	6.0	13.0	12.0	24.0	7.0	13.0
Very low (under 1)	6.0	13.0	5.0	14.0	9.0	21.0	14.0	30.0	8.0	20.0
Low (1–10)	32.0	36.0	33.0	42.0	35.0	38.0	39.0	29.0	35.0	37.0
Moderate (11–21)	18.0	20.0	26.0	19.0	24.0	15.0	18.0	10.0	23.0	16.0
Fairly high (22–35)	16.0	12.0	16.0	11.0	15.0	9.0	10.0	5.0	15.0	9.0
High (36–50)	9.0	4.0	7.0	3.0	6.0	2.0	4.0	1.0	7.0	2.0
Very high (51+)	10.0	5.0	6.0	2.0	5.0	2.0	3.0	1.0	6.0	2.0
Mean weekly units	20.3	9.5	17.6	7.2	15.6	5.9	11.0	3.5	16.0	6.3
Base = 100%	880.0	968.0	2612.0	3179.0	2214.0	2508.0	1445.0	1836.0	7151.0	8491.0

Source: ONS (1998a, p. 188).

TABLE 28.4
Alcohol consumption by gender and region

Region	Male mean weekly units	Female mean weekly units
North	19.1	5.9
Yorkshire and Humberside	16.8	6.6
North West	18.4	7.9
East Midlands	15.3	5.8
West Midlands	16.2	5.9
East Anglia	13.7	5.5
South East	15.2	6.2
Greater London	14.5	5.6
Outer Metropolitan	15.4	6.4
Outer South East	15.8	6.7
South West	15.0	6.1
England	16.1	6.3
Wales	15.0	6.8
Scotland	16.2	5.5
Great Britain	16.0	6.3

Source: ONS (1998*a*, p. 189).

Other general population surveys

A national survey of psychiatric morbidity was carried out by the OPCS in 1993 (OPCS, 1995). Population rates of dependence were 75 per 1000 for men and 21 per 1000 for women. In this survey, alcohol dependence was found to be less common among West Indian and African respondents and rare in Asian and Oriental respondents. Single people, unemployed people and unskilled manual workers renting property were more likely to be dependent. Regional differences were again evident, with North East Thames, Mersey Regional Health Authority and Scotland and Wales having higher levels of dependence.

Regional data

The 1992 Healthquest Survey collected data on a representative sample of South East Thames residents (*n*=40 162) using a postal questionnaire (valid response rate 57%; not representative of the whole population). The proportion of residents drinking above 'sensible limits' were below those reported for the GHS. However, significantly more men and women in the boroughs of Lambeth, Southwark & Lewisham (LSL) were drinking above sensible limits than in South East Thames as a whole (26.5% of men and 9.3% of women in the LSL area versus 17.1% of men and 6.1% of women in the region as a whole).

Alcohol-related mortality data

Table 28.5 shows deaths from alcohol-related causes for England and Wales in 1996 (ONS, 1998*b*). These deaths are probably an underestimate, because they do not include deaths from other causes where alcohol was a contributory factor.

Alcohol-related morbidity data

Excessive alcohol consumption is associated with a wide range of illnesses. It is estimated that approximately 20% of general hospital admissions have alcohol-related problems, many of which go undetected. In Scotland, there has been a decrease in mental illness admissions with a primary diagnosis of alcohol-related disorder over the past few decades, whereas general hospital discharges for alcohol

TABLE 28.5
Deaths from alcohol-related causes, England and Wales, 1996

Cause of death	*Male*	*Female*	*Total*
Alcohol psychosis	10	4	14
Alcohol dependence syndrome	172	78	250
Non-dependent use of alcohol	100	44	144
Alcoholic cardiomyopathy	116	24	140
Alcholic gastritis	3	2	5
Alcoholic fatty liver	41	28	69
Acute alcoholic hepatitis	64	38	102
Acute cirrhosis of the liver	569	250	819
Alcoholic liver damage (unspecified)	696	373	1069
Toxic effects of alcohol	102	50	152
Total	1873	891	2764
Chronic liver disease and cirrhosis	2261	1528	3789
Total including all liver disease and cirrhosis	2754	1730	4484

Source: ONS (1998*b*).

dependence, psychosis and misuse have increased since the 1980s. This probably reflects a shift from psychiatric to general hospital admissions as the number of beds in specialist alcohol units decreases. Table 28.6 presents data taken from the Hospital Episodes Statistics for England (Department of Health, 1995b), describing the number of admissions to all NHS hospitals in England by health region.

A recent study of 2988 acute general medical admissions to a South London teaching hospital found a 20% prevalence rate of substance misuse (mainly alcohol), 9% being identified by the admitting doctor, and 11% by means of a screening questionnaire (Canning *et al*, 1999). The alcohol misusers were more likely to be older and Irish. ICD–10 categories of the alcohol dependent (*n*=233) and alcohol misusing (*n*=204) patients are set out in Table 28.7.

Ideally, all local agencies caring for individuals with alcohol problems should be surveyed to obtain information about the number of clients seen and their socio-demographic profile. Such a survey should

TABLE 28.6
Hospital episodes of main alcohol-related diagnoses, by region

Health region	Alcohol dependence syndrome	Toxic effects of alcohol	Alcoholic psychoses	Chronic liver disease	Total
Northern	1433	262	428	979	3102
Yorkshire	1696	212	340	656	2904
Trent	1461	133	308	1077	2979
East Anglia	1081	59	136	369	1645
NW Thames	1386	98	651	665	2800
NE Thames	1238	77	428	1099	2842
SE Thames	1300	195	413	1144	3052
SW Thames	1387	66	422	727	2602
Wessex	1110	144	240	566	2060
Oxford	711	91	226	471	1499
South Western	1045	165	171	697	2078
West Midlands	2345	285	378	1864	4872
Mersey	2120	109	208	940	3377
North Western	2479	364	499	1150	4492
Special HAS	158	8	44	51	261
Total	20 950	2268	4892	12 455	40 565

Source: Department of Health, 1995b.

TABLE 28.7
ICD–10 diagnostic categories of all patients and substance misusers

ICD–10 categories	Alcohol dependent n=233 (%)	AUDIT positives n=204 (%)
Primary alcohol-related diagnosis	48 (21)	1 (1)
Secondary alcohol-related diagnosis	103 (44)	19 (9)
Neoplasm	5 (2)	6 (3)
Diseases of the circulatory system	16 (7)	63 (31)
Diseases of the respiratory system	15 (6)	44 (22)
Diseases of the digestive system	41 (18)	29 (14)
Injury, poisoning and other external causes	32 (14)	8 (4)

Source: Canning *et al*, 1999.

compare the estimated need for services with the levels of service provided by the agencies. The pyramid of need (Box 28.1) was constructed from 1996 data collected in the LSL Health Authority Area (the population in 1996 was 734 525).

Services available

Services for alcohol misuse and dependence have grown and diversified considerably over the past 30 years. They consist of a

---

Box 28.1
Pyramid of need – alcohol
Lambeth, Southwark & Lewisham Health Authority (population 734 525)

The pyramid below summarises some of the information about alcohol and its associated morbidity. The estimates are very approximate and the numbers given are intended to give an idea of the relative sizes of the conditions rather than their true extent.

Deaths from chronic liver disease and cirrhosis (62)
Hospital admissions for alcoholic liver disease (180)
Hospital admissions for mental/behavioural problems (634)
Consuming high levels of alcohol (21 789)
Drinking alcohol above sensible weekly limits (109 749)

Taken from Wilkinson (1996)

broad mix of statutory, voluntary and private agencies. In contrast with other mental health areas, alcohol services have a particularly strong voluntary (non-statutory) element, with a track record in providing flexible, accessible and innovative services. Alcohol services target a wide range of drinking problems and no longer focus only on the treatment of chronic dependence. Psychology has played an important role in this wider remit, particularly the development of theories of behavioural change, motivational enhancement therapy and brief intervention strategies. Generic services have developed alongside specialist services. Over the past 10 years, there has been a transformation in services, with a shift from in-patient provision to the development of community alcohol teams (CATs). This has arisen as a result of the separation of the roles of purchasers and providers, a public health perspective on alcohol problems and limited resources. Service providers have, in effect, had to become small businesses that are accountable to the purchasers and deliver value for money, providing treatments based on scientific evidence of effectiveness (Raistrick *et al*, 1999).

The current provision of core services includes the following: outreach work; screening for alcohol problems; brief interventions; short treatment packages; longer-term specialist treatment that includes detoxification and counselling services in day care and residential settings; self-help support groups; and support for the families of problem drinkers (Alcohol Concern, 1999).

Figure 28.2 illustrates the range of alcohol problems and the appropriate responses. Brief interventions are effective in 'at-risk' drinkers who have not yet developed serious problems. Specialist treatment is needed for individuals with serious problems or severe dependence.

The first national census for alcohol treatment agencies in the UK estimated that some 10 000 individuals were seen for treatment or advice regarding an alcohol problem on the census day (Luce *et al*, 1998). The non-statutory sector accounted for almost two-thirds of all clients seen on the census day, with most of the remaining clients (30%) being seen in the statutory sector (NHS).

Health education

In 1986, the health education authority (HEA) became the principal national statutory body responsible for developing public education programmes on alcohol misuse. The HEA has now been superseded by Health Promotion England and the Health Development Agency, the latter having a remit with an evaluation focus. Their work is carried out in collaboration with other national

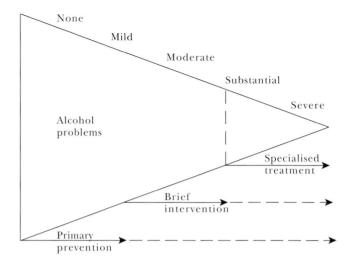

Fig. 28.2 Relationship between the severity of alcohol problems and the type of intervention needed (from Heather, 1995)

alcohol organisations, including Alcohol Concern. Local campaigns and public education schemes developed by health promotion units, alcohol services and other interested agencies complement this work (Alcohol Concern, 1999). Many drug reference groups (DRGs) and drug action teams (DATs) already incorporate alcohol into their remit.

Community action on prevention

Many opportunities directed at the prevention or reduction of alcohol-related problems exist at the community level. These include the provision of good practice guidance to local authorities and the police with particular emphasis on:

    (a) regulation of the number of outlets and their opening times;
    (b) enforcement of existing law on under-age drinking; and
    (c) the use of toughened glass in licensed premises.

Statutory social services

Local authority social services departments have been responsible for arranging and funding the social care needs of substance misusers since April 1993 (NHS and Community Care Act, 1990). This Act requires local authorities to assess the needs of the local population for alcohol (and drug) services, include such services in their community care plans, assess the social care needs of individual alcohol (and drug) misusers and arrange appropriate packages of care. There is, as yet, very little information in the public arena on the implementation of Community Care with this client group, and a review carried out in 1994 expressed concern about the need for service users to "jump through a number of hoops and express high levels of motivation before gaining access to a service" (Department of Health, Social Services Inspectorate, 1999).

Non-statutory social services

These organisations deal with alcohol misuse problems. While much of the work is excellent, staff are usually inadequately trained in the field.

Primary care services

Figure 28.3 illustrates the centrality of primary care within a community service model. Although primary care is the ideal setting for screening and early intervention, many GPs do not see this work as particularly rewarding. Local CATs and specialist teams within general practice potentially play an important role in supporting and facilitating better links with GPs.

General hospital

Most general hospitals lack a commitment to alcohol misuse and do not have systems to coordinate action hospital wide. Often, a lead is taken by an interested department or a particular consultant. Opportunities are widespread and include the provision of joint clinics, screening and intervention on hospital wards and in accident and emergency departments.

General psychiatry

Up to a fifth of admissions to psychiatric hospitals may be heavy drinkers (Bernadt & Murray, 1986). However, psychiatric registrars are poor at taking drinking histories (Farrell & David, 1988) and have negative attitudes towards patients with alcohol dependence (Farrell & Lewis, 1990). As general psychiatry focuses more on severe mental illness, so general psychiatrists are increasingly reluctant to treat individuals with

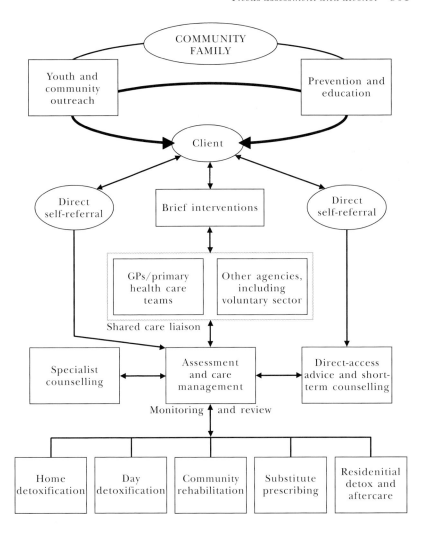

Fig. 28.3 The care pathway: a service model for the Southampton and South West Hampshire Joint Commissioning Board for Substance Misuse (with permission from Alcohol Concern, 1999).

alcohol problems. However, psychiatrists cannot ignore the psychiatric complications of alcohol dependence that can present to the psychiatric or general hospital and the increasingly important issue of comorbidity. The UK Alcohol Forum has recently produced guidelines for the management of alcohol problems in general psychiatry and primary care (UK Alcohol Forum, 2001).

Specialised NHS alcohol treatment services

Most specialised NHS agencies offer a range of services and collaborate with other statutory and non-statutory services. The main service components include:

- community and in-patient detoxification;
- out-patient treatment utilising relapse prevention and cognitive–behavioural strategies;
- introduction to Alcoholics Anonymous (AA);
- liaison with other community services; and
- referral to residential rehabilitation or hostels for longer-term treatment.

The overall tendency has been to move towards out-patient rather than in-patient care. Most centres have developed CATs that work closely with primary care and other generalists.

Many in-patient alcohol units have closed over the past 5–10 years and those that remain open largely offer a short-stay detoxification service. Some health authorities contract in-patient services across several districts; some have beds on general psychiatry or general medical wards. The closure of beds within dedicated alcoholism treatment units has meant the loss of critical functions such as training and research and development.

Community alcohol teams

CATs usually form part of the range of services offered by statutory and non-statutory specialist agencies. These teams are multi-disciplinary, but there is a tendency to employ more psychiatric nurses than members of other professions (social work, occupational therapy, psychology and psychiatry). Although the original remit of CATs was to facilitate front-line agencies rather than to offer treatment, most teams have now evolved into service agencies and work across substances. NHS teams are increasingly working with dual-diagnosis patients.

Specialised non-statutory services

The non-statutory sector makes an important contribution to services:

- Alcoholics Anonymous (AA) offers about 3000 meetings in England and Wales each week and has an active membership of some 60 000. AA is 'free' and highly accessible.
- Alcohol Counselling Services are usually run by local councils on alcoholism. Organisations such as the Alcohol Recovery Project, Turning Point and the Salvation Army offer halfway

houses and hostels, supported tenancies, day centres and detoxification facilities, and often concentrate on the needs of the homeless drinker and drunkenness offender.

Private health care organisations

Private health care organisations still have a general focus on in-patient treatment, but many are developing out-patient and family services.

The Criminal Justice System

The relationship between alcohol and crime is a complex one to which simple cause and effect explanations cannot be applied. Alcohol-related crime can be classified into that which is carried out 'under the influence' (either while intoxicated or during the withdrawal period), acquisitive crime (including prostitution) and domestic violence/abuse. Violent crime is associated with intoxication and its attendant aggression. The state of intoxication at the time of a crime does not prove that alcohol caused the crime but rather that it played a direct part in it. The police and probation and prison services all potentially have a role to play in the screening and brief interventions. Police officers should have a knowledge of drug and alcohol services in their local area and be in a position to refer directly, facilitate referral or at the very least hand out promotional material (Raistrick *et al*, 1999). In 1994, probation officers reported that 30% of their case-loads had severe problems with alcohol. They usually have a lengthy period of contact with the individual on probation, and are therefore in a position to facilitate behavioural change. As with social workers, training in alcohol-related skills and techniques should be an intrinsic part of the training programme.

Theoretically, the prison system is an ideal place in which to set up an alcohol treatment programme. The population is truly 'captive' and research suggests that many prisoners wish to abstain or to cut down on their drinking. Despite this, services in prisons are patchy and delivered mainly by probation officers, social workers, prison officers and Alcoholics Anonymous. A centrally coordinated package subject to evaluation should be considered (McMurran & Baldwin, 1989; McMurran & Hollin, 1989).

The Alcohol Concern Services Directory for 1998/99 lists a total of 544 specialist providers in England and Wales: 342 non-statutory; 144 statutory, 49 private and nine partnerships. There are no data available on the numbers of staff employed, their training or the total expenditure of the services (Raistrick *et al*, 1999).

Evidence of effectiveness of services and interventions

A great deal of knowledge about effective treatments has been amassed in recent years, and this has been associated with a move towards shorter community-based treatment packages (Institute of Medicine, 1990).

The main conclusion from this literature is that drinking problems are extremely diverse and need different types of treatment and help. Within the context of treatment, it is important that the individual retains the right to choose.

Prevention

The strongest evidence in this category relates to the affordability of alcohol. As the price of alcohol increases, so the per capita consumption falls. At the local level, two types of preventive strategy should be considered: public education and an improved preventive focus through existing services. Although there is no evidence to demonstrate that public education programmes are effective in influencing drinking behaviour in the short term, they do raise public awareness and can promote earlier self-referral and help-seeking behaviour. Although school-based approaches are popular, there is no strong evidence to support widespread adoption of such interventions. Health education should also aim to move alcohol misusers earlier into treatment by self-referral (media campaigns).

Advice given through primary care is effective in reducing individual levels of alcohol consumption and preventing alcohol-related harm. This is discussed in the next section.

Generalist treatment and brief interventions

Many health and other professionals regularly see problem drinkers during the course of their day-to-day work. Health professionals include GPs and practice nurses, general psychiatrists and community psychiatric nurses, hospital physicians and accident and emergency specialists. Other professionals include social workers and probation officers, the police, prison officers, occupational health physicians and nurses. Individuals drinking at hazardous and harmful levels are not readily identifiable, and may not even be aware that their drinking has the potential to cause harm. Generalists should take advantage of the opportunities to screen for alcohol problems when such individuals present to services for other reasons. Opportunistic screening should, therefore, be built into the infrastructure of all settings. In general practice, this might include new patient screening clinics, health-promotion and well-person clinics, management of chronic disease clinic, ante- and post-natal checks, and clinics for the elderly. Identification of hazardous and harmful drinking should be followed by brief intervention. This could consist of the following:

(a) an assessment of alcohol intake;
(b) information on hazardous/harmful drinking;
(c) clear advice, with booklets and details of local services; and
(d) an attempt to understand the triggers for drinking and negotiation of realistic aims.

Evidence suggests that such interventions are effective in reducing alcohol intake by 20% (Effective Health Care Bulletin, 1993; Wallace *et al*, 1998).

Primary care

Primary health care is ideally placed for opportunistic detection of hazardous and harmful drinking. In the UK, over 98% of the population is registered with a GP. During any year, a GP will see over 70% of their practice list, increasing to over 90% within a five-year period. Furthermore, heavy drinkers consult their GPs twice as often as light drinkers (see Deehan *et al* (1998) for a review). While brief interventions may reduce individual consumption by very little (and are more effective in women than in men), their public health value is potentially enormous. Wallace *et al* (1988) noted that if their results were applied to the UK, intervention by GPs could reduce the alcohol consumption of 250 000 men and 67 500 women currently drinking to excess, to moderate levels each year.

Despite evidence for their effectiveness in primary care, it is proving very difficult to persuade GPs to utilise brief interventions as part of routine practice, because of a perceived lack of training and lack of confidence (Deehan *et al*, 1996). Education and support from local specialists services have been identified as key factors in performance in this area.

Practice nurses are fully trained general or psychiatric nurses undertaking health promotion and chronic disease management within primary care. They routinely see every new patient registering with a practice and thus have a unique and legitimate opportunity to discuss lifestyle issues, including alcohol consumption. A recent national survey of the work of practice nurses with harmful and hazardous drinkers found that they detected as many problem drinkers as GPs, but were identifying them at an earlier stage in their drinking career (Deehan *et al*, 1996). They will clearly need support and training in order to expand this role and capitalise on the unique position they occupy with early problem drinkers.

The general hospital

It is estimated that 20% of all adult in-patients admitted to general hospital settings may be classified as hazardous or harmful drinkers, and are unlikely to be detected unless specifically assessed (Effective Health Care Bulletin, 1993; Canning *et al*, 1999). There is also evidence that brief interventions are effective in this setting (Chick *et al*, 1985). Several models of specialist alcohol liaison in the general hospital have been developed, and all aim to promote early intervention using a combination of feedback, advice and motivational support (Royal College of Physicians Working Party Report, 2001).

Accident and emergency departments

Heavy drinkers frequently present to accident and emergency services. One study reported that 40% of patients presenting had consumed alcohol before attending and 32% had a blood alcohol concentration of 80 mg % (Holt *et al*, 1980). Results of a brief intervention study in a London accident and emergency department suggested that referral to an alcohol health worker resulted in a significant reduction in alcohol consumption (Wright *et al*, 1998). Brief intervention strategies in the accident and emergency department should be integrated with intervention strategies in the hospital as a whole (i.e. hospital-wide alcohol policy as part of health promotion).

Social services

Alcohol is a significant aspect of the work in between 20% and 40% of all social work case-loads. The figure is likely to be higher in child abuse cases (see Raistrick *et al* (1999) for a review). Furthermore, parental alcohol misuse is the most important factor contributing to the reception of children into local authority care.

A recent study highlighted the range of social, health and personal difficulties of substance misusers referred to a substance misuse care management team (Clark, 1998). Clients had high levels of housing needs, unemployment, poor adjustment to childhood trauma, high levels of psychological distress/illness and poor general health. GPs played a very important role in supporting these individuals. The study commented on the lack of a valid needs assessment instrument examining composite need in these individuals, and recommended that such an instrument be developed.

Finally, the use of routine screening and brief interventions should be built into social work treatment, and a major training and research initiative is needed in this field.

Specialist treatment

Specialist treatment for alcohol problems should be seen as existing along a continuum with generalist interventions. It is important to recognise that specialist treatment within the alcohol field is not uniform. On the one hand, specialist treatment can refer to treatment by personnel who have a specific training in the area. On the other hand, the treatment might be delivered by a service that works exclusively with alcohol problems but does not employ specially trained staff.

Is treatment effective? Evidence suggests that any treatment for alcohol problems is better than no treatment. About two-thirds of individuals receiving treatment show some improvement, whereas one-third would have improved without treatment, or with minimal intervention (Babor, 1995). Evidence from the USA suggests that a combination of population-based environmental measures and individually based interventions can work together to achieve a large-scale reduction in alcohol-related harm. Holder *et al* (1995) calculated that for every US $10 000 invested in treatment, the managed care provider saves about US $30 000 on medical spending (Raistrick *et al*, 1999).

Treatment of the 'at-risk' drinker

Advice given in the primary care setting is the main treatment plank for this group. Wallace *et al* (1998) showed that at one-year follow-up, 47% of alcohol misusers who received advice from the GP reduced their drinking, compared with 25% of those who received no advice.

Treatment of the problem and dependent drinker

Advice

Brief advice may be as effective as more intensive treatment in this group and should not be overlooked.

Treatment intensity

Start with less intensive treatment. More intensive work should be reserved for:

- more severely dependent patients;
- the homeless and unsupported;

- drinkers with severe psychological or physical illness or drug misuse; and
- individuals who present a suicidal risk or who are a danger to other people.

Out-patient or in-patient care

Out-patient or community treatment is the initial treatment of choice for dependent drinkers. In-patient care should be reserved for individuals with:

- severe dependence;
- history of delirium tremens or withdrawal seizures;
- previous failed community detoxification; and
- unsupported home environment.

Detoxification

Many individuals with alcohol problems have not developed the alcohol dependence syndrome and will therefore not experience withdrawal symptoms when they stop drinking. A further group of patients with a mild or moderate degree of alcohol dependence may not suffer from appreciable withdrawal symptoms. However, severely alcohol-dependent individuals can experience a complicated or life-threatening condition on withdrawal. This diversity of withdrawal experiences means that different patients have different treatment needs. Many patients need no medication to come off alcohol. Many others can be safely managed as out-patients by a GP or CAT, with minimum drug cover. Only the minority of severely dependent patients will require admission to hospital. Contraindications to community detoxification are listed in the section on 'Out-patient or in-patient care' above.

Rehabilitation hostels and day programmes

These are usually aimed at people with significant social problems. There is little evidence to support their effectiveness, but they may provide a way out of a cycle of homelessness and excessive alcohol consumption and potentially help towards better long-term adjustments.

Alcoholics Anonymous and Al-Anon

Research on the effectiveness of AA has been difficult to carry out, but there is a perception that those who join have a better prognosis than those who do not.

Cost-effectiveness of treatment interventions

'At-risk' drinkers

The cost-effectiveness of brief interventions delivered by GPs and other generalists is high, the estimated cost per brief intervention being between £8 and £20 (Effective Health Care Bulletin, 1993).

Problem and dependent drinkers

The evidence for the cost-effectiveness of alcohol services has been reviewed by Edwards & Unnithan (1994) and Godfrey (1994). Low-cost interventions are as effective as more expensive treatments for many problem drinkers. Such interventions include simple advice, out-patient counselling and care. Residential detoxification and treatment on a routine basis are not cost-effective. In the first instance, detoxification should be managed through primary care or on an out-patient basis. In-patient treatment should be reserved for clients with complications. Specialised rehabilitation hostels are more cost-effective than general psychiatric hospitals or other hostels.

Outcome measures

'At-risk' drinkers

Outcomes can be measured individually in terms of a reduction in alcohol consumption to sensible levels after 6–12 months. Population outcomes can be measured in terms of average percentage reduction, or percentage of population drinking at sensible levels.

Drinkers with alcohol-related problems

Outcomes can be measured in terms of reduction in alcohol consumption, as above, and also in terms of reduction in the number of alcohol problems. Simple instruments such as the Alcohol Problems Questionnaire (Drummond, 1990) can be used to obtain a quantitative measure of the overall alcohol problems score.

Dependent drinkers

Outcome measures should be simple and able to evaluate improvements in drinking, health and social adjustment, rather than just dealing in a categorical way with drinking and abstinence.

Targets

The 'Health of the Nation' proposed that the proportion of men drinking more than 21 units per week in 1990 (28%) be reduced to 18% by 2005. The equivalent target for women drinking above 14 units per week was a reduction from 11% to 7% (Department of Health, 1992). These targets will not be met, because primary care initiatives have not been supported by alcohol policy measures such as increased taxation on alcohol.

Conclusions

- The provision of alcohol services should be based on need and effectiveness of treatment.
- Primary health care services should play a central role in providing treatment, but health authorities rather than primary care groups should have the principal planning role in relation to health service provision, in order to prevent fragmentation.
- Accessibility of services should be improved to facilitate their use by young people, women and ethnic minorities.
- The requirements of special groups should be reviewed, for example, dual diagnosis, polydrug users, the homeless and individuals in the criminal justice system.
- Training is the cornerstone to delivering effective treatments. Specialist and generic training should be reviewed.

References

ALCOHOL CONCERN (1997) *Measures for Measures. A Framework for Alcohol Policy*. London: Alcohol Concern.

—— (1999) *Proposals for a National Alcohol Strategy for England*. London: Alcohol Concern.

AMERICAN PSYCHIATRIC ASSOCIATION (1994) *Diagnostic and Statistical Manual of Mental Disorders (4th edition). DSM–IV*. Washington, DC: APA.

ANDERSON, P. (1995) Alcohol and risk of physical harm. In: *Alcohol and Public Policy: Evidence and Issues* (eds H. D. Holder & G. Edwards), pp. 82–113. Oxford: Oxford University Press.

BABOR, T. E. (1995) The social and public health significance of individually directed interventions. In: *Alcohol and Public Policy: Evidence and Issues* (eds H. D. Holder & G. Edwards). Oxford: Oxford University Press.

BERNADT, M. W. & MURRAY, R. M. (1986) Psychiatric disorder, drinking and alcoholism: what are the links. *British Journal of Psychiatry*, **148**, 393–400.

CANNING, U. P., KENNELL-WEBB, S. A., MARSHALL, E. J., *ET AL* (1999) Substance misuse in acute general medical admissions. *Quarterly Journal of Medicine*, **92**, 319–326.

CHICK, J., LLOYD, G. & GROMBIE, E. (1985) Counselling problem drinkers in medical wards: a controlled study. *British Medical Journal*, **290**, 965–967.

——, GODFREY, C., HORE, B. D., *ET AL* (1997) *Alcohol Dependence: A Clinical Problem*. London: Mosby-Wolfe Medical Communications.

CLARK, H. (1998) *Community Care for Substance Misusers*. A description of clients referred and assessed by a London Substance Misuse Care Management Team. Unpublished MSc thesis: University of London.

CUFFEL, B. (1992) Prevalence estimates of substance abuse in schizophrenia and their correlates. *Journal of Nervous and Mental Disorders*, **180**, 589–592.

DEEHAN, A., TEMPLETON, L., DRUMMOND, C., *ET AL* (1996) *The Detection and Management of Alcohol Misuse Patients in Primary Care: General Practitioners' Behaviour and Attitudes*. A report to the Department of Health. London: Institute of Psychiatry.

——, MARSHALL, E. J. & STRANG, J. (1998) Tackling alcohol misuse: opportunities and obstacles in primary care. *British Journal of General Practice*, **48**, 1779–1782.

DEPARTMENT OF HEALTH (1992) *The Health of the Nation: A Strategy for Health in England and Wales*. London: HMSO.

—— (1995a) *Sensible Drinking. The Report of an Inter-departmental Working Group*. London: Department of Health.

—— (1995b) *Hospital Episode Statistics, Volume 1: England: Financial Year 1993–4*. London: Government Statistical Service.

DEPARTMENT OF HEALTH, SOCIAL SERVICES INSPECTORATE (1999) *Inspection of Social Services for People who Misuse Alcohol and Drugs*. Overview Report. London: Department of Health.

DRUMMOND, D. C. (1990) The relationship between alcohol dependence and alcohol-related problems in a clinical population. *British Journal of Addiction*, **89**, 357–366.

EDWARDS, G. & UNNITHAN, S. (1994) Alcohol misuse. In: *Health Care Needs Assessment* (eds A. Stevens & J. Raftery), pp. 341–375. Oxford: Radcliffe Medical Press.

——, ANDERSON, P., BABOR, T. F., *ET AL* (1994) *Alcohol Policy and the Public Good*. Oxford: Oxford University Press.

EFFECTIVE HEALTH CARE BULLETIN (1993) Brief interventions and alcohol use. *Effective Health Care Bulletin*, **7**, 2–14.

FARRELL, M. P. & DAVID, A. S. (1988) Do psychiatric registrars take a proper drinking history? *British Medical Journal*, **296**, 395–396.

—— & LEWIS, G. (1990) Discrimination on grounds of diagnosis. *British Journal of Addiction*, **85**, 883–890.

GLASS, I. B. & JACKSON, P. (1988) Maudsley Hospital survey prevalence of alcohol problems and other psychiatric disorders in a hospital population. *British Journal of Addiction*, **83**, 1105–1111.

GLUCKSMAN, E. (1994) Alcohol and accidents. In: *Alcohol and Alcohol Problems* (eds G. Edwards & T. J. Peters), pp. 76–84. British Medical Bulletin 50. London: Churchill Livingstone.

GODFREY, C. (1994) Assessing the cost-effectiveness of alcohol services. *Journal of Mental Health*, **3**, 3–21.

—— (1995) *Treatment Approaches to Alcohol Problems*. WHO Reciprocal Publications European series, 65. Copenhagen: WHO Regional Office for Europe.

HEATHER, N. (1982) Alcohol dependence and problem drinking in Scottish young offenders. *British Journal of Alcohol and Alcoholism*, **17**, 145–154.

—— (1995) *Treatment Approaches to Alcohol Problems*. WHO Reciprocal Publications, European Series, no. 65. Copenhagen: WHO Regional Office for Europe.

HOLDER, H. D., STEWART, I. C., DIXON, J. M. J., *ET AL* (1980) Alcohol and the emergency service patient. *British Medical Journal*, **281**, 638–640.

——, MILLER, W. R. & CARINA, R. T. (1995) *Cost Savings of Substance Abuse Prevention in Managed Care*. Berkeley, CA: Center for Substance Abuse Prevention.

HOLT, S., STEWARD, I. C, DIXON, J. M. J., *ET AL* (1980) Alcohol and the emergency service patient. *British Medical Journal*, **281**, 638–640.

INSTITUTE OF MEDICINE (1990) *Broadening the Base of Treatment for Alcohol Problems*. Report of a study by a Committee of the Institute of Medicine, Division of Mental and Behavioural Medicine. Washington, DC: National Academy Press.

KREITMAN, N. (1986) Alcohol consumption and the prevention paradox. *British Journal of Addiction*, **81**, 353–363.

LUCE, A., HEATHER, N. & McCARTHY, S. (1998) *Census of Alcohol Treatment Agencies in the UK*. Report to the Society for the Study of Addiction. Newcastle upon Tyne: Centre for Drug and Alcohol Studies.

McMURRAN, M. & BALDWIN, S. (1989) Services for prisoners with alcohol-related problems: a survey of UK prisons. *British Journal of Addiction*, **84**, 1053–1088.

—— & HOLLIN, C. R. (1989) Drinking and delinquency: another look at young offenders and alcohol. *British Journal of Criminology*, **29**, 386–394.

MENEZES, P. R., JOHNSON, S., THORNICROFT, G., *ET AL* (1996) Drug and alcohol problems among individuals with severe mental illness in south London. *British Journal of Psychiatry*, **168**, 612–619.

NEWCOMBE, R., MEASHAM, F. & PARKER, H. (1995) A survey of drinking and deviant behaviour among 14–15 year olds in North West England. *Addiction Research*, **2**, 319–341.

NHS AND COMMUNITY CARE ACT (1990) London: HMSO.

OFFICE FOR NATIONAL STATISTICS (1998*a*) *Living in Britain: Results from the 1996 General Household Survey: A Survey carried out by Social Survey Division*. London: The Stationery Office.

—— (1998*b*) *Mortality Statistics, Cause: England and Wales*. London: The Stationery Office.

OFFICE OF POPULATION CENSUSES AND SURVEYS (1995) *The Prevalence of Psychiatric Morbidity Among Adults Living in Private Houses*. London: HMSO.

—— (1996) *Psychiatric Morbidity among Homeless People*. London: HMSO.

OSHER, F. C. & DRAKE R. E. (1996) Reversing a history of unmet needs: approaches to care for persons with co-occurring addictive and mental disorders. *American Journal of Orthopsychiatry*, **66**, 4–11.

RAISTRICK, D., HODGSON, R. & RITSON, B. (1999) *Tackling Alcohol Together. The Evidence Base for a UK Alcohol Policy*. London: Free Association Books.

REED, A., RAMSDEN, S., MARSHALL, J., *ET AL* (1992) Psychiatric morbidity and substance abuse among residents of a cold weather shelter. *British Medical Journal*, **304**, 1028–1029.

ROYAL COLLEGE OF PHYSICIANS (2001) *Alcohol – Can the NHS afford it? A Royal College of Physicians Working Party Report*. London: Royal College of Physicians.

ROYAL COLLEGE OF PHYSICIANS, PSYCHIATRISTS AND GENERAL PRACTITIONERS (1995) *Alcohol and the Heart in Perspective: Sensible Limits Reaffirmed*. London: Royal College of Physicians, Psychiatrists and General Practitioners.

ROYAL COLLEGE OF PSYCHIATRISTS (1986) *Alcohol – Our Favourite Drug*. London: Tavistock.

UK ALCOHOL FORUM (2001) *Guidelines for the Management of Alcohol Problems in Primary Care and General Psychiatry*.

WALLACE, P., CUTLER, S. & HAINES, A. (1998) Randomised controlled trial of general practitioner intervention in patients with excessive alcohol consumption. *British Medical Journal*, **297**, 663–668.

WEBB, E., ASHTON, C. H., KELLEY, P., *ET AL* (1996) Alcohol and drug use in UK university students. *Lancet*, **348**, 922–925.

WILKINSON, P. (1996) *Substance Misuse: The Joint Community Care Plan for Inner South East London: 1997/8. Needs Assessment for Alcohol and Drug Users in LSL*. London: Lambeth, Southwark and Lewisham Health Authority.

WORLD HEALTH ORGANIZATION (1992) *The ICD–10 Classification of Mental and Behavioural Disorders: Clinical Descriptions and Diagnostic Guidelines (10th edn). ICD–10*. Geneva: WHO.

WRIGHT, S., MORAN, L., MEYRICK, M., *ET AL* (1998) Intervention by an alcohol health worker in an Accident and Emergency Department. *Alcohol and Alcoholism*, **33**, 651–656.

Index

Compiled by **LINDA ENGLISH**

Aberrant Behaviour Checklist 381
ability to benefit 65
abuse of elderly 397
accessibility of services
  measures 97
  perceived 91
  as planning principle 114
  primary care 133, 412, 416
  in rural areas 437, 438–441
  users' perspective 192–193,
    195–196, 412, 416
acute care
  MILMIS study 244–249
  patient characteristics 254
  and priority setting 147, 148, 149
  and sector services 181
  use of MRC Needs for Care
    Assessment 286–287
Adaptive Behaviour Scale 382
admission rates 87–88
adolescents *see* children and
  adolescents
advocacy 191, 195, 448
agricultural chemicals 444
Alcoholics Anonymous 502, 508
alcohol misuse 486–512
  and accident and emergency
    departments 506
  alcohol-related morbidity/mortality
    data 495–497
  'at-risk' drinkers 489, 507, 509
  brief interventions/generalist
    treatment 504–505
  community alcohol teams 502
  cost-effectiveness of interventions
    509
  and criminal justice system 503

dependence 53–54, 487, 489, 490,
  507–508, 509
detoxification 508
effectiveness of services/
  interventions 504–507
in elderly 491
estimating levels of need 492–497
in ethnic minorities 490
general hospital services 500, 506
general psychiatry services 500–501
geographical variation in
  consumption 492
health targets 510
heavy drinking 486–487, 489
in homeless 53–54, 310–311, 319,
  491
outcome measures 509
polydrug use 492
population surveys 50, 53–54,
  492–494
prevention 499, 504
primary care services 500, 505–506,
  507
in prisons 492, 503
problem drinkers 486–487, 489,
  490, 507–508, 509
in psychiatric populations 491–492
public education 498–499, 504
regional data 494–495
services available 497–503
social services 499–500, 506–507
specialist treatment services 502–
  503, 507–508
sub-categories as target populations
  489–492
in women 490
in young people 491

amphetamines 455, 463
anorexia nervosa 472–485
antidepressants 134, 136, 139, 140–141, 479
anxiety disorders 140–141
assertive community treatment 330, 446
audit
defined 241–242
reasons for 242
use of psychiatric beds 241–260
Australia, health targets 35–40
for depression and related disorders 37–38
national mental health goals 36–37
for schizophrenia/other psychoses 38–39
for suicide reduction 39–40

Baltimore Homeless Study 320–321
Bangor Assessment of Need Profile (BANP) 294, 398
bed use, auditing 241–260
Britain
health targets 23–24
modelling of utilisation in Scotland 102–104
population surveys 25–26, 43–58, 128–129
rural areas in England 436–438
bulimia nervosa 472, 473, 474–475, 478–479, 481
burden of care
and families 343–346, 349–350
objective 344
subjective 344
and symptoms 349–350

Camberwell Assessment of Need (CAN) 9, 271, 291–303
and Care Programme Approach 162
and elderly 398
and ethnic minorities 425–426
and population assessment 110, 127
psychometric properties 299–300
training 300
translations 301
Camberwell Assessment of Need Clinical version (CAN–C) 295, 298–299, 300

Camberwell Assessment of Need for Adults with Developmental and Intellectual Disabilities (CANDID) 382–390
development process 383
reliability 384–390
validity studies 383–384
Camberwell Assessment of Need for the Elderly (CANE) 399–402
Camberwell Assessment of Need Research version (CAN–R) 295, 298–299, 300, 301
Camberwell Assessment of Need Short Appraisal (CANSAS) 295, 296–298, 300
Camberwell Needs for Care Survey 138–142
Cardinal Needs Schedule (CNS) 261–272, 294, 398
Autoneed computer program 264, 268, 270–271
as intervention 269–270
as outcome measure 268–269
reliability 265–266
stages 264–265
as survey instrument 269
validity 266–267
care
agents 5
continuity 180
coordination 7, 9, 180
and enabling 5
integration 180
measuring individual needs for 273–290
need for, defined 7–9, 274, 282
quality 10–11, 61–62, 73, 78
settings 5
terminology 5–7
Care Needs Assessment Pack for Dementia 399
Care Programme Approach (CPA)
elements 160
equity, needs assessment and 168–169
evaluation 163
and health targets 28–29
and individual needs assessment 162, 167–168
and needs in primary care 407–409
numbers and population need 166–167

numbers prioritised for care 163–166
origins 159–160
and population needs assessment
162–163
principles 160
and priority setting in policy and
practice 28–29, 159–170
and supervision register 161–162,
167–168
'tiered' 161–162
carers 280, 342–362
adjustment to illness 347–348
and burdensome symptoms 349–350
and Cardinal Needs Schedule 262,
263, 264, 265, 270–271
continuity of care needs 355
effects on social/leisure activities
346–347
of elderly 397, 402
emotional support needs 355
financial and employment problems
347
information needs 354, 448
measurement of family burden
343–346
mental health of 348–349
needs of 'peripheral' relatives 357
need to look after themselves 356
problem-solving needs 354–355
relations with mental health
professionals 350–351, 353–354
respite care needs 356
in rural areas 440, 448
specific needs for services 353–357
user satisfaction with involvement
of 413, 416
case management, for homeless 329, 330
case-mix approach 4
case registers 179
and assessment at district level
110–124
catchment areas 171–189, 228
charters 191–192
children and adolescents 363–378
alcohol misuse 491
at risk of mental disorder 371–372
concepts of mental health/ill
health 364–365
definition of need 364
eating disorders 475–476, 478
epidemiological data 368–371

evidence base for interventions
372–374
health targets 37
homeless 314–315, 326–327, 371
information utilisation 375–376
overall approach 366–367
policy context 367–368
present situation 366
purpose of needs assessment 365–366
service usage 375
stakeholder views 374–375
use of Cardinal Needs Schedule 271
with mentally ill parent 357
Client Service Receipt Inventory
(CSRI) 200, 203, 205–211, 220–221
Clifton Assessment Procedures for
the Elderly 398
cocaine 455, 463
cognitive–behavioural therapy 464–
465, 478
commissioning mental health services
commissioner's information
requirements 59–83
commissioner's intelligence
network 80–81
commissioner's role 62–64
commissioner's viewpoint on need
64–66
comparative assessment of need 68–69
corporate approach to needs
assessment 69–70
developing current routine
information 79–80
epidemiological assessment of need
67–68
five stages of commissioning
activity 63–64
future requirements 78–79
service description
quality 73
quantity 70–73
service monitoring
activity levels 77–78
health care quality and outcome 78
number and characteristics of
patients treated 76
population not treated 76
practical considerations 75–78
provider service description 77
resources 75–76
theoretical framework 73–75

common mental disorders 25, 423, 426–428
community alcohol teams 502
community care
  assessing systems of care for long-term mentally ill 225–240
  costs 17, 150, 205–219
  and local catchment areas 171, 173, 180
  and resource allocation 147–148, 150
Community Care Act 1992: 343, 354
community mental health teams 182–183
community support systems 229, 232
community surveys *see* epidemiological surveys
comorbidity (dual diagnosis) 311–312, 456, 491–492
comparative assessment of need 68–69
complaints procedures 192
confidentiality 191
contract management 64
contract types 73
corporate approach to needs assessment 69–70
costs
  basic rules 204–205
  and Client Service Receipt Inventory 200, 203, 205–211, 220–221
  and commissioning
    comparative data on 68, 69
    and service description 71
    and service monitoring 75–76
  of community care 17, 150, 205–219
  cost-effectiveness of alcohol treatments 509
  costing full care packages 214–215
  costing psychiatric interventions 200–224
  demands for information 201–203
  estimating unit costs for services 211–213
  financial problems of patients and carers 347
  and in-patients 149, 150
  long-run marginal opportunity cost 211
  and scarcity 200–204
  see also resource allocation

counselling 133, 136, 137, 448, 464–465
Crighton Royal Behaviour Scale 398
criminality 306, 457, 503
critical time intervention, for homeless 330–331, 333
cultural minorities *see* ethnic minorities

defining mental health needs 1–21
demand
  area-level analysis of determinants 90–91
  assessment at district level using psychiatric case register 110–124
  defined 9, 65, 111–112, 292
  and environmental factors 112
  supplier-induced 91
dementia 393–394, 395–396, 398–399
depression
  burden of symptoms 350
  carers' needs 346, 348, 350
  in elderly 394
  and health targets in Australia 37–38, 39
  influences on obtaining treatment 133–137, 139–141
  in NHS workforce 31–32
  surveys 25, 26
deprivation *see* socio-demographic indices of need
developing countries 441
diagnosis, and service utilisation 112
disability
  concepts 2–3
  prevention 4–5
  severity 3–4
Disability Assessment Schedule 382
district level
  assessing demand using case register 110–124
  district effects and utilisation 94, 101
  needs assessment using community surveys 125–143
  priority setting and service planning 144–158
drug misuse
  counselling services 464–465
  diagnostic definitions 457–458
  drug-related risks/harms 455–457
  drug types 455

in homeless 54, 309–312, 313–314, 315, 323, 326
needs assessment for services 454–471
polydrug use 492
prescribing services 461–464
residential services 465–466
services available and effectiveness 459–466
sub-categories 458
surveys 50, 54, 454–455
syringe exchange services 461
towards more integrated services 466–467
treatment tiers 459–461, 467–468
see also alcohol misuse
drug treatment
access to information 191
and ethnic minorities 422–423, 425
influences on receipt of 133–137, 139, 140–141
side-effects 413, 416
user satisfaction 413, 416

eating disorders 472–485
diagnosis and pathways to care 480
history of services 472–474
predicted demand for services 474–476
treatments 476–479
ecological fallacy 85, 90, 94, 104–105
effectiveness, of interventions/ services 65, 67–68, 114, 127
efficacy, of intervention/service 65, 414
efficiency, of services 114
elderly people 393–406
alcohol misuse 491
epidemiology of psychiatric morbidity 393–394
homeless 327–328, 395–396
needs 394–395
needs assessment 397–402
needs of special groups 395–397
use of MRC NCA 287, 397–398
employment
for drug misusers 457
problems of patients and carers 347
in rural areas 436–438
status, and neurotic disorders 49–50
status, influence on help-seeking and receipt of treatment 133, 136, 137

epidemiological surveys 11–12, 126
of alcohol misuse 492–497
of children and adolescents 368–371
of drug misuse 454–455
of eating disorders 474–476
of elderly 393–394
of ethnic minorities 426–429
information for commissioners 66, 67–68
of low-contact groups 275–277
national surveys 24–26, 43–58, 128–129, 492–494
and needs assessment at district level 125–143, 153
population surveys of morbidity and need 43–58
in rural areas 442–444
of service utilisation 86–88
Epidemiologic Catchment Area Survey 137–138
equity principle 129, 168–169, 201
ethnic minorities 420–434
alcohol misuse 490
conceptualisation of need 421–422
cultural context of core needs 425–426
elderly 397
and evidence-based psychiatry 422–423
local community needs 431–432
meeting needs through culturally competent action 423–424
and MRC NCA 288
ownership and ascription of need 425
and primary care 133
professionals and value systems 423
research and surveys as assessments of need 426–429
service needs 429–431
service usage 176, 375, 397
training for professionals 431
ethnographic surveys 428
evidence-based psychiatry
and children and adolescents 372–374
and ethnic minorities 422–423
and resource allocation 86–88
expressed emotion 347, 353, 354
extra-contractual referrals (ECRs) 73, 244, 248–249

families
    as carers *see* carers
    homeless 313–314, 326–327
farmers 444
focus groups 432
forensic units 253

general practice *see* primary care
group homes 254
group needs 11–17

hallucinogens 455
Hampshire Assessment for Living
    with Others 382
handicap concept 2–3
Health Action Zone areas 156
health benefit groups 76
health gain 4–5, 74
Health Improvement Programmes
    (HImPs) 60–61, 69–70
Health of the Nation Outcome Scales
    (HoNOS) 78, 80, 256, 390
Health of the Nation strategy 23–24
health service indicators (HSIs) 13, 69
health targets 4–5, 22–42
    alcohol misuse 510
    Australian experience 35–40
    continuing development of good
        practice 28–35
    developing comprehensive local
        services 27–28
    improving information and
        understanding 24–27
    international context 22–23
    UK experience 23–24
hearing-impaired children 372
heroin 455, 456, 461–464
high-contact groups, measuring need
    in 277–281
homeless people
    case management programmes 329,
        330
    characteristics affecting service
        provision 321–324
    consumer involvement 331
    continuum of residential stability
        concept 307
    criminalisation 306
    critical time intervention 330–331,
        333
    defining need at local level 332

distrust of authority 318, 322
    elderly 327–328, 395–396
    families 313–314, 326–327
    housing 329, 330, 333
    lack of collateral informants
        318–319
    lack of supports 322–323
    legal protection 331
    mental health services for 304–341
    mobile assertive treatment
        programmes 330
    mobility 317–318
    needs assessment 317–332
    physical illness 315–316, 323
    poverty 323–324
    practical problems in data collection
        317–319
    prevention of homelessness
        332–333
    principles of service provision 324
    problem of definition 305–307
    psychiatric disability 312–313
    psychiatric morbidity 53–54, 307–312
        in children 314
        schizophrenia and affective
            disorders 308–309
        substance misuse 53–54, 309–
            312, 313–314, 315, 319, 323,
            326, 491
        in women 313–314
        in youths 314–315
    quantitative/qualitative descriptions
        of need 319–321
    rehabilitation 331
    and research instruments 318, 319
    in rural areas 437
    safe havens 331
    sampling biases 317
    service models 328–331
    services integration 329–330
    shelter-based interventions 329
    special clinical services 328–329
    street outreach programmes 328
    surveys 46, 53–54
    target populations for services 324–328
    trauma and victimisation 316–317
    with severe mental illness 325–326
    youths 314–315, 327, 371
hostels 254, 305, 318
household surveys 45–46, 47, 48–51,
    128–129, 492

impairment concept 2
indirect indicators of need 110
individual needs assessment 261–303
  and Camberwell Assessment of
    Need 291–303
  and Cardinal Needs Schedule 261–
    272
  and Care Programme Approach 162,
    167–168
  for care and services 273–290
  definitions and terminology 2–5
information management 12–13, 17,
  79–80, 154
information needs
  of carers 354, 448
  of ethnic minorities 429
  of users 190–191, 414, 448
information requirements of
  commissioners 59–83
injecting drug misuse 311–312, 456–
  457, 461
in-patients
  alcohol misusers 508
  auditing use of psychiatric beds
    241–260
  costs 149, 150
  long-stay 254, 287–288, 396
  residential services for drug
    misusers 465–466
  with eating disorders 473, 476, 477
institutional surveys 46, 47–48, 52–53

key informant surveys 126–127, 225,
  230–236

learning disabilities
  assessment and diagnostic
    instruments 381
  and Cardinal Needs Schedule 270
  development of CANDID 382–390
  elderly people 396
  and mental health problems 379–392
  and needs assessment 380–382
  service needs instruments 382
  service provision 380
local authorities, service planning
  144–145, 156
local authority care, children in 371
local catchment areas for needs-led
  services 171–189
    clarifying service priorities 176–177

commissioning clinical teams
  182–183
dichotomies and development of
  sector services 181–182
effective delivery of community
  care 180
establishing sector boundaries
  173–174
factors influencing sector size
  174–176
information infrastructure
  177–179
inter-agency planning and
  organisation 179–180
needs for training 184
local services
  health targets and development of
    27–28
  priority setting during development
    144–158
long-stay patients 254, 287–288, 396
long-term care, and priority setting
  147, 148
long-term mental illness, assessing
  systems of care 225–240
long-term service agreements 79
low-contact groups, measuring need
  in 275–277

Manchester Scale 264
marital status 14, 49, 132, 134–136,
  137, 345–346
matrix model, for service planning
  and provision 1
medication *see* drug treatment
mental health information systems
  (MHISs) 12–13, 17, 79–80, 154
mental health needs, definitions 1–21
Mental Health Needs Index (MINI)
  166–167
mental health services
  for alcohol misuse 497–508
  assessing systems of care for long-
    term mentally ill 225–240
  commissioning 59–83
  conceptual model for planning and
    provision 1
  for drug misuse 459–469
  evaluation of ability to meet needs
    225–260
  for homeless 304–341

mental health services (*cont'd*)
  influence of organisation on met/
    unmet needs 113–115
  local catchment areas for needs-led
    services 171–189
  measuring individual needs for
    273–290
  priority setting in development of
    local services 144–158
  resource allocation 84–109,
    148–150
  rural areas 435–453
  terminology 5–7
  user-run 194–195
  see also planning; utilisation
mental health targets *see* health targets
Mental Illness Specific Grant 150
methadone 461–464
MILMIS (Monitoring Inner London
  Mental Illness Services) 244–249
Mini Finland Health Survey 138
minimum data-set 12, 13, 77, 80
morbidity
  alcohol-related 495–497
  and comparative assessment of
    need 68–69
  in elderly 393–394
  in homeless 307–308
  population surveys 43–58
  resource allocation and predictive
    models 84–88
  in rural areas 442–444
mortality
  alcohol-related 495
  changing patterns 85–86
  and comparative assessment of need
    68–69
  and resource allocation 84–86
MRC Needs for Care Assessment (MRC
  NCA) 271, 280–289, 293–294
    and acute populations 286–287
    and carers 351
    community version 127, 138, 139
    and elderly 287, 397–398
    and ethnic minorities 288
    and individuals out of contact
      with services 287, 318
    and long-stay in-patients 287–288
    measurement principles 282–285
    model of care and definition of
      need 281–282, 292, 293

  modifications to 263
  problems with 261–263
  training and manpower
    requirements 285–286
MRC Social Behaviour Schedule 351
multi-disciplinary teams 182–183

National Health Service (NHS)
  occupational stress in staff 31–32
  re-organisation 60–62
National Health Service and
  Community Care Act 1990 155–157,
    200–201, 380, 390, 499–500
national health targets *see* health
  targets
National Institute for Clinical
  Excellence (NICE) 61–62
National Psychiatric Morbidity Surveys
  of Great Britain 25–26, 128–129
National Service Framework (NSF) for
  Mental Health 5, 28, 61
national survey programmes 24–26,
  43–58, 128–129, 492–494
need(s)
  for care 7–9, 274, 282
  from commissioner's viewpoint
    64–66
  comparative 125, 292
  defined 8–9, 273–275, 281–282,
    291–293, 364, 381
  expressed 125, 292
  future need 285
  hierarchy of 292
  legitimate/illegitimate 93, 106–108
  normative 125, 262, 292
  perceived 125
  for services 7–9, 274
needs assessment, definitions and
  terminology 1–21
needs assessment techniques 9,
  261–303
needs-led assessment 291, 380
neurotic disorders
  contact with health professionals
    51, 130–133
  receipt of treatment 136, 141
  surveys 25, 26, 32, 48–50, 51, 52,
    53, 56, 129–137
no meetable need 274–275, 284–285
non-statutory services 439–440, 448,
  497, 502–503

occupational mental health 30–32
offenders
    use of Cardinal Needs Schedule 271
    young 371
Office of Population Censuses and
    Surveys (OPCS) survey programme
    25–26, 44–57, 494
older people *see* elderly people
opioids 455, 456, 461–464, 465, 466
outcome, defined 65
outcome measurement
    and alcohol misuse interventions
        509
    and Camberwell Assessment of
        Need 298, 299
    and Cardinal Needs Schedule
        268–269
    and commissioning 68–69, 78
    and health targets 23, 27
outreach programmes 328
over-provision 9, 285

patients *see* user perspective on needs
period prevalence admission rate 87–88
personality disorders 55, 312
physical illness
    in alcohol misusers 496–497
    in homeless 315–316, 323
    influence on help seeking and
        receipt of treatment 130, 134
planning
    advantages of sectorisation 174
    incrementalist approach 145–146
    joint 144–145, 154–155, 179–180
    matrix model 1
    principles 113–114, 150–153, 171
    priority setting in development of
        local services 144–158
    rationalist approach 146
polydrug use 492
population needs
    and ability to benefit 65
    and Care Programme Approach
        162–163, 166–167
    measurement 43–143
population surveys *see* epidemiological
    surveys
post-traumatic stress disorder 312
prevention
    of alcohol misuse 499, 504
    of disability 4–5, 17

and health targets 32–35, 37–39
of suicide 24, 33–35, 39, 444
primary care 407–419
    alcohol misuse services 500, 505–
        506, 507
    drug misuse services 463–464, 469
    eating disorders referrals 480
    eliciting real and perceived needs
        407–409
    groups (PCGs) 62, 156, 182, 407,
        409, 469
    and health targets 29–30
    help-seeking behaviour 130–133,
        428–429
    influences on receipt of treatment
        133–137, 141–142
    in rural areas 439
    and sectorisation 181–182
    trusts (PCTs) 62, 156, 182, 432
    user satisfaction surveys 409–417
principles
    equity 129, 168–169, 201
    and service planning 113–114,
        150–153, 171
priority setting 14–17
    and Care Programme Approach
        28–29, 159–170
    in development of local services
        144–158
        client groups 153
        establishing principles/goals/
            vision 150–153
        impact of legislation 155–157
        interpretation of local
            information 153–154
        maintaining flexibility and
            responsiveness 157–158
        participation and consultation
            154–155
        resources 148–150
        target groups 152
        type of function needed 153
        understanding current focus of
            service 147–148
    and sector planning 176–177
prisons
    alcohol misuse in 492, 503
    and health targets 32
    surveys 46–47, 55–56, 57
Program for Assertive Community
    Treatment (PACT) 330

provision
    data on 68, 69
    defined 9
Psychiatric Assessment Schedule for
    Adults with Developmental
    Disabilities 381
psychiatric bed use, auditing 241–260
psychiatric case registers (PCRs) 179
    and assessment of demand at
        district level 110–124
        individual and district level needs
            assessment 111–112
        influence of service organisation
            on met/unmet needs 113–115
        longitudinal study of planned/
            unplanned contacts 115–120
psychiatric reprovision, economic
    evaluation 206, 212–213, 215–219
psychiatric services *see* mental health
    services
psychological treatments
    counselling 133, 136, 137, 448,
        464–465
    for eating disorders 477–479, 481
    influences on receipt of 133–137
    in rural areas 448
Psychopathology Instrument for
    Mentally Retarded Adults 381
psychosis
    family burden 349
    health targets 38–39
    population surveys 25–26, 46, 47,
        51, 52, 53, 54–55, 56
Psychosis Screening Questionnaire 47
public education 26–27, 142, 498–
    499, 504
public safety 151–152

quality of care/services 10–11
    and commissioning 61–62, 73, 78
    and sectors 174
quality of life 10–11

REHAB scale 264
Reiss Screen For Maladaptive
    Behaviour 381
relatives *see* carers
Relatives' Cardinal Needs Schedule
    (RCNS) 270–271
residential care, auditing patient
    characteristics 249–258

resource allocation 84–109
    conclusions and further
        developments 104–105
    data used to develop model 96–98
    development of model 88–96
        area-level analysis 90–91
        individual-level analysis 88–90
        modelling process with real data
            91–94
        rationale for procedure 88–94
        second stage 94–96
    evidence-based 86–88
    historical approach 86
    modelling approach 86
    normative approach 86
    and predictive models of morbidity
        84–88
        changing patterns of mortality
            85–86
    original Resource Allocation
        Working Party approach 84–85
    and priority setting 148–150
    regression approach 86
    in Scotland 102–104
    statistical modelling 98–104
respite care 356
Revised Clinical Interview Schedule
    (CIS-R) 47, 129
Robert Wood Johnson (RWJ)
    Foundation Program on Chronic
    Mental Illness 225–240
        background 225–226
        design of national evaluation
            229–230
        development of key informant
            survey 230–235
        findings from key informant
            survey 235–236
        other needs assessment methods
            236–239
        relevance of model to UK
            situation 228–229
rural mental health services, needs
    assessment for 435–453
        challenges and opportunities
            445–447
        examples of local solutions 447–449
        meeting health needs 445–449
        nature and epidemiology of
            mental illness 442–444
        nature of rural areas 435–436

rural areas in England 436–438
rural services 437–441.

safe havens, for homeless 331
safety
public 151–152
of users 192
satisfaction of users, with primary care
services 410–417
Schedules for Clinical Assessment in
Neuropsychiatry 47, 138
schizophrenia
carers' needs 345, 346, 353
in ethnic minorities 397, 426, 428
health targets 38–39
in homeless 308–309
surveys 52
Scotland, modelling of utilisation in
102–104
sectorised services 171–189
segmental approach, to service
organisation 113–114
service-based assessment 291
services *see* mental health services
severe mental illness
assessing systems of care in urban
settings 225–240
and Camberwell Assessment of
Need 294–295
and Care Programme Approach 29,
159, 168
needs assessment for relatives
270–271
and priority setting 29, 152, 159,
168, 176–177
services for homeless 325–326
unmet need 76
severity of disablement 3–4
severity of illness
influence on help seeking and
receipt of treatment 129, 130,
134, 136–137, 141
in rural areas 442
and utilisation 112
siblings 357
single mothers, homeless 313
social care services
and alcohol misuse 499–500, 506–507
and learning disabilities 380
and priority setting 147–148, 150,
152

social disablement
concept 2–4, 281–282, 283
influence on help seeking and
receipt of treatment 129–130,
137
prevention 4
surveys 51, 56–57
social exclusion 306
social isolation 14, 193, 322, 346–347
socio-demographic indices of need
13–14, 126
and homeless 321
and local catchment areas 175–176
and resource allocation 85–86,
88, 96–97
South Verona longitudinal case
register study 115–123
South West London Total Purchasing
Pilot (SWLTPP) 409, 410
statistical modelling, to predict
utilisation 86, 88–108
stigma and discrimination 36, 346,
347, 417
stress
occupational 31–32
and prevention 32–33
substance misuse *see* alcohol misuse;
drug misuse
substance misuse teams (SMTs) 467
suicide/suicidality 88
in farmers 444
health targets 24, 33–35, 39–40
prevention 24, 33–35, 39, 444
surveys 25, 26, 50, 56, 57
supervision register 161–162, 163,
164, 167–168
supply
defined 65, 292
endogeneity and variables 91–92,
93, 99
interrelationship with need and
utilisation 91–94
legitimate/illegitimate 93–94
surveys *see* epidemiological surveys
syringe exchange services 461
systemic approach, to service
organisation 113–114
systems of care
assessment for long-term mentally
ill 225–240
configuration 128

targets *see* health targets
Tayside Profile for Dementia
   Planning 399
training and education
   in community-based services 184
   in primary care 29, 141–142
   for professionals working with
      ethnic minorities 431
transport, in rural areas 437, 445–446
treatment(s)
   access to information 191
   for alcohol misuse 504–509
   for children and adolescents
      372–374
   for eating disorders 476–479
   and ethnic minorities 422–423, 425
   influences on receipt of 133–142
   user satisfaction in primary care
      413–414
   see also drug treatment

United Kingdom *see* Britain
United States, assessing systems of care
   for long-term mentally ill 225–240
unmet need
   data from community surveys
      128–142
   defined 9, 274, 275, 282
   and resource allocation 104
   and service monitoring by
      commissioners 76
unplanned contacts, longitudinal case
   register study 115–123
urban areas
   assessing systems of care for long-
      term mentally ill 225–240
   concentration of services in
      437–438
   and demand 112
user perspective on needs 190–199
   access to information 190–191
   access to specialist help 195–196
   advocacy 195
   availability of services 192–193
   child and adolescent services
      374–375
   ethnic minorities 421–422, 432
   flexibility and responsiveness to
      needs 194
   integrated services 196–197
   meaningful activities 196

monitoring user participation
   197–198
practical help 193
presence of charter 191–192
and research instruments 262, 263,
   264
services for homeless 331
user-run services 194–195
user satisfaction survey of primary
   care services 409–417
utilisation
   children and adolescents 375
   and comparative assessment of
      need 68, 69
   data collection using CSRI schedule
      205–211
   defined 9
   and diagnosis 112
   ethnic minorities 176, 375, 397
   and filters 90
   and illness severity 112
   modelling of interrelationship with
      need and supply 86, 88–108
   surveys 51, 86–88, 126

Verona Service Satisfaction Scale–54
   (VSSS–54) 410, 412
Vineland Social Maturity Scale 382
violence, against homeless 316–317
violent patients 253, 258
voluntary sector 414, 430–431,
   439–440, 497

want, defined 65
women
   alcohol misuse in 490
   carers 346, 352
   eating disorders in 475–476
   homeless 313–314
workplace, and health targets 30–32
World Health Organization
   Health for All by the Year 2000
      22–23
   Illness, Disability and Handicap
      (IDH) classification 2–3
   International Classification of
      Impairments, Disabilities and
      Handicaps (ICIDH) 3

young people *see* children and
   adolescents

CL

362.
209
41
MEA